Prolonged and Long-Term Mechanical Ventilation in Children

Atsushi Kawaguchi • Marti Pons Odena
Robert J. Graham
Editors

Prolonged and Long-Term Mechanical Ventilation in Children

Springer

Editors
Atsushi Kawaguchi
Division of Pediatric Critical Care, Department of Pediatrics
School of Medicine,
St Marianna University,
Kawasaki, Kanagawa, Japan

Marti Pons Odena
Department of Pediatric Intensive Care
Hospital Sant Joan de Déu
Barcelona, Barcelona, Spain

Robert J. Graham
Department of Anesthesiology, Critical Care and Pain Medicine, Division of Critical Care Medicine
Boston Children's Hospital
Boston, MA, USA

ISBN 978-981-97-8902-3 ISBN 978-981-97-8903-0 (eBook)
https://doi.org/10.1007/978-981-97-8903-0

This Springer imprint is published by the registered company Springer Nature Singapore Pte Ltd.
The registered company address is: 152 Beach Road, #21-01/04 Gateway East, Singapore 189721, Singapore

Preface

The journey of pediatric care for children requiring prolonged and long-term mechanical ventilation is complex, evolving, and often challenging for clinicians, patients, and families alike. Advances in medical science have saved countless young lives; yet, with this success comes the responsibility to support children who, due to the intricacies of their conditions, depend on continuous ventilatory assistance.

This book, *Prolonged and Long-Term Mechanical Ventilation in Children*, reflects our commitment to advancing this vital area of pediatric care. It offers a comprehensive overview of the epidemiology, management strategies, and therapeutic approaches for children who require mechanical ventilation, either temporarily or for extended periods. Informed by the latest research and practical experience from specialized healthcare providers in this field worldwide, this book offers invaluable insights for a diverse audience. Pediatricians, intensivists, home care providers, and other healthcare professionals involved in the care of children on prolonged and long-term ventilation will find practical guidance and a well-rounded understanding of both the challenges and advancements central to pediatric ventilatory support.

The contributors to this book are specialized healthcare providers who have dedicated their work to understanding and advancing the care for ventilated children. Their collective expertise creates a much-needed resource that addresses the unique complexities of pediatric ventilatory support, from managing tracheostomies to transitioning patients from hospital to home care.

It is our hope that this book will serve as both a reference and a source of inspiration, encouraging further collaboration, research, and the development of protocols that will ultimately improve the lives of children and their families.

Kawasaki, Japan | Atsushi Kawaguchi

Contents

Prolonged Mechanical Ventilation, Need for Definition

Michaël Sauthier and Philippe Jouvet

1 Introduction

Mechanical ventilation is one of the most common treatments in pediatric intensive care units (PICUs). Most of the time, the support is intended for a short period, usually a few days [1, 2]. However, a small proportion of patients require the support to be prolonged over a few weeks and sometimes months [3, 4]. This proportion seems to increase in the last decade due to patients getting more complex with more comorbidities and due to technology advances allowing better support [3–5]. Despite representing a minority of the admissions, these patients may utilize more than half of the resources of a PICU. An audit in the United Kingdom showed that 10% of the patients used nearly 60% of the PICU bed days [6]. Moreover, prolonged invasive ventilation (i.e., using an endotracheal tube or tracheostomy) time is associated with several complications, such as increased PICU length of stay, post-extubation upper airway obstruction, nutritional deficiency, neurological complications, weaning failure, supplementary oxygen at home, and death [1, 4, 7–10].

Even if prolonged mechanical ventilation (PMV) is a common concept among clinicians, no accepted consensus exists to define it in children. "Prolonged" is often used in the sense of "longer than expected." However, the expectation largely differs from the context it is used. For example, a patient still intubated 6 hours after the end of the surgery may be considered as "prolonged" [11], but it would be more than 3 months for a team specialized in home ventilation [12]. Moreover,

M. Sauthier (✉) · P. Jouvet
Department of Pediatrics, Critical Care Unit, CHU Sainte-Justine, QC, Canada
e-mail: michael.sauthier@umontreal.ca; philippe.jouvet.med@ssss.gouv.qc.ca

A. Kawaguchi et al. (eds.), *Prolonged and Long-Term Mechanical Ventilation in Children*, https://doi.org/10.1007/978-981-97-8903-0_1

"mechanical ventilation" usually refers to invasive ventilation (endotracheal tube or tracheostomy) and often noninvasive ventilation too, but respiratory support is more and more diversified (e.g., high flow nasal cannula and negative pressure ventilation) and what "mechanical" exactly covers is not yet well defined and accepted. This lack of standardization makes the clinical studies incomparable, restraining any scientific progress. In this chapter, we present the different components that should be included in the definition and the rationale for them.

2 Different Components of the Definition

2.1 Ventilation Duration

The main criterion to define PMV is ventilation duration [1]. In 2005, a consensus conference led by the National Association for Medical Direction of Respiratory Care (NAMDRC) set the first adult definition for PMV. To reach the definition, patients had to be ventilated for 21 days or more using invasive or noninvasive ventilation (facial or nasal mask) [13]. Days with less than 6 hours of ventilation or only a nocturnal application of the support were excluded. No other ventilation modalities, such as high-flow nasal cannula (HFNC), were mentioned at this time. Despite this consensus, numerous adult studies have used other definitions [14]. Another frequent threshold to define PMV is patients supported for more than 96 hours, because many databases using the International Classification of Disease (ICD) had a code specifically for that duration (code 96.72 in version 9 and 5A1955Z in version 10). Hence, this cutoff has been frequently used in studies [1, 14].

In 2017, we published a pediatric definition proposition of PMV based on the 21-day NAMDRC definition [1]. This definition integrates more than just ventilation duration (discussed below). Based on a 2021 pediatric systematic review of the literature [7], 9 studies (544 patients) used the 7-day cutoff, 3 studies (1009 patients) used the 14-day cutoff, and 3 studies (1286 patients) used the 21-day cutoff. Authors concluded that there was no evidence to determine clear cutoffs of ventilation duration for the definition of PMV in children. Moreover, the proportion of extubation followed an inverse exponential curve, where about 75% of the patients were extubated before 7 days of ventilation, 90% before 14 days, and 95% before 21 days (Fig. 1) [15, 16]. Thus, the difference between 14 and 21 days was small, and both seemed to be a reasonable threshold to establish PMV (Fig. 2).

Very few studies discussed the implication of interruptions of the ventilation in the calculation of the ventilation time [15, 17]. For example, if a patient is ventilated for 11 days who failed an extubation 36 hours later and needed to be reintubated for another 13 days, would that patient be identified as having PMV? Weaning success is usually defined for invasive ventilation when no reintubation was required in the next 48–72 hours [13, 18]. In case of tracheostomy, tube decannulation in addition to stopping ventilation support is generally not required to be considered as a

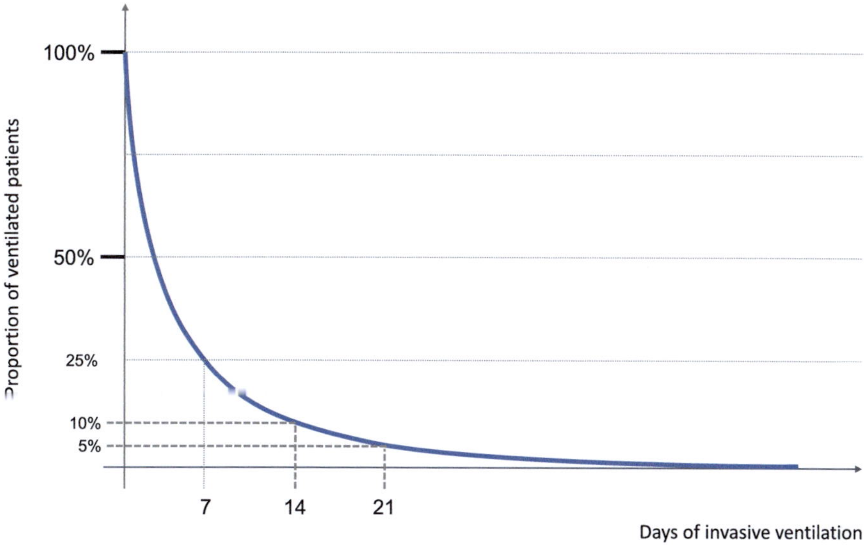

Fig. 1 Proportion of pediatric patients on invasive mechanical ventilation

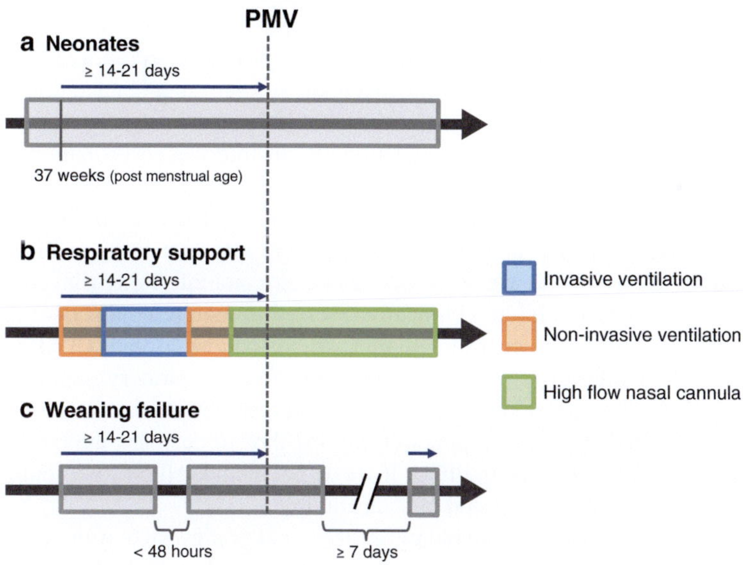

Fig. 2 One of the possible pediatric definitions of prolonged mechanical ventilation (PMV). High-flow nasal cannula inclusion is still debated

weaning success [13]. However, the longer the ventilation support is, the longer the interruption should be to guarantee success [18]. The NAMDRC suggested 7 days to consider the extubation to be a success in case of PMV. However, for small interruptions, the 2017 pediatric PMV proposition definition suggested that interruptions of less than 48 h should still be counted in the same ventilation episode. Thus, in the example above, total ventilation time would be 25.5 days (11 + 1.5 + 13) and would qualify for PMV.

The NAMDRC definition explicitly excluded nocturnal use only of ventilation, and this criterion was also retained in the 2017 pediatric proposition of definition. Most will agree that sleep obstructive apnea is not an ICU illness. However, this is less obvious when young patients may spend a significant proportion of their day asleep. Moreover, even if ventilation support was used during sleep only, children still require much more monitoring than adults and probably have a worse outcome than those who are not ventilated during this period.

2.2 *Ventilation Modality*

Ventilation modalities can be divided into two major categories: invasive and noninvasive ventilation (NIV). Invasive ventilation refers to subglottic devices (endotracheal tubes and tracheostomy). Noninvasive ventilation devices are external interfaces coupled to a ventilator to assist breathing while the patient is awake [19]. Traditionally, it was defined by external masks adjusted on the face (nasal mask, nose and mouth mask, or full-face mask). Helmets are another interface that has been more popular in Europe, mainly Italy, and can provide effective and high-level noninvasive support [20]. It provides accurate oxygen supplementation and is appropriate for long-term use by preventing skin lesions and pressure ulcers on the face [19, 20]. However, noise is a concern with this interface, especially when the airflow is high [20].

In the last decade, high-flow nasal cannula (HFNC) has been more and more popular among clinicians mainly because they are effective in hypoxemia [21], comfortable, and simple to use [19]. A 2022 pediatric noninferiority trial concludes that "among acutely ill children clinically assessed to require noninvasive respiratory support in a pediatric critical care unit, HFNC compared with CPAP met the criterion for noninferiority in time to liberation from respiratory support" [22]. Excluding high-flow nasal cannula would exclude patients in the weaning phase. Also, use of HFNC for several hours during the day, to decrease the burden of a mask, is more and more used in PICU. If we do not include HFNC, we could artificially decrease the weaning period of such children.

The NAMDRC suggested including invasive and noninvasive in the definition, and the 2017 pediatric proposition definition opened the door to the HFNC because of its presumed comparative effectiveness at this time to conventional NIV. However, again, no consensus definition clearly stated which mode should be included or not. However, counting every ventilated day to assess if patients qualify for PMV or not may be reasonable for heterogeneous forms of supports, and one must be extremely careful when comparing patients and populations using different modalities.

2.3 Age

Children ventilated in PICU are very diversified with extremes of age (preterm newborns to adults). Former preterm infants and term infants are similar in size and in the ventilation devices used, but very different in lung maturation and diseases. Therefore, studying PMV in infants is a challenge, especially when both term and preterms are admitted in the same unit. In a heterogeneous cohort of preterm and term infants, the 2017 pediatric definition proposition suggested that only the ventilated days after 37 weeks' postmenstrual age should be counted to standardize children by ages. Of course, this results in not counting the ventilation period before the term is reached and would underestimate the ventilation burden in this population, but in a study that we published, this did not have a great impact on outcomes [2].

2.4 Underlying Conditions and Complication Risk

A 2021 systematic search of the literature showed that the most frequent cutoffs used in the literature (7, 14, 21, and 30 or more days of ventilation) are associated with different conditions [7]. The PMV group defined as 7 days or more of ventilation was not specific. It was associated with tracheobronchomalacia, younger age, healthcare-associated infections, noninfectious pulmonary complications, malnutrition, positive hydric balance, multiviral infections, bacterial lower respiratory tract infection, extubation failure, critical illness myopathy, and neuropathy. The PMV group defined as more than 14 days of ventilation was associated with multiple organ system dysfunction, extubation failure, and tracheostomy. Those ventilated for more than 21 days were associated with chronic comorbidities (cardiac and genetic), use of vasoactive drugs, and multiple antibiotic administration.

3 How Can We Obtain a Reliable Definition?

3.1 Standardize the Ventilation Data Collection

Defining and studying PMV minimally require to be able to measure ventilation duration. As described above, there are many ventilation modalities, and multiple changes for each patient can occur. Even using electronic health records with continuous data recording, a technology that is far from widely available, we observed [23] that two major limitations can be observed: (1) manually entered data by caregivers are at risk of entry errors. They are also less precise on the start or stop time of the therapies, especially when caregivers are busy. Moreover, small changes and trials at the bedside may not be recorded. (2) Some modern PICUs can automatically record all the data (pressure, volume, ventilation mode along with all the monitoring and therapeutic data) in a high temporal resolution database (HTRD) at a high frequency (>1 data point per minute) (Fig. 3) [23]. This method has many advantages, in particular to be able to store and to precisely recreate the complete stay of a patient and do multiple analyses retrospectively with minimal loss of data [24]. It can also be done at a much lower cost than a prospective study. However, even if the database is rich, new problems can arise. For example, as the intentions of the caregivers are generally not recorded, other data sources are required to understand if the ventilation interruption was planned or not (e.g., unplanned extubation) or the reason for the ventilatory support modification (e.g., NIV failure). Moreover, interruptions in the data continuous flow occurred when patients were temporarily moved to another unit without this technology (for example, medical imagery or operating room). It also requires a highly trained team of experts to manage and analyze the data.

There is a significant variability between units worldwide. Some centers have more patients and thus are more probably exposed to PMV; others may have access to higher quality data, while some others may have different resources dedicated to PMV. All these differences between centers might significantly impact how PMV is identified and compared to in a single-center.

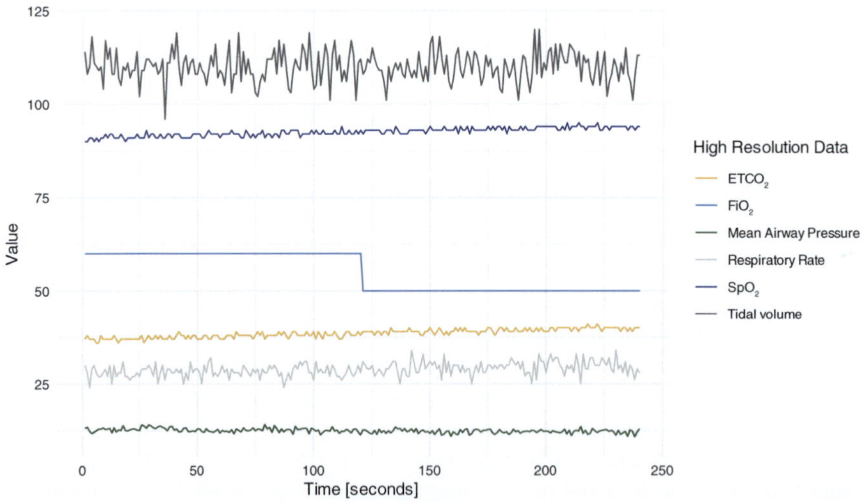

Fig. 3 Example of continuous high-resolution data

3.2 *Increases Data on the Children Outcomes Depending on Ventilation Duration*

PMV is a relatively rare entity, but evidence suggests that it uses a high level of resources and it is increasing. To better understand it and eventually improve care, a large international cross-sectional study started in 2019 (LongVentKids study, ClinicalTrials.gov Identifier: NCT04112459) that aims to describe PMV occurrence care provided in PICU. In 2022, it involved 263 centers from 42 countries. Another study, the "Long Term Ventilation," a study supported by the National Confidential Enquiry into Patient Outcome and Death in the United Kingdom, aimed "to identify remediable factors in the care of patients before their 25th birthday who are receiving, or have received, long-term ventilation." These two studies will give more data on the link between ventilation duration and outcomes. This will refine the population on which we should focus the PMV definition to improve the children outcome. However, in neonates, we already demonstrated that more than 21 days of ventilation results in a high burden at 18-month corrected age including a death rate of 29%, 41% still with respiratory support and high rate of neurological impairment, and 55% of the children were not exclusively orally fed [2].

3.3 *Create an Expert Panel and an International Consensus Conference*

A consensus conference is a pragmatic and efficient solution to establish guidelines for a rare matter where there is a lack of randomized controlled data [25]. In 2015, the Pediatric Acute Lung Injury Consensus Conference (PALICC) published the first recommendations for pediatric acute respiratory distress syndrome (P-ARDS) [26]. It involved 27 experts who met three times in 2 years. Each subgroup reviewed the literature to define P-ARDS and to make recommendations regarding treatment and future research priorities. All members then voted on all recommendations, and those without a strong agreement were sent back to the respective subgroup of revision. The second agreement was then noted. This methodology was repeated for the revision of P-ARDS recommendations (PALICC-2) and is a model that would be totally applicable to establish recommendations for pediatric PMV.

4 Conclusion

There is a clear need for consensual, unified, and integrated definition of PMV in children. The challenge is significant, but much work has already been done in that field. In the meantime, we propose to use the definition detailed in Fig. 2; if not, we recommend to clearly define the four components of the definition (duration, modality, age, and diseases) used in any clinical study.

References

1. Sauthier M, Rose L, Jouvet P. Pediatric prolonged mechanical ventilation: considerations for definitional criteria. Respir Care. 2016;62:49–53.
2. Sauthier M, Sauthier N, Gallant KB, Lodygensky GA, Kawaguchi A, Emeriaud G, Jouvet P. Long-term mechanical ventilation in neonates: a 10-year overview and predictive model. Front Pediatr. 2021;9:689190.
3. Traiber C, Piva JP, Fritsher CC, Garcia PCR, Lago PM, Trotta EA, Ricachinevsky CP, Bueno FU, Baecker V, Lisboa BD. Profile and consequences of children requiring prolonged mechanical ventilation in three Brazilian pediatric intensive care units. Pediatr Crit Care Med. 2009;10:375–80.
4. Lone NI, Walsh TS. Prolonged mechanical ventilation in critically ill patients: epidemiology, outcomes and modelling the potential cost consequences of establishing a regional weaning unit. Crit Care. 2011;15:R102.
5. Zilberberg MD, Shorr AF. Prolonged acute mechanical ventilation and hospital bed utilization in 2020 in the United States: implications for budgets, plant and personnel planning. BMC Health Serv Res. 2008;8:242.
6. Network PICA. November 2016 annual report, 2016. https://www.picanet.org.uk/wp-content/uploads/sites/25/2018/05/PICANet_Annual_Report_Tables_and_Figures_2016.pdf. Accessed 26 July 2022.
7. Colleti J, Azevedo RT, Caino FR, Araujo OR. Prolonged mechanical ventilation in children: review of the definition. Pediatr Crit Care Med. 2021;22:e588–93.
8. Rivera R, Tibballs J. Complications of endotracheal intubation and mechanical ventilation in infants and children. Crit Care Med. 1992;20:193–9.
9. Mutlu GM, Factor P. Complications of mechanical ventilation. Respir Care Clin North Am. 2000;6:213–52.
10. Principi T, Fraser DD, Morrison GC, Farsi SA, Carrelas JF, Maurice EA, Kornecki A. Complications of mechanical ventilation in the pediatric population. Pediatr Pulm. 2011;46:452–7.
11. Ribeiro T, Magalhães P, Andrade L, Silva B, Duarte MB. Factors associated with prolonged mechanical ventilation in children undergoing cardiac surgery. Neonatol Paediatr Intens Care. 2015;46(suppl 59):PA1870.
12. Amin R, Sayal P, Syed F, Chaves A, Moraes TJ, MacLusky I. Pediatric long-term home mechanical ventilation: twenty years of follow-up from one Canadian center. Pediatr Pulm. 2014;49:816–24.
13. MacIntyre NR, Epstein SK, Carson S, Scheinhorn D, Christopher K, Muldoon S, Care NA for MD of R. Management of patients requiring prolonged mechanical ventilation report of a NAMDRC consensus conference. Chest. 2005;128:3937–54.
14. Rose L, McGinlay M, Amin R, et al. Variation in definition of prolonged mechanical ventilation. Respir Care. 2017;62:1324–32.
15. Payen V, Jouvet P, Lacroix J, Ducruet T, Gauvin F. Risk factors associated with increased length of mechanical ventilation in children. Pediatr Crit Care Med. 2012;13:152–7.
16. Wakeham MK, Kuhn EM, Lee KJ, McCrory MC, Scanlon MC. Use of tracheostomy in the PICU among patients requiring prolonged mechanical ventilation. Intens Care Med. 2014;40:863–70.

17. Farias JA, Fernández A, Monteverde E, et al. Mechanical ventilation in pediatric intensive care units during the season for acute lower respiratory infection. Pediatr Crit Care Med. 2012;13:158–64.
18. MacIntyre NR, Cook DJ, Ely EW, et al. Evidence-based guidelines for weaning and discontinuing ventilatory support a collective task force facilitated by the American College of Chest Physicians; the American Association for Respiratory Care; and the American College of Critical Care Medicine. Chest. 2001;120:375S–95S.
19. Rittayamai N, Grieco DL, Brochard L. Noninvasive respiratory support in intensive care medicine. Intens Care Med. 2022:1–4.
20. Mu S-C, Chien Y-H, Lai P-Z, Chao K-Y. Helmet ventilation for pediatric patients during the COVID-19 pandemic: a narrative review. Front Pediatr. 2022;10:839476.
21. Frat J-P, Thille AW, Mercat A, et al. High-flow oxygen through nasal cannula in acute hypoxemic respiratory failure. New Engl J Med. 2015;372:2185–96.
22. Ramnarayan P, Richards-Belle A, Drikite L, et al. Effect of high-flow nasal cannula therapy vs continuous positive airway pressure therapy on liberation from respiratory support in acutely ill children admitted to pediatric critical care units. JAMA. 2022;328:162–72.
23. Brossier D, Taani RE, Sauthier M, Roumeliotis N, Emeriaud G, Jouvet P. Creating a high-frequency electronic database in the PICU. Pediatr Crit Care Med. 2018;19:e189–98.
24. Mathieu A, Brossier D, Sauthier M, Taani RE, Goyer I, Emeriaud G, Jouvet P. Creating a high resolution electronic database in the pediatric intensive care unit: validation phase. Ann Intensive Care. 2018;8:63.
25. Bembea MM, Jouvet P, Willson D, Thomas NJ, Group PALICC. Methodology of the pediatric acute lung injury consensus conference. Pediatr Crit Care Med. 2015;16:S1–5.
26. Khemani RG, Smith LS, Zimmerman JJ, Erickson S, Group PALICC. Pediatric acute respiratory distress syndrome. Pediatr Crit Care Med. 2015;16:S23–40.

History and Epidemiology of PMVed Children (Including Home-Ventilated Children)

Takahiro Kido and Atsushi Kawaguchi

1 Introduction

Prolonged mechanical ventilation (PMV) has been made possible by medical advances during the twentieth century, but it can cause problems such as respiratory muscle weakness and formation of atelectasis. In addition, PMV may raise socio-medical or economic issues, such as the impact of bed occupancy for chronically PMVed patients on acute medical care and its costs. The definition and perception of the word "prolonged" depend on how these issues are raised and can vary from as short as a few days to as long as several months, which is discussed in more detail in the other chapter. The wide variation in definitions and management may be due to the lack of consistent epidemiological information and evidence-based practice guidelines on weaning, extubation, tracheostomy, and management of PMVed cases. In this chapter, we will describe how the concept of PMV has evolved to date in the context of the history of ventilator development, including the epidemiological information on PMV available today.

T. Kido
University of Tsukuba Hospital, Tsukuba, Japan
e-mail: kido.takahiro.xj@alumni.tsukuba.ac.jp

A. Kawaguchi (✉)
Division of Pediatric Critical Care, Department of Pediatrics, St. Marianna University, Kawasaki, Japan
e-mail: atsushi.kawaguchi@marianna-u.ac.jp

A. Kawaguchi et al. (eds.), *Prolonged and Long-Term Mechanical Ventilation in Children*, https://doi.org/10.1007/978-981-97-8903-0_2

2 History of PMV

2.1 Dawn of Artificial Ventilator: Iron Lung

The idea of artificially supporting breathing in people who have stopped breathing or are breathing inadequately has been around since the 1800s. Many of these procedures were performed manually by applying positive pressure through the trachea during surgical anesthesia. However, due to the risk of pneumothorax and problems with prolonged use of manual methods, negative-pressure ventilators were developed for long-term use in patients with respiratory failure and for management in hospital wards [1]. In 1928, Shaw and Drinker's "iron lung" was first commercialized for children with polio [2]. Many polio patients took several weeks to recover and often required prolonged ventilation.

2.2 The Emergence of Invasive Mechanical Ventilation: Polio Epidemic (1952–)

Until the 1950s, negative-pressure ventilators dominated the development of respiratory management, so the noninvasive ventilation was the first respiratory support to be applied at a large scale. However, these devices were inefficient in terms of space and cost because they were huge and required a lot of energy to operate [3]. During the 1952 polio epidemic, there was a shortage of iron lungs, and many patients were treated with manual positive-pressure ventilation through the trachea, as in surgery. The prognosis was unexpectedly better for those managed with manual positive-pressure ventilation than for those placed in an iron lung, and the mainstream of ventilator management gradually shifted to positive-pressure ventilation. It forced the development of intensive care medicine and the associated technology [1, 4].

In addition to initial concerns about airway damage from positive pressure (now known as barotrauma), the disadvantages associated with prolonged positive-pressure ventilation (specifically volutrauma in the 1970s and biotrauma since the 1990s) have gradually been recognized, and the technical aspects of ventilatory management have evolved in response [5].

2.3 The Era of NIV (Noninvasive Ventilation with Positive Airway Pressure)

Prior to the iron lung described above, mask ventilation had been used during surgery, but not for long-term management in adult cohorts [2]. Sullivan et al. first reported the efficacy of masked continuous positive airway pressure (CPAP) in the management of obstructive sleep apnea syndrome in 1981 [6], and masked CPAP began to be studied primarily as a treatment for chronic conditions. Around 1990, its efficacy in avoiding intubation in acute respiratory failure and in postoperative management after extubation was widely studied and recognized as a practical option [7, 8]. In pediatric cohorts, this began with its introduction in muscular dystrophy and other neurological disorders to avoid or delay tracheostomy [9] and later on was generalized to prevent reintubation in different scenarios. Today, in addition to CPAP, it includes the biphasic positive-pressure mode, collectively referred to as noninvasive positive-pressure ventilation (NIPPV). NIPPV is increasingly being used in a variety of settings, but the long-term use of NIPPV poses a new problem. In children, the most commonly reported complication of long-term NIPPV is skin damage associated with mask wear. Other concerns include nasal symptoms (e.g., sinusitis) and effects on facial development [10] as well as aerodigestive considerations with aerophagia contributing to aspiration risk and impaired respiratory mechanics with abdominal distention. In recent years, high-flow nasal therapy (HFNT) has become available in addition to NIPPV with several studies trying to find its non-inferiority to NIV [11, 12].

2.4 *Transitions in Scope and Targeted Issues in PMV*

In the 1950s and 1960s, when mechanical ventilators were first developed, PMV was reported in the context of "success stories" in achieving long-term respiratory management [13, 14]. While experience had been gained in adults with various diseases and poisonings other than polio [15, 16], reports of neonatal respiratory distress syndrome were also widespread in the pediatric field [17]. In the 1970s, the disadvantages of prolonged positive-pressure ventilation, such as lung damage and ventilator-associated pneumonia (VAP), began to be recognized [18, 19]. It was recognized as something to be "avoided" [20], and recent studies have mainly evaluated PMV for its negative aspects [21].

In the 1980s and 1990s, studies began to address PMV in critically ill or injured children in the PICU [22], and it began to be recognized as a health policy and economic issue due to increasing medical costs [23, 24]. Studies have tried to find a better way of weaning [25, 26], and in some countries, dedicated units for PMVed patients have to be established. For example, it is known as long-term acute care hospital (LTACH) in the United States and regional weaning center (RWC) in Europe [27–30].

Additionally, pulmonologists started to develop follow-up programs mainly for neuromuscular patients so as to implement long-term ventilation before clinical decompensation and patient's admission in intensive care. At the beginning of the twenty-first century, there was a growing awareness of the many disadvantages associated with long-term mechanical ventilation, and concepts such as post-intensive care syndrome (PICS) and ICU-acquired weakness (ICU-AW) began to receive attention [31, 32]. Efforts to address PMV have also become more important, and there is now a need for international studies on a larger scale, taking into account the heterogeneity of target cohorts and practice settings.

In adult cohorts, diagnostic criteria for PMV have been developed by the National Association for Medical Direction of Respiratory Care (NAMDRC) and the European Respiratory Society (ERS) (see another chapter), and in recent years, epidemiological studies have begun to be conducted on the basis of these criteria. Although there has been active discussion about PMV in children since around 2010 [33], it has not been investigated whether the same definition can be used in adults [34, 35]. The results of these studies may provide further insight into the definition of PMV in children and treatment strategies in the future.

3 Epidemiology

3.1 Epidemiology in Acute Care Settings

Reports on the epidemiology of PMV in acute care settings are limited. A Canadian single-center study reported that 2.9% of all PICU admissions were defined as PMV [36]. The UK multicenter PICU database also showed a rate of around 3% defining PMV [37]. A large US registry reported that the proportion of ventilator-dependent patients was approximately 13% of all ventilator-dependent children in the PICU [38], giving an estimated rate of 2–3% of all PICU admissions. All PICU studies included here define PMV as ≥21 days of invasive ventilation.

Studies in NICUs have reported that the incidence of PMV varies widely depending on the patient population. A Korean national registry reported that 20% of very-low-birth-weight infants (<1500 g) had PMV [39]. In addition, a single-center report from the United States reported that 40% of infants with a birth weight of 700–1000 g and 73% of infants with a birth weight of 500–699 g required PMV (both defined as >4 weeks of invasive MV) [40]. Similarly, infants born at less than 28 weeks' gestation have been reported to have a median MV of 45 days [41]. Thus, there is a clear difference in the incidence of PMV in the NICU according to birth weight or gestational age. In studies of infants admitted to the NICU after surgery, the definition of PMV is much shorter. After gastrointestinal surgery 25.6% (>7 days) and after cardiac surgery 35.4% (>72 h) have been reported [42, 43]. A study of PMV in all infants admitted to the NICU reported a frequency of 3% (>21 days of invasive or noninvasive ventilation), similar to that in the PICU [44].

3.2 Epidemiology of HMV (Home Mechanical Ventilation)

Although the exact number of children dependent on HMV worldwide is unknown, many countries have reported a sharp increase in the number of patients discharged home on chronic ventilators. The estimated rate of pediatric HMV in Utah, USA, is reported to be 6.3 per 100,000 children [45], with almost similar reports from Korea [46]. These figures are slightly lower than the prevalence in adults [45–47]. They also share the common feature of having a lower percentage of NIPPV than adults, i.e., a higher percentage of tracheostomy management. Data from medical expenditure reported by individual hospitals in Japan show that the number of children is approximately 19.4 per 100,000 [48]. Again, this epidemiology is likely to be strongly influenced by the healthcare system and the current state of healthcare in each region and country.

Longitudinal studies report that both invasive and noninvasive HMV have increased in all countries over the past 10–20 years and that the increase has been rapid [49–52]. Although bias is likely due to survey methods that lack complete coverage, such as questionnaires and single-institution surveys, similar results have been obtained using high-quality survey methods, such as insurance claims data [46, 53]. The reason for the rapid increase in HMVs may simply be an increase in the number of new patients, but the fact that some conditions now allow long-term survival with home ventilation is likely to be an important factor. For example, many neurological diseases, such as SMA, now have a life expectancy of over 20 years due to improved respiratory support [54, 55]. HMV has also been introduced for many other diseases or medical conditions (Table 1). The long-term survival of children with HMV, in addition to the aforementioned medical costs and bed occupancy, poses a new problem of transition to adult care.

3.3 Regional Epidemiology of PMV

As PMV is closely linked to the health insurance system and associated medical resources, its epidemiology varies widely from country to country and region to region. The percentage of PICU admissions in high-income countries is generally 2–3%, as shown above. In contrast, in low- and middle-income countries, the percentage of PICU admissions tends to be higher, with considerable variation between reports (2.5% in Brazil [58], 1.8% in India [59], 9% in Argentina [60], and 33% in China [61]).

There are several main reasons for the wide variation between reports. One is that there is a great deal of national and regional variation in the weaning process of respiratory management and the timing of tracheostomy [62, 63]. Another is that long-term care cannot be designed around breathing alone, as there are complex factors in the background of children requiring PMV, such as systemic illness and immaturity, in addition to respiratory problems [64]. These complex factors include social factors such as national health services or local social care support (e.g., home care program).

HMV, like PMV in hospitals, consumes many medical resources and costs. A study shows a correlation between HMV and GDP, and the percentage of HMV use per population and GDP per capita are positively correlated. Furthermore, the same report found that the rapid increase in the number of HMV patients over a 10–20-year period described above only occurred in high-income countries [65].

Table 1 List of reported diseases or medical condition which have been managed with HMV currently

Group	Disease Name			
upper airway obstruction	trisomy 21	craniofacial abnormality (Pierre-Robin syndrome etc)	laryngomalacia	
	Obesity(including Prader-Willi)	Tumor		
Neuromuscular/ musculoskeletal	Spinal muscular atrophy	Muscular dystrophy (congenital, Duchenne, myotonic)	Congenital myopathy	Pompe's disease
	Hereditary sensory motor neuropathy	Myasthenia gravis	Bilateral diaphragmatic palsy	
Pulmonary	Cystic fibrosis	Chronic lung disease	Lung fibrosis	Obliterate bronchiolitis
Central nervous system	Sleep disordered sleeping	Congenital hypoventilation syndrome, ROHHAD syndrome	Hypoxic ischemic injury	Brain tumor sequelae
Multiple medical conditions	Cardiac disease	Cerebral palsy		
Other medical conditions	Chest wall disease	Rett syndrome		

Refs. [56, 57]

Few studies have tracked how many people survive long-term after PMV in the PICU and how many stay at home. The Brazilian PICU study mentioned above reported that of children with PMV, approximately 50% survived to discharge from the PICU and 6% were discharged home [37]. There are several reports that children with PMV occupy a large proportion of hospital beds because they are not discharged smoothly [66, 67]. A study that looks at all aspects of acute, chronic, and home care is desirable to see whether an appropriate care environment is provided for children and whether appropriate medical resources are allocated.

4 Summary

Mechanical ventilation is an indispensable part of current pediatric care, both in the acute and chronic phases of treatment. Research and clinical management of prolonged or long-term ventilation have largely focused on liberation and managing ventilators in the acute phase. However, the rapid increase in the number of cases has not been adequately matched by sociomedical research, such as epidemiological studies, management guidelines, and policies. There is a need to better understand the environment of children who require prolonged or long-term ventilation, including the medical environment in each healthcare environment and medical advances, and to gather information and provide timely care.

References

1. Romero-Ávila P, Márquez-Espinós C, Cabrera Afonso JR. Historical development of the anesthetic machine: from Morton to the integration of the mechanical ventilator. Brazilian J Anesthesiol. 2021;71:148–61.
2. Nixon JA. Drinker's "Iron Lung" and other artificial respirators. Bristol Med Chir J (1883). 1938;55:239–44.
3. Wunsch H. Chapter 5: Deadly start. In The autumn ghost. Part I: The spector rises (pp. 56–61). ISBN 9781771649452.
4. Reisner-Sénélar L. The birth of intensive care medicine: Björn Ibsen's records. Intensive Care Med. 2011;37(7):1084–6. https://doi.org/10.1007/s00134-011-2235-z. Epub 2011 May 25. PMID: 21611906.
5. Slutsky AS. History of mechanical ventilation. From vesalius to ventilator-induced lung injury. Am J Respir Crit Care Med. 2015;191:1106–15.
6. Sullivan CE, Issa FG, Berthon-Jones M, Eves L. Reversal of obstructive sleep apnoea by continuous positive airway pressure applied through the nares. Lancet. 1981;1:862–5.
7. Meduri GU, Conoscenti CC, Menashe P, Nair S. Noninvasive face mask ventilation in patients with acute respiratory failure. Chest. 1989;95:865–70.
8. Stock MC, Downs JB, Corkran ML. Pulmonary function before and after prolonged continuous positive airway pressure by mask. Crit Care Med. 1984;12:973–4.
9. Segall D. Noninvasive nasal mask-assisted ventilation in respiratory failure of Duchenne muscular dystrophy. Chest. 1988;93:1298–300.
10. Castro-Codesal ML, Dehaan K, Featherstone R, et al. Long-term non-invasive ventilation therapies in children: a scoping review. Sleep Med Rev. 2018;37:148–58.
11. Ramnarayan P, Richards-Belle A, Drikite L. Airway pressure therapy on liberation from respiratory support in acutely ill children admitted to pediatric critical care units. A randomized clinical trial. JAMA. 2022;328(2):162–72.
12. Milési C, Essouri S, Pouyau R. High flow nasal cannula (HFNC) versus nasal continuous positive airway pressure (nCPAP) for the initial respiratory management of acute viral bronchiolitis in young infants: a multicenter randomized controlled trial (TRAMONTANE study). Intensive Care Med. 2017;43(2):209–16.
13. Drinker P, Shaw LA. AN APPARATUS FOR THE PROLONGED ADMINISTRATION OF ARTIFICIAL RESPIRATION: I. A design for adults and children. J Clin Invest. 1929;7:229–47.
14. Sykes MK. Prolonged intubation in neonatal tetanus. Anaesthesia. 1960;15:394–400.
15. Amaha K. Studies on prolonged artificial respiration. 1. Treatment of medical patients with respiratory insufficiency. Masui. 1967;16:952–60.
16. Pearn JH. Survival after snake-bite with prolonged neurotoxic envenomation. Med J Aust. 1971;2:259–61.
17. Tunstall ME, Cater JI, Thomson JS, Mitchell RG. Ventilating the lungs of newborn infants for prolonged periods. Arch Dis Child. 1968;43:486–97.
18. Banerjee CK, Girling DJ, Wigglesworth JS. Pulmonary fibroplasia in newborn babies treated with oxygen and artificial ventilation. Arch Dis Child. 1972;47:509–18.
19. Gillbe CE, Salt JC, Branthwaite MA. Pulmonary function after prolonged mechanical ventilation with high concentrations of oxygen. Thorax. 1980;35:907–13.

20. Glover WJ. Artificial ventilation, prolonged endotracheal intubation and tracheostomy in paediatric surgery. Postgrad Med J. 1972;48:507–13.
21. Kanter RK, Bove EL, Tobin JR, Zimmerman JJ. Prolonged mechanical ventilation of infants after open heart surgery. Crit Care Med. 1986;14:211–4.
22. Schreiner MS, Downes JJ, Kettrick RG, Ise C, Voit R. Chronic respiratory failure in infants with prolonged ventilator dependency. JAMA. 1987;258:3398–404.
23. Davis H 2nd, Lefrak SS, Miller D, Malt S. Prolonged mechanically assisted ventilation. An analysis of outcome and charges. JAMA. 1980;243:43–5.
24. Thoner J. Outcome and costs of intensive care. A follow-up study on patients requiring prolonged mechanical ventilation. Acta Anaesthesiol Scand. 1987;31:693–8.
25. Morganroth ML, Morganroth JL, Nett LM, Petty TL. Criteria for weaning from prolonged mechanical ventilation. Arch Intern Med. 1984;144:1012–6.
26. Okamoto K, Iwamasa H, Dogomori H, Morioka T. Evaluation of conventional weaning criteria in patients with acute respiratory failure. J Anesth. 1990;4:213–8.
27. Lone NI, Walsh TS. Prolonged mechanical ventilation in critically ill patients: epidemiology, outcomes and modelling the potential cost consequences of establishing a regional weaning unit. Crit Care. 2011;15:R102.
28. Zilberberg MD, Luippold RS, Sulsky S, Shorr AF. Prolonged acute mechanical ventilation, hospital resource utilization, and mortality in the United States. Crit Care Med. 2008;36:724–30.
29. Seneff MG, Wagner D, Thompson D, Honeycutt C, Silver MR. The impact of long-term acute-care facilities on the outcome and cost of care for patients undergoing prolonged mechanical ventilation. Crit Care Med. 2000;28:342–50.
30. Scheinhorn DJ, Chao DC, Stearn-Hassenpflug M, LaBree LD, Heltsley DJ. Post-ICU mechanical ventilation: treatment of 1,123 patients at a regional weaning center. Chest. 1997;111:1654–9.
31. Harvey MA, Davidson JE. Postintensive care syndrome: right care, right now…and later. Crit Care Med. 2016;44:381–5.
32. Vasilevskis EE, Ely EW, Speroff T, Pun BT, Boehm L, Dittus RS. Reducing iatrogenic risks: ICU-acquired delirium and weakness--crossing the quality chasm. Chest. 2010;138:1224–33.
33. Sauthier M, Rose L, Jouvet P. Pediatric prolonged mechanical ventilation: considerations for definitional criteria. Respir Care. 2017;62:49–53.
34. Thomas M, Greenough A, Morton M. Prolonged ventilation and intact survival in very low birth weight infants. Eur J Pediatr. 2003;162:65–7.
35. Voiriot G, Oualha M, Pierre A, et al. Chronic critical illness and post-intensive care syndrome: from pathophysiology to clinical challenges. Ann Intensive Care. 2022;12:58.
36. Payen V, Jouvet P, Lacroix J, Ducruet T, Gauvin F. Risk factors associated with increased length of mechanical ventilation in children. Pediatr Crit Care Med J Soc Crit Care Med World Fed Pediatr Intensive Crit Care Soc. 2012;13:152–7.
37. Fleming SJ, Lamming CR, Evans A, Morris KP, Draper ES, Parslow RC. G372 prolonged invasive ventilation in paediatric intensive care: children resident in England and Wales, 2004–2013. Arch Dis Child. 2015;100:A152 LP-A152.
38. Wakeham MK, Kuhn EM, Lee KJ, McCrory MC, Scanlon MC. Use of tracheostomy in the PICU among patients requiring prolonged mechanical ventilation. Intensive Care Med. 2014;40:863–70.
39. Choi Y-B, Lee J, Park J, Jun YH. Impact of prolonged mechanical ventilation in very low birth weight infants: results from a National Cohort Study. J Pediatr. 2018;194:34–39.e3.
40. Reyes ZC, Claure N, Tauscher MK, D'Ugard C, Vanbuskirk S, Bancalari E. Randomized, controlled trial comparing synchronized intermittent mandatory ventilation and synchronized intermittent mandatory ventilation plus pressure support in preterm infants. Pediatrics. 2006;118:1409–17.
41. Williams E, Dassios T, Arnold K, Hickey A, Greenough A. Prolonged ventilation and postnatal growth of preterm infants. J Perinat Med. 2019;48:82–6.

42. Wang H, Gauda EB, Chiu PPL, Moore AM. Risk factors for prolonged mechanical ventilation in neonates following gastrointestinal surgery. Transl Pediatr. 2022;11:617–24.
43. Shi S, Zhao Z, Liu X, Shu Q, Tan L, Lin R, Shi Z, Fang X. Perioperative risk factors for prolonged mechanical ventilation following cardiac surgery in neonates and young infants. Chest. 2008;134:768–74.
44. Sauthier M, Sauthier N, Bergeron Gallant K, Lodygensky GA, Kawaguchi A, Emeriaud G, Jouvet P. Long-term mechanical ventilation in neonates: a 10-year overview and predictive model. Front Pediatr. 2021;9:689190.
45. Gowans M, Keenan HT, Bratton SL. The population prevalence of children receiving invasive home ventilation in Utah. Pediatr Pulmonol. 2007;42:231–6.
46. Il KH, Cho JH, Park SY, et al. Home mechanical ventilation use in South Korea based on National Health Insurance Service Data. Respir Care. 2019;64:528–35.
47. Lloyd-Owen SJ, Donaldson GC, Ambrosino N, Escarabill J, Farre R, Fauroux B, Robert D, Schoenhofer B, Simonds AK, Wedzicha JA. Patterns of home mechanical ventilation use in Europe: results from the Eurovent survey. Eur Respir J. 2005;25:1025–31.
48. Nakamura T. Current status and future aspects of home care medicine for children with medical complexity. Organ Biol. 2019;27:21–30.
49. Amin R, Sayal P, Syed F, Chaves A, Moraes TJ, MacLusky I. Pediatric long-term home mechanical ventilation: twenty years of follow-up from one Canadian center. Pediatr Pulmonol. 2014;49:816–24.
50. Palfrey JS, Haynie M, Porter S, Fenton T, Cooperman-Vincent P, Shaw D, Johnson B, Bierle T, Walker DK. Prevalence of medical technology assistance among children in Massachusetts in 1987 and 1990. Public Health Rep. 1994;109:226–33.
51. Graham RJ, Fleegler EW, Robinson WM. Chronic ventilator need in the community: a 2005 pediatric census of Massachusetts. Pediatrics. 2007;119:e1280–7.
52. Edwards EA, Hsiao K, Nixon GM. Paediatric home ventilatory support: the Auckland experience. J Paediatr Child Health. 2005;41:652–8.
53. Racca F, Berta G, Sequi M, et al. Long-term home ventilation of children in Italy: a national survey. Pediatr Pulmonol. 2011;46:566–72.
54. Young HK, Lowe A, Fitzgerald DA, Seton C, Waters KA, Kenny E, Hynan LS, Iannaccone ST, North KN, Ryan MM. Outcome of noninvasive ventilation in children with neuromuscular disease. Neurology. 2007;68:198–201.
55. Gilgoff RL, Gilgoff IS. Long-term follow-up of home mechanical ventilation in young children with spinal cord injury and neuromuscular conditions. J Pediatr. 2003;142:476–80.
56. Chatwin M, Tan H-L, Bush A, Rosenthal M, Simonds AK. Long term non-invasive ventilation in children: impact on survival and transition to adult care. PLoS One. 2015;10:e0125839.
57. Fauroux B, Boffa C, Desguerre I, Estournet B, Trang H. Long-term noninvasive mechanical ventilation for children at home: a national survey. Pediatr Pulmonol. 2003;35:119–25.
58. Traiber C, Piva JP, Fritsher CC, Garcia PCR, Lago PM, Trotta EA, Ricachinevsky CP, Bueno FU, Baecker V, Lisboa BD. Profile and consequences of children requiring prolonged mechanical ventilation in three Brazilian pediatric intensive care units. Pediatr Crit Care Med. 2009;10:375–80.
59. Karthikeyan B, Kadhiravan T, Deepanjali S, Swaminathan RP. Case-mix, care processes, and outcomes in medically-ill patients receiving mechanical ventilation in a low-resource setting from Southern India: a prospective clinical case series. PLoS One. 2015;10:e0135336.
60. Monteverde E, Fernández A, Poterala R, Vidal N, Siaba Serrate A, Castelani P, Albano L, Podestá F, Farias JA. Characterization of pediatric patients receiving prolonged mechanical ventilation. Pediatr Crit Care Med. 2011;12:e287–91.
61. Liu Y, Wang Q, Hu J, Zhou F, Liu C, Li J, Fu Y, Dang H. Characteristics and risk factors of children requiring prolonged mechanical ventilation vs. non-prolonged mechanical ventilation in the PICU: a prospective single-center study. Front Pediatr. 2022;10:830075.

62. Rose L, McKim D, Katz S, Leasa D, Nonoyama M, Pedersen C, Avendano M, Goldstein R. Institutional care for long-term mechanical ventilation in Canada: a national survey. Can Respir J. 2014;21:357–62.
63. Esteban A, Anzueto A, Alía I, et al. How is mechanical ventilation employed in the intensive care unit? An international utilization review. Am J Respir Crit Care Med. 2000;161:1450–8.
64. O'Brien S, Nadel S, Almossawi O, Inwald DP. The impact of chronic health conditions on length of stay and mortality in a general PICU. Pediatr Crit Care Med. 2017;18:1–7.
65. Toussaint M, Wijkstra PJ, McKim D, Benditt J, Winck JC, Nasiłowski J, Borel J-C. Building a home ventilation programme: population, equipment, delivery and cost. Thorax. 2022;77:1140–8.
66. Maynard R, Christensen E, Cady R, Jacob A, Ouellette Y, Podgorski H, Schiltz B, Schwantes S, Wheeler W. Home health care availability and discharge delays in children with medical complexity. Pediatrics. 2019;143(1):e20181951.
67. Sobotka SA, Foster C, Lynch E, Hird-McCorry L, Goodman DM. Attributable delay of discharge for children with long-term mechanical ventilation. J Pediatr. 2019;212:166–71.

Overview, Management Strategy of Prolonged and Long-Term Mechanical Ventilation in Children

Geovanny F. Perez

Prolonged and long-term mechanical ventilation are challenging to study since the terms have been used interchangeably to describe children that require mechanical ventilation beyond the acute phase. For example, long-term ventilation, chronic ventilator support, dependent ventilator support, and home ventilation are terms that are used to describe patients requiring some type of mechanical method for respiratory support after discharge from the hospital [1–4]. On the other hand, prolonged ventilation is generally used to describe patients in the intensive care unit that need ventilatory support beyond an expected period of time [5]. Thus, it is crucial to try to clarify the differences between both.

1 Definitions

There is a lack of consistent definition of what is considered prolonged mechanical ventilation in the pediatric population. In 2005, the National Association for Medical Direction of Respiratory Care (NAMDRC) defined prolonged mechanical ventilation (PMV) for adults as mechanical ventilation for more than 21 consecutive days for >6 h/d of invasive and/or noninvasive methods of delivery. In pediatrics, many definitions have been used in the literature to describe PMV, ranging from 2–7 days to 21–28 days, tracheostomy use, or home care management [6]. In 2017, Sauthier M et al. recommended defining pediatric PMV as >21 consecutive days (after 37 weeks' postmenstrual age) of ventilation for >6 h/d considering invasive ventilation and NIV and including short interruption [7]. This is the first time that

G. F. Perez (✉)
Division of Pulmonary and Sleep Medicine, Oishei Children's Hospital, Jacobs School of Medicine and Biomedical Sciences, Buffalo, NY, USA
e-mail: gperez9@buffalo.edu

A. Kawaguchi et al. (eds.), *Prolonged and Long-Term Mechanical Ventilation in Children*, https://doi.org/10.1007/978-981-97-8903-0_3

gestational age was included in the definition, which is a relevant factor for the pediatric population; however, it also has some gaps, such as the role of high-flow nasal cannula (HFNC) as a PMV modality. The lack of a PMV consensus definition can affect medical decisions, such as tracheostomy placement and transfer to sub-acute care. For instance, ventilation for >21 days is used as an indication for transfer to long-term acute care or step-down unit in the adult population. Likewise, the threshold for tracheostomy is a crucial aspect that has not been well studied in children. In adults, early tracheostomy (<7 days) has been shown to be associated with lower rates of ventilator-associated pneumonia, shorter days of mechanical ventilation, and ICU stay [8, 9]. Recent studies have shown similar results in the pediatric population where early tracheostomy, <14 days, was associated with decreased length of stay and ventilator days and with no effect on mortality [10]. Tracheostomy and PMV outcomes in infants, particularly those with bronchopulmonary dysplasia (BDP), are challenging to study. Several outcomes are used to evaluate the effectiveness of tracheostomy. In infants with BPD, the neurodevelopmental assessment is widely used as an outcome measure at 2 years of age. Infants with BPD needing tracheostomy for ventilatory support have overall worse neurodevelopmental outcomes. However, a large retrospective study from the Child Health and Human Development Neonatal Research Network showed better neurodevelopmental outcomes when a tracheostomy was placed earlier, defined as <120 days of life [11]. Tracheostomy placement in the severe BPD population is also associated with improved linear growth, physical and occupational therapy tolerance, and a faster wean of sedation [11, 12].

2 Home Mechanical Ventilation

Home mechanical ventilation (HMV) is the use of any mechanical method of respiratory support in the patient's home, continuously or intermittently, provided invasively through the tracheostomy or noninvasively through any other type of interface [13–15]. The use of HMV has become widespread in recent years due to medical and technological advances, which have contributed to the increased survival of critical patients [16, 17]. In addition, better diagnostic tools and new therapeutics such as gene therapy or enzyme replacement therapy have changed the natural history of several otherwise deemed fatal disorders [18, 19]. The development of new user-friendly devices for home use and the increased awareness of the patient's autonomy and right to be an active member of society have pushed the narrative and ethical considerations for the benefit of HMV [20]. Also, the creation of specialized multidisciplinary units for the follow-up of patients with HMV has improved survival, morbidity, and quality of life. Additionally, HMV can produce psychosocial improvements for patients and their families and contribute to more efficient use of the financial resources of the healthcare system [21–23].

For the purpose of this review, the term long-term ventilation (LTV) will be used for patients that require home ventilator support independently if it was started in the hospital setting and then transitioned to a subacute unit or home. Also, we will consider NIV only for bi-level positive-pressure ventilation and not for continuous positive-pressure ventilation (CPPV).

3 Goals of LTV

Most simplistically, the main goal of LTV is to correct abnormal gas exchange, improve ventilation, and reduce the work of breathing. However, the goals of LTV go beyond the correction of a physiologic impartment and should include (1) enhancement of quality of life, (2) prolonging life without compromising quality, (3) promoting growth and providing energy for activities that will allow children to achieve their developmental potential [15], and (4) providing cost-effective care [15, 24–26].

It is essential to consider that children that require LTV are fragile and often need complex care—but with committed and well-educated families and support (i.e., nurses, aids), they can attend school and live rich and joyful lives [27, 28].

4 LTV Indications

Children requiring LTV are a very heterogeneous group varying across different functional statuses and prognoses. Table 1 summarizes the prognosis among the most common respiratory disorders in children. In general, children that need LTV can be divided into six groups:

– Children with disorders that affect the respiratory drive: congenital central hypoventilation syndrome (CCHS), Chiari malformations, and brain tumors.

Table 1 Long-term ventilation indications and prognosis

	Onset	Disease	Prognosis/ ventilation
Respiratory drive	Congenital	CCHS [29]	Long term
Thoracic problems	Congenital/ acquired	Scoliosis, pectus excavatum [30]	Variable
Neuromuscular	Congenital	SMA [19, 31], CM [32, 33], DMD [34]	Variable
Parenchymal disorders	Congenital	ABCA3, ACD [35]	Poor prognosis
Development	Congenital	BPD [36]	Good prognosis
Upper airway	Acquired	OSA [37, 38]	Variable

CCHS congenital central hypoventilation syndrome, *SMA* spinal muscular atrophy, *CM* congenital myopathy, *DMD* Duchenne muscular dystrophy, *ABCA3* surfactant protein mutation, *ACD* alveolar-capillary dysplasia, *BPD* bronchopulmonary dysplasia, *OSA* obstructive sleep apnea

- Children with thoracic/spine problems: scoliosis and pectus excavatum.
- Children with neuromuscular disorders: spinal muscular atrophy, congenital myopathies, and muscular dystrophies.
- Children with parenchymal lung disorders/diffuse lung disorders: surfactant protein mutations and alveolar-capillary dysplasia.
- Children with disorders of development: bronchopulmonary dysplasia/chronic lung disease of prematurity.
- Children with disorders of the upper airway: severe upper airway obstruction associated with craniofacial abnormalities (Pierre Robin, Crouzon). Children with static encephalopathy, who, over time, develop upper airway obstruction that is initially treated with NIV and later can require LTV.

5 Clinical Scenarios

There are different clinical scenarios for when to start LTV.

- Management of hypoventilation: This is the most common clinical indication. Children with progressive respiratory disorders will first develop nighttime respiratory disturbances associated with REM sleep before progressing to daytime respiratory failure. This is most commonly seen in children with neuromuscular disorders, such as Duchenne muscular dystrophy, but is also seen in the vast majority of respiratory diseases, like severe scoliosis and interstitial lung disorders [4, 17, 30, 39–41].
- *Transitory use*: LTV is considered for children whose respiratory disorder is expected to improve over time. For instance, children with severe bronchopulmonary dysplasia require LTV until lung growth and alveolarization improve and respiratory support is discontinued [36, 42]. LTV can also be considered a bridge for lung transplantation in patients with diffuse lung disease (i.e., ABCA3) or patients with cystic fibrosis [43–45].
- *Prolongation of life*: This is the clearest indication for LTM. A child with end-stage respiratory failure has a limited life expectancy; thus, long-term ventilation is the only treatment option—infants with congenital central hypoventilation syndrome (CCHS) [29, 46].
- *Parental wishes*: This is perhaps one of the most controversial indications. Ideally, the decision to start LTV will be agreed upon between the medical team, parents, and the child when appropriate. However, this is not always the case. Often, the medical team does not recommend starting LTV due to the progressive nature of disorders where LTV will not improve quality of life but prolonged life. The final decision, particularly in the USA, is on parental wishes. In other geographic areas with different healthcare systems, the decision to start LTV relies more on the medical team or an ethics comitee [47–51]. A clinical scenario is a patient with severe hypoxic brain injury with no respiratory drive. Initiation of LTV, in this case, will prolong life but will not significantly impact the overall

outcome. Also, quality of life can be affected due to the potential complications related to frequent medical procedures and hospitalizations.

- *Palliative care*: In patients with any respiratory disorder, primary or secondary, LMV can facilitate the transition to home where the child can be cared for and die in a familiar environment per the family's wishes [52–57].

Despite the different indications and clinical scenarios, the most common indications for PMV in the pediatric population include chronic lung disease, neurological impairment, and upper airway anomalies [58].

6 Principles of Mechanical Ventilation

Describing the principles of mechanical ventilation in detail is beyond the scope of this review. However, we will review some basic principles of ventilator support that are important in LTV. Regardless of the indication for ventilator support, three main parameters are applied to all settings. In addition, new algorithms may provide modifications to improve synchrony or increased/variable support throughout time or during sickness.

These parameters are the trigger variable, the target or limit variable, and the termination or cycle variable.

Trigger variable The trigger variable defines how a ventilator breath is initiated. The ventilator breath can be initiated by (1) pressure, (2) flow, and (3) time. The changes in pressure and flow are due to a patient's effort; thus, these are patient-triggered breaths. Time-mandatory breaths are initiated by the ventilator. A common problem in patients with neuromuscular weakness or infants is their inability to trigger the ventilator despite new devices having very sensitive triggers to patient effort [3, 59, 60]. For this reason, it is recommended that a backup rate is always set [59]. The starting backup rate is equal to or slightly less than the spontaneous sleeping respiratory rate and can be calculated by subtracting 2–4 breaths from the patient's awake respiratory rate [1, 3, 4, 59, 60].

Limit This is the maximal limit set up on the ventilator. The limit variable can be (1) pressure limited (i.e., peak inspiratory pressure (PIP) or pressure control above the PEEP), (2) volume limited (a set tidal volume), or (3) time limited (the inspiratory time during a flow-cycle breath). Pressure-limited ventilation compensates for non-intentional leaks better than volume-limited ventilation; thus, it tends to be the choice for LTV [7, 61–64]. It also has the advantage of not requiring frequent adjustments due to the patient linear growth, compared with volume-limited ventilation, where the TV needs to be adjusted over time. However, a disadvantage of pressure-limited ventilation is that volumes will be affected by changes in respiratory mechanics, such as changes in resistance due to airway secretions or compliance with respiratory infections [61, 65]. During respiratory illnesses, children on LTV often need increased ventilator support, which requires management in the acute care setting or office. However, frequently, the changes in ventilator settings are minimal and, if done at home, could allow the child to recover without admission to the hospital. Therefore, new hybrid modes of ventilation that adjust the pressure to achieve a set volume limit or minute ventilation have been developed [66, 67]. These modes have the advantage of auto-adjusting the pressure limits within a certain range (upper and lower limits), thus allowing for changes in ventilator support during respiratory illness but also due to typical day-to-day variations.

Cycle This term refers to the change from the inspiratory to the expiratory phases. A breath can be time, flow, or pressure cycled. A time-cycle breath is defined as when the breath is terminated after the inspiratory time is reached. A breath is flow cycled when the ventilator detects the end of the patient's inspiration/flow and terminates the breath [65]. Leaks can affect cycling; the inspiratory phase will continue if the leak flow is greater than the ventilator's flow-cycle setup. Most new home ventilators have the advantage of setting flow-cycle criteria, which could help mitigate issues with leaks [1, 3, 59, 60, 68].

Other aspects of LTV and setting a home ventilator are essential, such as the type of circuit (active vs. passive, single vs. dual limb), blending oxygen, and battery. All of them play a role in patient adjustment and comfort [63]. In addition, new devices provide ventilatory support and can also function as a suction device, oxygen concentrators, cough assistance, and nebulizer [69]. Since patients on LTV often have comorbidities that require therapies with multiple devices, these new devices can facilitate home care.

7 Nighttime Ventilation

Due to changes in muscle tone, respiratory problems are usually first seen during sleep and progress to daytime-related symptoms in most respiratory disorders [34, 70–74]. When nighttime respiratory failure is present, the treatment of choice is noninvasive ventilation (e.g., bi-level positive airway pressure (BPAP)) in children without contraindications and who can wear/tolerate a facial interface.

8 Screening for Sleep-Disordered Breathing

Symptoms of sleep-disordered breathing (SDB) and nocturnal hypoventilation may include the more classic snoring, witnessed apneas, or gasping respirations to more subtle morning headaches, poor concentration, nocturnal sweating, restlessness, sleep disturbance, fatigue, and poor appetite that can lead to failure to thrive. Patients with symptoms of SDB warrant further evaluation and management; however, many individuals are often asymptomatic [32, 39, 73, 75, 76].

Without ideal clinical predictors for SDB, vital capacity (VC) is the most predictive measure currently implemented. For patients who can perform spirometry, a VC less than 40% predicted is highly suggestive of nocturnal hypoventilation with hypercapnia [34, 77, 78]. With VC less than 40% predicted, individuals may already have chronic respiratory failure. Intending to identify patients before progressing to chronic respiratory failure, screening patients with VC less than 60% predicted is a sensitive marker of SDB [79, 80].

For asymptomatic patients who cannot perform pulmonary function tests, screening for SDB relies on history and a physical exam. Furthermore, using available questionnaires like the Sleep-Disordered Breathing in Neuromuscular Disease Questionnaire (SiNQ-5) may be beneficial [81]. Further testing should also be considered when patients develop deterioration in baseline muscle strength.

9 Diagnosing Sleep-Disordered Breathing

The gold standard for assessing SDB is polysomnography (PSG) [32, 70, 82]. A complete PSG with accompanying measurement of CO_2 values (end tidal or transcutaneous) is the test of choice. Nocturnal pulse oximetry can be considered a screening test in the absence of access to PSG [34, 40]. There are no standardized definitions as to what constitutes abnormal oximetry in the context of hypoventilation. The presence of clusters of desaturations, or a "saw-tooth pattern," can be a sign of early obstructive apnea or hypopneas in REM sleep in NMD [40, 83].

Transcutaneous capnography ($TcCO_2$) is emerging as a tool for assessing nocturnal respiratory failure. This appears to identify individuals with nocturnal hypoventilation who otherwise have normal nocturnal oximetry and normal daytime blood gases. This testing, however, is not universally available in the outpatient setting. Independent of SDB, healthcare professionals should be monitoring for awake hypercarbia. During regular office visits, CO_2 levels should be checked by either $EtCO_2$ or $TcCO_2$ analyses [84]. Capillary or venous blood gases can be performed if less invasive measures are unavailable or more precise CO_2 measurements are required.

10 Initiating Respiratory Support

The long-term benefits of respiratory support in progressive respiratory disorders such as neuromuscular disorders are well established. Respiratory support for nocturnal respiratory failure has demonstrated multiple benefits, including decreased mortality, unplanned hospitalizations, daytime hypercarbia, and overall daytime symptom improvement [70]. Delayed initiation of respiratory support can increase the risk for worsened pulmonary function, nutritional deterioration, and progressive respiratory failure [4].

Daytime respiratory failure, characterized by awake hypercarbia with or without accompanying hypoxia, tends to develop slowly and follows the appearance of nocturnal hypoventilation and/or recurrent respiratory exacerbations [85]. The development of daytime hypercarbia is an indication for the initiation of ventilatory support, if not already initiated. Left untreated, awake hypercarbia is associated with a poor prognosis [17].

11 Noninvasive Ventilatory Support

Noninvasive ventilation (NIV) is the most common ventilatory support modality for treating nighttime respiratory failure [86]. The main goals of NIV support are (a) to rest the respiratory muscles, (b) to improve the sensitivity of the respiratory center to CO_2, (c) to improve pulmonary mechanics, and (d) to improve sleep architecture.

Nocturnal NIV allows the muscles to rest and recover with a subsequent improvement in inspiratory muscle function and gas exchange during the day [87–89]. It also prevents hypoventilation, thus restoring the sensitivity of the respiratory center to CO_2 and improving ventilation and gas exchange during the day [70, 88]. Furthermore, it has also been proposed that NIV improves lung function through the recruitment of atelectatic areas, increasing lung compliance and improving ventilation-perfusion relationships.

NIV improves sleep architecture and reduces sleep fragmentation, thus improving overall sleep efficiency. Moreover, NIV improves the most common symptoms of SDB, such as hypersomnolence, fatigue, morning headache, cognitive dysfunction, and dyspnea, mainly related to sleep disruption secondary to apneas [70, 82].

Treatment success with NIV depends on several factors, including correct patient selection, appropriate medical indication, the patient's ability to cooperate, adequate support (including nursing), a proper fitting interface, and family education.

12 Interface

Proper mask fitting is critical for the acceptance of NIV therapy [90]. A poorly fitted interface can lead to physical discomfort and suboptimal ventilator support, leading to poor tolerance and treatment failure. With acclimation and support, nasal interfaces are ultimately well tolerated and effective. They have less static dead space, allow the patient to expectorate any coughed-up mucus, and provide access to the mouth for suctioning of secretions. They may also be less claustrophobic than oronasal or full-face masks [91–94]. The nasal interface is also safer than a full-face mask for patients that are not supervised when asleep. If the pressure circuit becomes occluded accidentally, the patient can mouth breathe until attended. Nasal interfaces may be less useful in acute decompensations when patients have significant nasal congestion and are mouth breathing.

A challenge of mask fitting is air leaks resulting from the inadequate fit between the skin and the mask or from an open mouth. Leaks reduce alveolar ventilation and synchronization between the patient and the machine, leading to suboptimal support. Continuous monitoring and leak compensation are common features of most NIV devices [95, 96]. Headgear helps maintain the mask in an optimal position. Finding optimal headgear sizes in infants or patients with microcephaly can be challenging; thus, custom modifications are usually required.

Noninvasive ventilation modes and settings: For a child with a compromised respiratory system, alveoli may not adequately inflate due to weakness of respiratory muscles, airway obstruction, and injury to lung tissue leading to hypoventilation. The type of NIV generally recommended for respiratory failure with hypercapnia is bi-level positive airway pressure (BPAP). BPAP provides constant positive pressure at two different settings, one for inspiration (inspiratory positive airway pressure) and another for expiration (expiratory positive airway pressure).

The IPAP and rate are adjusted to deliver adequate ventilatory support, and the EPAP helps to maintain patency of the upper airway. The settings are titrated based on individual patients' needs. Ideally, a titration study is performed to assess key polysomnographic parameters (pressures and gas exchange) to integrate these into decision-making. For children with respiratory muscle weakness and infants, it is recommended that a backup rate is set, as they may be unable to trigger the device [3, 59, 60]. Besides setting the trigger, limit, and cycling, NIV devices have other important parameters that can affect ventilation and comfort, including rise time, ramp cycle, and heated humidification.

There are new algorithms that combine different modes of ventilation that can target minute ventilation or tidal volumes (i.e., AVAPS, iVAPS). These hybrid modes have theoretical advantages over standard fixed-pressure NIV; however, the data on its use in pediatrics is sparse, and recommendations are often extrapolated from adult populations [66, 67, 97, 98].

12.1 Contraindications to and Considerations for NIV

There are a few important considerations prior to the initiation of NIV [30]:

- Behavioral problems that could compromise adherence to therapy.
- Skin lesions/trauma at the site of mask apposition.
- The inability of a community-based durable medical equipment (DME) provider or hospital to provide or manage this type of support.
- NIV use of more than 16 h per day. Prolonged use may increase the risk of complications and side effects such as skin breakdown and midface hypoplasia and possibly increase the risk of morbidity.
- Patient/parent discussions about switching to invasive ventilation with a tracheostomy are indicated, as this is a quality-of-life decision.

- Bulbar muscle weakness associated with swallowing dysfunction will increase the risk of aspiration.
- The only absolute contraindication is respiratory failure that is not controlled by NIV.

13 Tracheostomy

Noninvasive ventilation (NIV) has gained increasing popularity over invasive ventilation via tracheostomy (LT-IMV) to correct hypoventilation and sleep-disordered breathing in patients with chronic respiratory failure in the last two decades [2, 27, 99, 100]. Nevertheless, long-term mechanical ventilation via tracheotomy continues to be used commonly in cases of respiratory failure where NIV or other modalities are contraindicated, impractical, or not the patient's preference. There are no formal globally accepted indications for tracheostomy, and practice does vary considerably, ranging from clinical judgment to results from a complete polysomnogram [27]. In children, LT-IMV is considered for those who require ventilatory assistance continuously, who are too young to be able to perform mouthpiece ventilation, and those for whom continuous nasal ventilation interferes with development or is considered too challenging to achieve by caregivers. Older children with cerebral palsy who develop upper airway obstruction typically require tracheostomy placement when NIV proves ineffective at overcoming the obstruction or the child needs positive-pressure support during waking hours to overcome airway obstruction [37, 101]. Children with congenital neuromuscular disorders, such as infants with congenital myopathies, or spinal muscular atrophy that causes profound weakness in infancy, are typically those patients considered for LT-IMV [33, 102]. In addition to severe extrathoracic airway obstruction preventing adequate airflow through the natural airway, the general indications for long-term ventilatory support via tracheostomy include (1) glottic dysfunction that predisposes to recurrent aspiration and interferes with cough clearance despite assistance; (2) development of recurrent pneumonia despite the use of aggressive cough augmentation; (3) persistent hypercapnia despite optimal use of NIV; (4) patient preference; and (5) lack of healthcare providers experienced in the use of continuous NIV [72]. When chronic respiratory failure ensues after an acute illness for which invasive ventilation is required, tracheostomy placement is typically offered to adults if the need for invasive ventilator support is expected to be longer than 1–3 weeks. Available evidence suggests the superiority of early (<10 days) over late tracheostomy in such situations [10, 103, 104]. In children, however, tracheostomy placement for support of prolonged mechanical ventilation is often not offered until several weeks of mechanical ventilation via an endotracheal tube have passed [105–107].

Tracheostomy prevalence in mechanically ventilated adults in the ICU is around 10% and increasing [108, 109]. Of those, about 25% are discharged tracheostomized with preserved spontaneous breathing. The incidence of tracheostomy use in pediatric ICUs is slightly lower, and children who undergo tracheostomy placement often have several comorbidities and are considered medically complex [105, 106]. The lack of suitable interfaces and machines with adequate trigger and cycle sensitivities is likely a contributing factor for the use of LT-IMV over NIV in the smallest and weakest patients. The prevalence of LT-IMV has varied a great deal over time and differs from one country to another [110–117]. European data from 2005 reported a mean prevalence of LT-IMV of 0.9 per 100,000, with the highest prevalence in France and the Scandinavian countries and most frequently applied in neuromuscular conditions as compared to thoracic and lung diseases [118]. The prevalence of all LT-IMV in Massachusetts at the same time was 7.1–8.3 per 100,000, of whom 75% received LT-IMV [119]. A survey of the same region involving only children cared for outside of an acute care hospital showed that 49% of the 197 subjects received LT-IMV via tracheostomy; 53 of the 97 children receiving LT-IMV had an underlying neurological or neuromuscular condition [120]. Recent national data from Canada reported a mean prevalence covering a wide span of 2.9/100,000 for LT-IMV, most frequently applied in patients suffering from ALS, muscular dystrophy, spinal cord injuries, or central hypoventilation [27]. The prevalence in Denmark exceeds 6/100,000. The fraction of individuals requiring LT-IMV via tracheostomy has been reported to be around 30% among patients with neuromuscular disease [121].

The advantages of tracheostomy include reduced risk of aspiration (when using cuffed tubes), better secretion clearance, possibility for airway inspection, reduction of dead space, and a reduction of resistive loads by 50–80% [122, 123]. Among adults treated with both NIV and LT-IMV, approximately 1/3 preferred tracheostomy for clearance of secretions during acute respiratory tract infections. Those who had switched from NIV to tracheostomy preferred the latter for sleep, comfort, and security [124]. In contrast, the respondents preferred NIV when considering swallowing, appearance, and ease of care. A number of adverse effects, sometimes fatal, from LT-IMV have been reported [125–127]. Tracheo-broncho-malacia is a potentially fatal complication with an incidence of over 20% and has been documented even when uncuffed cannulas were used [128]. Other disadvantages of tracheostomies include more complex and costly care, loss of glottic control with the inability to perform breath stacking, gram-negative bacterial colonization, traumatic tracheo-innominate or tracheo-esophageal fistula formation, occlusion of the tube by secretions, granuloma formation within the airway, and inadvertent displacement of the tube [129–131].

Following the emergence of centers for home mechanical ventilation in the early 1990s using almost exclusively LT-IMV, the 15-year survival changed from 52% to 77%, and mortality per 100 years at risk decreased from 4.7 to 2.6 in a group of Danish boys suffering from DMD [132]. Swedish data documented from a mean period of T-LTMV for 26 years that life expectancy was not reduced compared to the expected length of life in a heterogeneous group of patients [133]. Similar trends have also been shown in other countries, such as Japan and France [134, 135]. A meta-analysis of patients on LT-IMV showed similar mortality outcomes among the acute care setting and home or centers for home mechanical ventilation, as well as low ventilator failure rate [136]. The data highlights the increased trends and safety of home LT-IMV.

The incidence of pneumonia was low despite marked colonization [137] as was the hospitalization rate [133]. Quality of life while on LT-IMV has been reported as good in several studies [138, 139]. In contrast, Bach and coworkers showed that 22 men with DMD supported by LT-IMV experienced higher hospitalization rates and days of hospitalization compared with 24 men with DMD supported by NIV who used a protocol of oxyhemoglobin saturation monitoring to direct airway clearance [71].

LT-IMV was recently considered the preferred mode of ventilation for individuals suffering from ALS and resulted in an increased survival vs. no treatment. Similar results with ALS patients emerged from a Danish study where days of survival with no treatment, with NIV exclusively, with LT-IMV exclusively, and with NIV followed by LT-IMV were 699, 788, 1031, and 1734 days, respectively. Improved survival has also been shown in patients suffering from poliomyelitis [140, 141]. Among infants and children with SMA type 1 from four Italian centers, survival probability was significantly greater at 24 and 48 months in those supported with LT-IMV compared with those receiving NIV [31]. The approach to such patients is not uniform, however, with marked regional differences in the frequency of use of LT-IMV: whereas LT-IMV is commonly used to support infants with SMA type 1 in France, for instance, it is almost never used for those patients in Australia [142, 143]. Furthermore, Bach and coworkers have advocated for a noninvasive approach to infants with SMA type 1 who require continuous ventilatory support [144]. Nevertheless, it is important to note that no carefully controlled trials directly comparing outcomes of groups of patients with the neuromuscular disease treated with T-LTMV versus NIV have been done.

Although the area of LT-IMV has developed rapidly during recent decades, many challenges remain unsolved. Goals for the future should include national plans and creation of standards for this area, including:

- Establishment of guidelines and structured education for caregiver education regarding tracheostomy care and general respiratory assessments.
- Development of best practice guidelines regarding suctioning technique, type of catheter (close vs. open suction), duration of intervals between tube changes, stoma care, and skin care.
- Well-designed prospective studies that compare morbidity, mortality, and quality of life of patients supported by LT-IMV and NIV.
- Focus on phonation (where possible) and communication.
- Focus on the reduction of adverse effects, including infections, lesions, and leakage.
- Development of standards for facilities dedicated to LT-IMV.
- Creation of standards for monitoring and quality assurance of this treatment modality.

14 Summary

Long-term ventilation has increased in popularity over the last decades. It is an effective treatment option that can increase survival and provides adequate quality of life. However, it also has significant limitations including increased morbidity and healthcare cost and requires significant support at home. Therefore, the decision to explore ventilatory options should be carefully made between the family and their care team. Important considerations include the overall disease prognosis and course of the disease.

References

1. Amin R, Al-Saleh S, Narang I. Domiciliary noninvasive positive airway pressure therapy in children. Pediatr Pulmonol. 2016;51(4):335–48.
2. Fauroux B, Boffa C, Desguerre I, Estournet B, Trang H. Long-term noninvasive mechanical ventilation for children at home: a national survey. Pediatr Pulmonol. 2003;35(2):119–25.
3. Pavone M, Verrillo E, Caldarelli V, Ullmann N, Cutrera R. Non-invasive positive pressure ventilation in children. Early Hum Dev. 2013;89(Suppl 3):S25–31.
4. Simonds AK. Nocturnal ventilation in neuromuscular disease—when and how? Monaldi Arch Chest Dis. 2002;57(5–6):273–6.
5. MacIntyre NR, Epstein SK, Carson S, Scheinhorn D, Christopher K, Muldoon S. Management of patients requiring prolonged mechanical ventilation: report of a NAMDRC consensus conference. Chest. 2005;128(6):3937–54.
6. Rose L, McGinlay M, Amin R, et al. Variation in definition of prolonged mechanical ventilation. Respir Care. 2017;62(10):1324–32.
7. Sauthier M, Rose L, Jouvet P. Pediatric prolonged mechanical ventilation: considerations for definitional criteria. Respir Care. 2017;62(1):49–53.
8. Chorath K, Hoang A, Rajasekaran K, Moreira A. Association of Early vs late tracheostomy placement with pneumonia and ventilator days in critically ill patients: a meta-analysis. JAMA Otolaryngol Head Neck Surg. 2021;147(5):450–9.
9. Marra A, Vargas M, Buonanno P, Iacovazzo C, Coviello A, Servillo G. Early vs. late tracheostomy in patients with traumatic brain injury: systematic review and meta-analysis. J Clin Med. 2021;10(15):3319.
10. de Araujo OR, Azevedo RT, de Oliveira FRC, Colleti JJ. Tracheostomy practices in children on mechanical ventilation: a systematic review and meta-analysis. J Pediatr. 2022;98(2):126–35.
11. DeMauro SB, D'Agostino JA, Bann C, et al. Developmental outcomes of very preterm infants with tracheostomies. J Pediatr. 2014;164(6):1303–10.e2.
12. Luo J, Shepard S, Nilan K, et al. Improved growth and developmental activity post tracheostomy in preterm infants with severe BPD. Pediatr Pulmonol. 2018;53(9):1237–44.
13. McKim DA, Road J, Avendano M, et al. Home mechanical ventilation: a Canadian thoracic society clinical practice guideline. Can Respir J. 2011;18(4):197–215.
14. Simonds AK. Home mechanical ventilation: an overview. Ann Am Thorac Soc. 2016;13(11):2035–44.
15. Sterni LM, Collaco JM, Baker CD, et al. An official American Thoracic Society clinical practice guideline: pediatric chronic home invasive ventilation. Am J Respir Crit Care Med. 2016;193(8):e16–35.
16. Gilgoff RL, Gilgoff IS. Long-term follow-up of home mechanical ventilation in young children with spinal cord injury and neuromuscular conditions. J Pediatr. 2003;142(5):476–80.

17. Vianello A, Bevilacqua M, Salvador V, Cardaioli C, Vincenti E. Long-term nasal intermittent positive pressure ventilation in advanced Duchenne's muscular dystrophy. Chest. 1994;105(2):445–8.
18. Flotte TR, Gessler DJ. Gene therapy for rare neurological disorders. Clin Pharmacol Ther. 2022;111(4):743–57.
19. Reilly A, Chehade L, Kothary R. Curing SMA: are we there yet? Gene Ther. 2022;30(1–2):8–17.
20. Aas S, Wasserman D. Bodily rights in personal ventilators? J Appl Philos. 2022;39(1):73–86.
21. Klingshirn H, Gerken L, Hofmann K, et al. Comparing the quality of care for long-term ventilated individuals at home versus in shared living communities: a convergent parallel mixed-methods study. BMC Nurs. 2022;21(1):224.
22. Toussaint M, Wijkstra PJ, McKim D, et al. Building a home ventilation programme: population, equipment, delivery and cost. Thorax. 2022;77(11):1140–8.
23. Mattson J, Lunnelie J, Löfholm T, Andersson ES, Aune RE, Björling G. Quality of life in children with home mechanical ventilation – a scoping review. SAGE Open Nurs. 2022;8:23779608221094522.
24. Jardine E, Wallis C. Core guidelines for the discharge home of the child on long-term assisted ventilation in the United Kingdom. UK working party on paediatric long term ventilation. Thorax. 1998;53(9):762–7.
25. Tan LT, Nathan AM, Jayanath S, et al. Health-related quality of life and developmental outcome of children on home mechanical ventilation in a developing country: a cross-sectional study. Pediatr Pulmonol. 2020;55(12):3477–86.
26. Chawla J, Edwards EA, Griffiths AL, et al. Ventilatory support at home for children: a joint position paper from the Thoracic Society of Australia and New Zealand/Australasian Sleep Association. Respirology. 2021;26(10):920–37.
27. Rose L, McKim DA, Katz SL, et al. Home mechanical ventilation in Canada: a national survey. Respir Care. 2015;60(5):695–704.
28. Seear M, Kapur A, Wensley D, Morrison K, Behroozi A. The quality of life of home-ventilated children and their primary caregivers plus the associated social and economic burdens: a prospective study. Arch Dis Child. 2016;101(7):620–7.
29. Kasi AS, Li H, Harford KL, et al. Congenital central hypoventilation syndrome: optimizing care with a multidisciplinary approach. J Multidiscip Healthc. 2022;15:455–69.
30. Shneerson JM, Simonds AK. Noninvasive ventilation for chest wall and neuromuscular disorders. Eur Respir J. 2002;20(2):480–7.
31. Gregoretti C, Ottonello G, Chiarini Testa MB, et al. Survival of patients with spinal muscular atrophy type 1. Pediatrics. 2013;131(5):e1509–14.
32. Aboussouan LS. Sleep-disordered breathing in neuromuscular disease. Am J Respir Crit Care Med. 2015;191(9):979–89.
33. Lawlor MW, Dowling JJ. X-linked myotubular myopathy. Neuromuscul Disord. 2021;31(10):1004–12.
34. Birnkrant DJ, Bushby K, Bann CM, et al. Diagnosis and management of Duchenne muscular dystrophy, part 2: respiratory, cardiac, bone health, and orthopaedic management. Lancet Neurol. 2018;17(4):347–61.
35. Bush A, Gilbert C, Gregory J, Nicholson AG, Semple T, Pabary R. Interstitial lung disease in infancy. Early Hum Dev. 2020;150:105186.
36. Cristea AI, Carroll AE, Davis SD, Swigonski NL, Ackerman VL. Outcomes of children with severe bronchopulmonary dysplasia who were ventilator dependent at home. Pediatrics. 2013;132(3):e727–34.
37. Kontorinis G, Thevasagayam MS, Bateman ND. Airway obstruction in children with cerebral palsy: need for tracheostomy? Int J Pediatr Otorhinolaryngol. 2013;77(10):1647–50.
38. Garg RK, Afifi AM, Garland CB, Sanchez R, Mount DL. Pediatric obstructive sleep apnea: consensus, controversy, and craniofacial considerations. Plast Reconstr Surg. 2017;140(5):987–97.

39. Katz SL. Assessment of sleep-disordered breathing in pediatric neuromuscular diseases. Pediatrics. 2009;123(Suppl 4):S222–5.
40. Hull J, Aniapravan R, Chan E, et al. British Thoracic Society guideline for respiratory management of children with neuromuscular weakness. Thorax. 2012;67(Suppl 1):i1–40.
41. No Authors Listed. Clinical indications for noninvasive positive pressure ventilation in chronic respiratory failure due to restrictive lung disease, COPD, and nocturnal hypoventilation—a consensus conference report. Chest. 1999;116(2):521–34.
42. Baker CD. Long-term ventilation for children with chronic lung disease of infancy. Curr Opin Pediatr. 2019;31(3):357–66.
43. Toprak D, Midyat L, Freiberger D, Boyer D, Fynn-Thompson F, Visner G. Outcomes of mechanical support in a pediatric lung transplant center. Pediatr Pulmonol. 2017;52(3):360–6.
44. Flight WG, Shaw J, Johnson S, et al. Long-term non-invasive ventilation in cystic fibrosis—experience over two decades. J Cyst Fibros. 2012;11(3):187–92.
45. Madden BP, Kariyawasam H, Siddiqi AJ, Machin A, Pryor JA, Hodson ME. Noninvasive ventilation in cystic fibrosis patients with acute or chronic respiratory failure. Eur Respir J. 2002;19(2):310–3.
46. Trang H, Samuels M, Ceccherini I, et al. Guidelines for diagnosis and management of congenital central hypoventilation syndrome. Orphanet J Rare Dis. 2020;15(1):252.
47. Hopkins KA, Ott MA, Salih Z, Bosslet GT, Lantos J. When adolescent and parents disagree on medical plan, who gets to decide? Pediatrics. 2019;144(2):e20190291.
48. Bucher HU, Klein SD, Hendriks MJ, et al. Decision-making at the limit of viability: differing perceptions and opinions between neonatal physicians and nurses. BMC Pediatr. 2018;18(1):81.
49. Devictor DJ, Nguyen DT. Forgoing life-sustaining treatments in children: a comparison between northern and southern European pediatric intensive care units. Pediatr Crit Care Med. 2004;5(3):211–5.
50. Carey JC. Perspectives on the care and management of infants with trisomy 18 and trisomy 13: striving for balance. Curr Opin Pediatr. 2012;24(6):672–8.
51. Lantos JD. Ethical problems in decision making in the neonatal ICU. N Engl J Med. 2018;379(19):1851–60.
52. Krivec U, Caggiano S. Noninvasive ventilation in palliative care and ethical dilemma. Front Pediatr. 2020;8:483.
53. Mercadante S, Giarratano A, Cortegiani A, Gregoretti C. Application of palliative ventilation: potential and clinical evidence in palliative care. Support Care Cancer. 2017;25(7):2035–9.
54. Loganathan P, Simpson J, Boutcher P, Cooper A, Jackson A, Benson RJ. Home Extubation in a neonate. Pediatrics. 2018;142:1.
55. Laddie J, Craig F, Brierley J, Kelly P, Bluebond-Langner M. Withdrawal of ventilatory support outside the intensive care unit: guidance for practice. Arch Dis Child. 2014;99(9):812–6.
56. Davies JD. Noninvasive respiratory support at the end of life. Respir Care. 2019;64(6):701–11.
57. Wenzel D, Bleazard L, Pepper CJ, Wilson E, Faull C. Non-invasive advanced respiratory support in end-of-life care and symptom management: systematic review. BMJ Support Palliat Care. 2022;13(e3):e547–53.
58. Berry JG, Graham DA, Graham RJ, et al. Predictors of clinical outcomes and hospital resource use of children after tracheotomy. Pediatrics. 2009;124(2):563–72.
59. Berry RB, Chediak A, Brown LK, et al. Best clinical practices for the sleep center adjustment of noninvasive positive pressure ventilation (NPPV) in stable chronic alveolar hypoventilation syndromes. J Clin Sleep Med. 2010;6(5):491–509.
60. Khirani S, Louis B, Leroux K, Ramirez A, Lofaso F, Fauroux B. Improvement of the trigger of a ventilator for non-invasive ventilation in children: bench and clinical study. Clin Respir J. 2016;10(5):559–66.
61. De Luca A, Sall FS, Khoury A. Leak compensation algorithms: the key remedy to noninvasive ventilation failure? Respir Care. 2017;62(1):135–6.

62. Rabec C, Rodenstein D, Leger P, Rouault S, Perrin C, Gonzalez-Bermejo J. Ventilator modes and settings during non-invasive ventilation: effects on respiratory events and implications for their identification. Thorax. 2011;66(2):170–8.
63. Gregoretti C, Navalesi P, Ghannadian S, Carlucci A, Pelosi P. Choosing a ventilator for home mechanical ventilation. Breathe. 2013;9(5):394–409. https://doi.org/10.1183/20734735.042312.
64. Hess DR, Branson RD. Know your ventilator to beat the leak. Chest. 2012;142(2):274–5.
65. Chatburn RL, El-Khatib M, Mireles-Cabodevila E. A taxonomy for mechanical ventilation: 10 fundamental maxims. Respir Care. 2014;59(11):1747–63.
66. Rabec C, Emeriaud G, Amadeo A, Fauroux B, Georges M. New modes in non-invasive ventilation. Paediatr Respir Rev. 2016;18:73–84.
67. Selim BJ, Wolfe L, Coleman JM 3rd, Dewan NA. Initiation of noninvasive ventilation for sleep related hypoventilation disorders: advanced modes and devices. Chest. 2018;153(1):251–65.
68. Hess DR. Noninvasive ventilation in neuromuscular disease: equipment and application. Respir Care. 2006;51(8):896–911. discussion 2.
69. Sherwood SA, Martins BR, Ashworth L. Evaluation of a multifunction ventilator compared to a commonly used ventilator in pressure control ventilation. Respir Care. 2021;58(11):1911–22.
70. Annane D, Orlikowski D, Chevret S. Nocturnal mechanical ventilation for chronic hypoventilation in patients with neuromuscular and chest wall disorders. Cochrane Database Syst Rev. 2014;2014(12):Cd001941.
71. Bach JR, Ishikawa Y, Kim H. Prevention of pulmonary morbidity for patients with Duchenne muscular dystrophy. Chest. 1997;112(4):1024–8.
72. Benditt JO. Full-time noninvasive ventilation: possible and desirable. Respir Care. 2006;51(9):1005–12. discussion 12-5.
73. Dhand UK, Dhand R. Sleep disorders in neuromuscular diseases. Curr Opin Pulm Med. 2006;12(6):402–8.
74. Fauroux B, Abel F, Amaddeo A, et al. ERS statement on paediatric long-term noninvasive respiratory support. Eur Respir J. 2022;59(6):2101404.
75. Carroll JL, McColley SA, Marcus CL, Curtis S, Loughlin GM. Inability of clinical history to distinguish primary snoring from obstructive sleep apnea syndrome in children. Chest. 1995;108(3):610–8.
76. Katz SL, Gaboury I, Keilty K, et al. Nocturnal hypoventilation: predictors and outcomes in childhood progressive neuromuscular disease. Arch Dis Child. 2010;95(12):998–1003.
77. Lyager S, Steffensen B, Juhl B. Indicators of need for mechanical ventilation in Duchenne muscular dystrophy and spinal muscular atrophy. Chest. 1995;108(3):779–85.
78. Toussaint M, Steens M, Soudon P. Lung function accurately predicts hypercapnia in patients with Duchenne muscular dystrophy. Chest. 2007;131(2):368–75.
79. Mellies U, Ragette R, Schwake C, Boehm H, Voit T, Teschler H. Daytime predictors of sleep disordered breathing in children and adolescents with neuromuscular disorders. Neuromuscul Disord. 2003;13(2):123–8.
80. Ragette R, Mellies U, Schwake C, Voit T, Teschler H. Patterns and predictors of sleep disordered breathing in primary myopathies. Thorax. 2002;57(8):724–8.
81. Zhang C, Ramsay M, Drakatos P, Steier J. The clinical usefulness of a self-administered questionnaire for sleep-disordered breathing in patients with neuromuscular disease. J Thorac Dis. 2018;10(Suppl 1):S153–s9.
82. Annane D, Quera-Salva MA, Lofaso F, et al. Mechanisms underlying effects of nocturnal ventilation on daytime blood gases in neuromuscular diseases. Eur Respir J. 1999;13(1):157–62.
83. White JE, Drinnan MJ, Smithson AJ, Griffiths CJ, Gibson GJ. Respiratory muscle activity and oxygenation during sleep in patients with muscle weakness. Eur Respir J. 1995;8(5):807–14.
84. Georges M, Nguyen-Baranoff D, Griffon L, et al. Usefulness of transcutaneous PCO_2 to assess nocturnal hypoventilation in restrictive lung disorders. Respirology. 2016;21(7):1300–6.
85. Panitch HB. Diurnal hypercapnia in patients with neuromuscular disease. Paediatr Respir Rev. 2010;11(1):3–8.

86. Schönhofer B, Sortor-Leger S. Equipment needs for noninvasive mechanical ventilation. Eur Respir J. 2002;20(4):1029–36.
87. Goldstein RS, De Rosie JA, Avendano MA, Dolmage TE. Influence of noninvasive positive pressure ventilation on inspiratory muscles. Chest. 1991;99(2):408–15.
88. Rochester DF, Esau SA. Assessment of ventilatory function in patients with neuromuscular disease. Clin Chest Med. 1994;15(4):751–63.
89. Nickol AH, Hart N, Hopkinson NS, Moxham J, Simonds A, Polkey MI. Mechanisms of improvement of respiratory failure in patients with restrictive thoracic disease treated with non-invasive ventilation. Thorax. 2005;60(9):754–60.
90. Ward S, Chatwin M, Heather S, Simonds AK. Randomised controlled trial of non-invasive ventilation (NIV) for nocturnal hypoventilation in neuromuscular and chest wall disease patients with daytime normocapnia. Thorax. 2005;60(12):1019–24.
91. Fernandez R, Cabrera C, Rubinos G, et al. Nasal versus oronasal mask in home mechanical ventilation: the preference of patients as a strategy for choosing the interface. Respir Care. 2012;57(9):1413–7.
92. Elliott MW. The interface: crucial for successful noninvasive ventilation. Eur Respir J. 2004;23(1):7–8.
93. Bettinzoli M, Taranto-Montemurro L, Messineo L, et al. Oronasal masks require higher levels of positive airway pressure than nasal masks to treat obstructive sleep apnea. Sleep Breath. 2014;18(4):845–9.
94. Masolini M, Castellani C, Degli Innocenti C, et al. Interfaces for non invasive ventilation in children. ERJ Open Res. 2020;6(suppl 4):48. https://doi.org/10.1183/23120541.RFMVC-2020.48.
95. Arnal J-M, Thevenin C-P, Couzinou B, Texereau J, Garnero A. Setting up home noninvasive ventilation. Chron Respir Dis. 2019;16:1479973119844090.
96. Park S, Suh E-S. Home mechanical ventilation: back to basics. Acute Crit Care. 2020;35(3):131–41.
97. Saddi V, Thambipillay G, Martin B, Blecher G, Teng A. Pediatric average volume assured pressure support. Front Pediatr. 2022;10:868625.
98. Sunkonkit K, Al-Saleh S, Chiang J, et al. Volume-assured pressure support mode for noninvasive ventilation: can it improve overnight adherence in children with neuromuscular disease? Sleep Breath. 2021;25(4):1843–50.
99. Bach JR, Alba AS, Saporito LR. Intermittent positive pressure ventilation via the mouth as an alternative to tracheostomy for 257 ventilator users. Chest. 1993;103(1):174–82.
100. Simonds AK. Nasal ventilation in progressive neuromuscular disease: experience in adults and adolescents. Monaldi Arch Chest Dis. 2000;55(3):237–41.
101. Wilkinson DJ, Baikie G, Berkowitz RG, Reddihough DS. Awake upper airway obstruction in children with spastic quadriplegic cerebral palsy. J Paediatr Child Health. 2006;42(1–2):44–8.
102. Hjartarson HT, Nathorst-Böös K, Sejersen T. Disease modifying therapies for the Management of Children with spinal muscular atrophy (5q SMA): an update on the emerging evidence. Drug Des Devel Ther. 2022;16:1865–83.
103. Andriolo BN, Andriolo RB, Saconato H, Atallah ÁN, Valente O. Early versus late tracheostomy for critically ill patients. Cochrane Database Syst Rev. 2015;1(1):Cd007271.
104. Huang H, Li Y, Ariani F, Chen X, Lin J. Timing of tracheostomy in critically ill patients: a meta-analysis. PLoS One. 2014;9(3):e92981.
105. Liu C, Heffernan C, Saluja S, et al. Indications, hospital course, and complexity of patients undergoing tracheostomy at a tertiary care pediatric hospital. Otolaryngol Head Neck Surg. 2014;151(2):232–9.
106. Wakeham MK, Kuhn EM, Lee KJ, McCrory MC, Scanlon MC. Use of tracheostomy in the PICU among patients requiring prolonged mechanical ventilation. Intensive Care Med. 2014;40(6):863–70.

107. Sarkar M, Roychowdhoury S, Bhakta S, Raut S, Nandi M. Tracheostomy before 14 days: is it associated with better outcomes in pediatric patients on prolonged mechanical ventilation? Indian J Crit Care Med. 2021;25(4):435–40.
108. Mehta AB, Syeda SN, Bajpayee L, Cooke CR, Walkey AJ, Wiener RS. Trends in tracheostomy for mechanically ventilated patients in the United States, 1993–2012. Am J Respir Crit Care Med. 2015;192(4):446–54.
109. Abril MK, Berkowitz DM, Chen Y, Waller LA, Martin GS, Kempker JA. The epidemiology of adult tracheostomy in the United States 2002–2017: a serial cross-sectional study. Crit Care Explor. 2021;3(9):e0523.
110. Frutos-Vivar F, Esteban A, Apezteguía C, et al. Outcome of mechanically ventilated patients who require a tracheostomy. Crit Care Med. 2005;33(2):290–8.
111. Benson RC, Hardy KA, Gildengorin G, Hsia D. International survey of physician recommendation for tracheostomy for spinal muscular atrophy type I. Pediatr Pulmonol. 2012;47(6):606–11.
112. Chau SK, Yung AW, Lee SL. Long-term management for ventilator-assisted children in Hong Kong: 2 decades' experience. Respir Care. 2017;62(1):54–64.
113. Amin R, Sayal P, Syed F, Chaves A, Moraes TJ, MacLusky I. Pediatric long-term home mechanical ventilation: twenty years of follow-up from one Canadian center. Pediatr Pulmonol. 2014;49(8):816–24.
114. Czajkowska-Malinowska M, Bartolik K, Nasiłowski J, Kania A. Development of home mechanical ventilation in Poland in 2009-2019 based on the data of the National Health Fund. J Clin Med. 2022;11(8):2098.
115. Pavone M, Verrillo E, Onofri A, Caggiano S, Chiarini Testa MB, Cutrera R. Characteristics and outcomes in children on long-term mechanical ventilation: the experience of a pediatric tertiary center in Rome. Ital J Pediatr. 2020;46(1):12.
116. Park M, Jang H, Sol IS, et al. Pediatric home mechanical ventilation in Korea: the present situation and future strategy. J Korean Med Sci. 2019;34(42):e268.
117. Saiphoklang N, Kanitsap A, Ruchiwit P, Pirompanich P, Sricharoenchai T, Cooper CB. Patient characteristics and outcomes of a home mechanical ventilation program in a developing country. Lung India. 2019;36(3):207–11.
118. Lloyd-Owen SJ, Donaldson GC, Ambrosino N, et al. Patterns of home mechanical ventilation use in Europe: results from the Eurovent survey. Eur Respir J. 2005;25(6):1025–31.
119. Divo MJ, Murray S, Cortopassi F, Celli BR. Prolonged mechanical ventilation in Massachusetts: the 2006 prevalence survey. Respir Care. 2010;55(12):1693–8.
120. Graham RJ, Fleegler EW, Robinson WM. Chronic ventilator need in the community: a 2005 pediatric census of Massachusetts. Pediatrics. 2007;119(6):e1280–7.
121. Lofaso F, Prigent H, Tiffreau V, et al. Long-term mechanical ventilation equipment for neuromuscular patients: meeting the expectations of patients and prescribers. Respir Care. 2014;59(1):97–106.
122. Chadda K, Louis B, Benaïssa L, et al. Physiological effects of decannulation in tracheostomized patients. Intensive Care Med. 2002;28(12):1761–7.
123. Epstein SK. Anatomy and physiology of tracheostomy. Respir Care. 2005;50(4):476–82.
124. Bach JR. A comparison of long-term ventilatory support alternatives from the perspective of the patient and care giver. Chest. 1993;104(6):1702–6.
125. Deutsch ES. Tracheostomy: pediatric considerations. Respir Care. 2010;55(8):1082–90.
126. Dhand R, Johnson JC. Care of the chronic tracheostomy. Respir Care. 2006;51(9):984–1001. discussion 2-4
127. O'Connor HH, White AC. Tracheostomy decannulation. Respir Care. 2010;55(8):1076–81.
128. Baydur A, Kanel G. Tracheobronchomalacia and tracheal hemorrhage in patients with Duchenne muscular dystrophy receiving long-term ventilation with uncuffed tracheostomies. Chest. 2003;123(4):1307–11.
129. Al-Samri M, Mitchell I, Drummond DS, Bjornson C. Tracheostomy in children: a population-based experience over 17 years. Pediatr Pulmonol. 2010;45(5):487–93.

130. Fernandez-Bussy S, Mahajan B, Folch E, Caviedes I, Guerrero J, Majid A. Tracheostomy tube placement: early and late complications. J Bronchol Interv Pulmonol. 2015;22(4):357–64.
131. Morar P, Singh V, Jones AS, Hughes J, van Saene R. Impact of tracheotomy on colonization and infection of lower airways in children requiring long-term ventilation: a prospective observational cohort study. Chest. 1998;113(1):77–85.
132. Jeppesen J, Green A, Steffensen BF, Rahbek J. The Duchenne muscular dystrophy population in Denmark, 1977–2001: prevalence, incidence and survival in relation to the introduction of ventilator use. Neuromuscul Disord. 2003;13(10):804–12.
133. Björling G, Johansson UB, Andersson G, Schedin U, Markström A, Frostell C. A retrospective survey of outpatients with long-term tracheostomy. Acta Anaesthesiol Scand. 2006;50(4):399–406.
134. Saito T, Tatara K, Kawai M. Changes in clinical condition and causes of death of inpatients with Duchenne muscular dystrophy in Japan from 1999 to 2012. Rinsho Shinkeigaku. 2014;54(10):783–90.
135. Boussaïd G, Lofaso F, Santos DB, et al. Impact of invasive ventilation on survival when non-invasive ventilation is ineffective in patients with Duchenne muscular dystrophy: a prospective cohort. Respir Med. 2016;115:26–32.
136. Sison SM, Sivakumar GK, Caufield-Noll C, Greenough WB 3rd, Oh ES, Galiatsatos P. Mortality outcomes of patients on chronic mechanical ventilation in different care settings: a systematic review. Heliyon. 2021;7(2):e06230.
137. Harlid R, Andersson G, Frostell CG, Jörbeck HJ, Ortqvist AB. Respiratory tract colonization and infection in patients with chronic tracheostomy. A one-year study in patients living at home. Am J Respir Crit Care Med. 1996;154(1):124–9.
138. Markström A, Sundell K, Lysdahl M, Andersson G, Schedin U, Klang B. Quality-of-life evaluation of patients with neuromuscular and skeletal diseases treated with noninvasive and invasive home mechanical ventilation. Chest. 2002;122(5):1695–700.
139. Narayanaswami P, Bertorini TE, Pourmand R, Horner LH. Long-term tracheostomy ventilation in neuromuscular diseases: patient acceptance and quality of life. Neurorehabil Neural Repair. 2000;14(2):135–9.
140. Meinesz AF, Wijkstra PJ, Zijlstra JG, Albers MJ, Köter GH. From the poliomyelitis epidemic to the founding of artificial respiration centres, intensive care units and centres for home mechanical ventilation. Ned Tijdschr Geneeskd. 2006;150(8):444–9.
141. Mellem H, Bendz B. Artificial ventilation in the home. Experiences from a department of pulmonary medicine, Ullevål hospital. Tidsskr Nor Laegeforen. 1995;115(6):699–702.
142. Rul B, Carnevale F, Estournet B, Rudler M, Hervé C. Tracheotomy and children with spinal muscular atrophy type 1: ethical considerations in the French context. Nurs Ethics. 2012;19(3):408–18.
143. Tassie B, Isaacs D, Kilham H, Kerridge I. Management of children with spinal muscular atrophy type 1 in Australia. J Paediatr Child Health. 2013;49(10):815–9.
144. Bach JR, Niranjan V, Weaver B. Spinal muscular atrophy type 1: a noninvasive respiratory management approach. Chest. 2000;117(4):1100–5.

Oxygen Therapy for Prolonged and Long-Term Mechanical Ventilation in Children

Florent Baudin

In children with prolonged and long-term mechanical ventilation (PMV), supplemental oxygen is a frequent additional therapy. Supplemental oxygen can be used to increase inspired fraction of oxygen during mechanical ventilation but also as simple therapy between periods of ventilation. Most clinical conditions in children differ from those in adults, and there is no specific recommendation for the use of oxygen in children with PMV. However, some guidelines and expert opinions are available for home oxygen therapy in infants and children, and these may be used, in part, for children with PMV [1–3].

1 Physiology of Oxygen

In standard conditions, two atoms of the element oxygen bind to form dioxygen (O_2), a colorless and odorless gas that makes up 20.9% of air. In clinical practice, as herein, the term "oxygen" is frequently used instead of dioxygen to designate the gas used for medical application or in human physiology.

Oxygen (i.e., dioxygen, O_2) is transported in the blood dissolved in the plasma (~2%) or bound to hemoglobin (~98%). Each hemoglobin molecule can carry four O_2 molecules, and the proportion of binding sites occupied by oxygen is expressed as oxygen (O_2) saturation. Oxygen saturation can be measured either

F. Baudin (✉)
Hospices Civils de Lyon, Département d'anesthésie-réanimation, Hôpital Femme Mère Enfant, Bron, France

Agressions Pulmonaires et Circulatoires dans le Sepsis (APCSe), VetAgro Sup, Universités de Lyon, Lyon, France
e-mail: florent.baudin@chu-lyon.fr

A. Kawaguchi et al. (eds.), *Prolonged and Long-Term Mechanical Ventilation in Children*, https://doi.org/10.1007/978-981-97-8903-0_4

invasively by arterial blood gas analysis (SaO_2) or noninvasively by pulse oximetry (SpO_2). The partial pressure of oxygen (O_2) measured by arterial blood gas analysis (PaO_2) measures only O_2 dissolved in the plasma and not the part bound to hemoglobin. There is a dynamic equilibrium between the two forms described by the hemoglobin-oxygen dissociation curve that is sigmoidal [4]; at high PaO_2, large changes in pressure lead to only small changes in oxygen saturation, whereas with oxygen saturation <90%, a small change in PaO_2 results in a large change in oxygen saturation. For this reason, in order to estimate PaO_2 using noninvasive measurement (SpO_2), it is recommended not to exceed 97% SpO_2 when using supplemental oxygen [5]. The hemoglobin-oxygen dissociation curve is also dependent on temperature, pH, and 2,3-diphosphoglycerate (2,3-DPG) concentration; the affinity of hemoglobin for oxygen is increased (left shift of dissociation curve) at lower temperatures, lower CO_2 concentration, lower 2,3-DPG concentration, and higher pH.

2 Definition of Hypoxemia

Hypoxemia is defined as a low level of oxygen in the blood, and hypoxia as insufficient oxygen in tissues in order to ensure a normal cell and organ function. Hypoxemia can occur by only five mechanisms: decrease of inspired partial pressure of oxygen, hypoventilation, right-to-left shunt, diffusion impairment, or ventilation/perfusion mismatch. In children with PMV, the latter two are the two most frequent mechanisms of hypoxemia that lead to the use of oxygen therapy.

2.1 *Threshold*

The measurement of PaO_2 is not recommended for the diagnosis of chronic hypoxemia in children; noninvasive pulse oximetry (SpO_2) is sufficient. Oxygen saturation is normally (at or near sea level) between 97 and 99% and should be above 94% as defined by the World Health Organization [6]. In children living at high altitude, saturation is lower because of a lower inspired partial pressure of oxygen. In 2019, the American Thoracic Society Assembly on Pediatrics [1] published a systematic review and found that the mean SpO_2 in children <1 years of age was 97.8% (SD ± 1.4%), and in those ≥1 year of age, this was 97.6% (SD ± 0.7%); the experts determined that a low SpO_2 for a duration of 2 weeks in a clinically stable condition was sufficient evidence for the chronicity of hypoxemia. They defined chronic hypoxemia as spending 5% of the recording time with $SpO_2 \leq 90\%$ for children aged <1 year and $SpO_2 \leq 93\%$ for children aged ≥1 year. Intermittent measurement of SpO_2 may also be used for the diagnosis, in which case hypoxemia is defined as three independent measurements with $SpO_2 \leq 90\%$ for children aged <1 year and $SpO_2 \leq 93\%$ for children aged ≥1 year. However, normal intermittent measurement cannot totally exclude chronic hypoxemia.

2.2 Consequences of Chronic Hypoxemia

Chronic hypoxemia in infancy and childhood can lead to long-term severe organ dysfunctions and has been associated with deleterious consequences on pulmonary circulation, growth, sleep, and neurological development [7]. The mechanisms have been studied in patients with chronic neonatal lung disease or in children with cystic fibrosis or sickle cell disease in whom it is reported that hypoxemia is associated with arterial pulmonary vasoconstriction and affects vascular and alveolar development [8–10]. It is of note that the correction of hypoxemia may improve physiological condition and the right ventricle function [8]. In addition, in children with severe obstructive sleep apnea, as well as in neonates and infants with congenital heart disease (CHD), adverse neurodevelopmental outcome is reported to be associated with hypoxemic episodes [11, 12], and hypoxemic events may also affect growth and lead to sleep disorders by increasing the risk of central apneas [13].

3 Indication for Oxygen Therapy

It is difficult to make very strong recommendations as to the indications for oxygen therapy in children with PMVed. Based on the previous guidelines on home oxygen therapy in children [1, 3], which share some of the indications of mechanical ventilation, it is possible to identify some subgroups of patients that may benefit from oxygen therapy but with a low quality of evidence (Table 1).

Table 1 Main indications of oxygen therapy for prolonged and long-term mechanical ventilation in children (CPAP: continuous positive airway pressure; NIV: noninvasive ventilation)

Respiratory condition	Indication for oxygen therapy	Comment
Chronic neonatal lung disease	As primary or in addition to CPAP/NIV	Prevent pulmonary hypertension Promote growth Improve neurodevelopment To allow hospital discharge
Pulmonary hypertension	Without congenital heart disease	Not recommended at first in children with congenital heart disease because oxygen will impact hemodynamics and physiology
Obstructive sleep apnea	Only in patients who do not tolerate CPAP/NIV	Sleep-related oxygen (nocturnal and naps)
Chronic hypoventilation	When ventilator support is not possible	Sleep-related oxygen (nocturnal and naps)
Interstitial lung disease	Severe chronic hypoxemia	To allow hospital discharge
Sickle cell disease	Persistent nocturnal hypoxemia	Reduce risk of stroke, painful crises, and pulmonary hypertension
Cystic fibrosis	Severe chronic hypoxemia	May improve school attendance To obtain symptomatic relief
Palliative care	To obtain symptomatic relief	

Oxygen may also be used as intermittent emergency therapy in children without chronic hypoxemia (i.e., without continuous oxygen) but requiring mechanical ventilation who present intercurrent infection (fever, respiratory tract infection, etc.).

4 Equipment and Monitoring

Evidence on the optimal equipment and monitoring in children requiring long-term oxygen is lacking; most recommendations are based on expert opinions [1, 14]. However, pediatric pulmonologists or intensivists, or other specialists with extensive experience in chronic lung disease, should prescribe oxygen therapy. In addition, parents have to be educated on equipment, on the disease, and on emergency care, and a parent-held discharge plan is recommended to ensure a safe transition from hospital to home.

4.1 Provision of Oxygen

Oxygen concentrators are one of the main systems used at home and allow a delivery flow that is most commonly between 1 L and 5 L/min. Stationary devices require source of electricity, and therefore a backup generator or alternative source of oxygen (cylinders) should be associated. Tanks and cylinders are easier to transport but are limited by the duration of oxygen delivery, particularly in case of a high flow of oxygen. All children should have portable equipment (portable concentrators with battery or low-weight cylinders) to allow transport and movement [14]. In infants, low-flow meters are necessary to deliver flow <1 L/min. In cases where a home ventilator is not used, humidification of oxygen should be provided for a flow >1 L/min [3], and it is generally recommended for children with tracheostomy using a heat-moisture exchanger with oxygen attachment. For home ventilators, it is necessary to have the dedicated connector to supply oxygen directly on the ventilator or to add a T-piece on the circuit.

4.2 Monitoring

There is no evidence for the routine use of pulse oximeter at home; however, and especially in children with prolonged and long-term mechanical ventilation, experts endorse its use [1]. A pulse oximeter helps to identify hypoxemic events (during feeding or during intercurrent respiratory tract infections). Alarms should be adjusted according to the respiratory conditions to alert caregivers on life-threating event by avoiding the nuisance of frequent alarms. Caregivers should also be able to interpret the accuracy and validity of the value of pulse oximeters, based on the clinical status, to not make a decision only on the level of SpO_2. Pulse oximeters can also provide important information for the follow-up of these children.

4.3 Follow-Up and Weaning

It is recommended that at least a community nurse or a nurse specialist visit the child and the family at home in the 24 h following discharge and that a regular follow-up is organized [1, 3]. Improvement in respiratory condition is frequent in infants with chronic lung disease, and weaning of oxygen should be considered early. There are no formal criteria available to discontinue the patient's oxygen therapy, and readiness assessment should be based on a combination of several factors: respiratory conditions (period of stable condition), growth, and oxygen saturation measurement wakeful and nocturnal with the same goals that prompted imitation of oxygen therapy [1]. Weaning of oxygen can be evaluated either by decreasing the flow or by withdrawing supplemental oxygen during daytime activity or during mechanical ventilation. There is no evidence of the superiority of one modality over the other, and it should be based on experience and local protocol, respiratory condition, and daily duration of mechanical ventilation. Oxygen equipment should be left in the home for at least 2–3 months after weaning from oxygen therapy (longer during the winter period) [3].

5 High-Flow Nasal Therapy

High-flow nasal therapy (HFNT) allows the delivery of a flow greater than the inspiratory flow of the patient (up to 60–100 L/min). In contrast to conventional oxygen therapy, gas flow rate and FiO_2 can be adjusted independently [15, 16]. HFNT is safe and easy to use and is increasingly employed in neonatal and pediatric intensive care, but also now in ward patients [17, 18].

5.1 Mechanism of Action (Fig. 1)

HFNT provides a flow rate that matches the inspiratory flow and warmed and humidified gas flow to reduce metabolic work for gas conditioning and improve mucociliary clearance, for washout of the nasopharyngeal dead space and improving CO_2 removal, and generates a positive expiratory pressure [16]. The level of positive distending pressure for lung recruitment is highly dependent on the flow rate and whether the mouth is open or closed [19–21].

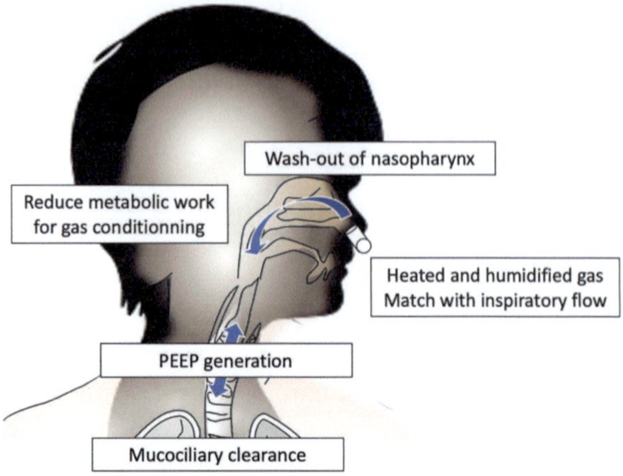

Fig. 1 Mechanism of action of high-flow nasal therapy. *PEEP* positive end expiratory pressure

5.2 Equipment

HFNT can be provided by three types of devices: specific devices with integrated humidification, ventilators with a dedicated module for high-flow therapy, or an air/oxygen blender connected to a system to humidify and heat the gas [22]. Home HFNT is possible only with electric high-flow devices with integrated humidification (for example, Airvo 2, Fisher & Paykel Healthcare, Auckland, New Zealand; HVT2.0, Vapotherm, Exeter, USA; TNI20, TNI Medical, Würzburg, Germany) or with home ventilator with external humidification. Additional oxygen has to be applied using cylinders or concentrator at home with a dedicated connection on the device. For the patient equipment, the cannula should not be strictly occlusive, and the size should be 75% lower than the nares' internal diameter in order to prevent air leak syndrome complications [15, 22, 23].

5.3 Settings

FiO_2 should be adjusted according to the target SpO_2 thresholds. The weight-adjusted flow rate is proportionally higher in neonates and in infants than in children or in adolescents. Flow rate is set to 8 L/min (~3 L/kg/min) in neonates, about 2 L/kg/min in infants, and 1 L/kg/min in children to reach the same level as that recommended in adults (50–70 L/min) [24, 25]. For chronic lung disease, there is no recommendation for flow setting, and they are mainly based on that used in neonatal and pediatric intensive care units.

5.4 *Clinical Evidence of HFNT for Prolonged and Long-Term Mechanical Ventilation in Children*

Data on the use of HFNT for children with chronic respiratory conditions are very limited. The main indications described in the literature are children with chronic neonatal lung disease and children with obstructive sleep apnea (OSA) who do not tolerate nasal continuous positive airway pressure (CPAP) [23, 26–29]. For instance, a case series has described the use of HFNT in children with CHD and miscellaneous respiratory problems [30], and one small study, including 12 patients, compared HFNT to CPAP in children with OSA and described comparable results on the apnea-hypopnea index [28]. Furthermore, in a retrospective study, Steindor et al. found that weaning success of HFNT at home was higher in infants with bronchopulmonary dysplasia than for other indications, although these infants required supplemental oxygen more often during HFNT [23]. The level of evidence remains currently limited to the use of long-term HFNT, but it appears as a suitable alternative for children in whom other ventilatory support is not tolerated.

6 Supplemental Oxygen During Air Travel

Air travel exposes children to decreased air pressure and lower-than-normal oxygen levels.

6.1 *Effect of Air Travel*

The main effect of increasing altitude is a decrease in barometric pressure. Regulatory government agencies require that commercial aircraft be pressurized to simulate an altitude below 8000 ft (2438 m), and the minimal allowed barometric pressure is approximately 564 mmHg (760 mmHg at sea level) [31]. The inspired fraction of oxygen is stable at 20.9%, but the drop in barometric pressure leads to a decrease of the inspired partial pressure of oxygen [32]. Therefore, children with prolonged and long-term mechanical ventilation may need oxygen supplementation in-flight, even if they do not use oxygen at home.

6.2 *Patients at Risk of In-Flight Hypoxemia*

The British Thoracic Society and Canadian Paediatric Society recommend that infants under 1 year with a history of neonatal chronic respiratory problems, children with chronic lung diseases with forced expiratory volume <50%, and infants and children who have had long-term oxygen within the last 6 months should have hypoxia altitude simulation testing [33, 34]. In children who are oxygen dependent at sea level or children with SpO_2 <85 or <90% during hypoxia altitude simulation testing depending on age (<1 or ≥1 year of age), supplemental oxygen during flight is recommended. Finally, it is recommended to refrain from air travel for 1 week after birth in term children.

6.3 Oxygen Delivery System for Air Travel

Most of the companies and aviation regulations prohibit patients from carrying oxygen cylinders aboard commercial aircraft. However, oxygen supplemental can be safely administered by a battery-powered portable oxygen concentrator throughout the flight [31, 35]. Portable oxygen concentrator provides up to 3–4 L/minute of oxygen flow, and it is recommended to bring batteries for 1.5 times the duration of the flight [31, 33, 34]. Air travel with ventilator support or with a higher oxygen flow rate is much more complicated and may require a medical escort. Therefore, the use of oxygen and/or respiratory devices has to be requested well in advance (at least 2 or 3 weeks before travel).

7 Conclusion

Oxygen therapy for prolonged and long-term mechanical ventilation in children is a challenge in infants and children with chronic respiratory diseases. HFNT is an emerging respiratory support at home as an alternative of CPAP in noncompliant children or in children with less severe disease. Air travel for children with prolonged and long-term mechanical ventilation should be well in advance anticipated because of the complexity of the logistic.

Financial Support This study was not funded.

Conflict of Interest Statement FB is a consultant for Fisher & Paykel Healthcare.

References

1. Hayes D, Wilson KC, Krivchenia K, Hawkins SMM, Balfour-Lynn IM, Gozal D, et al. Home oxygen therapy for children. An official American Thoracic Society clinical practice guideline. Am J Resp Crit Care. 2019;199:e5–23. https://doi.org/10.1164/rccm.201812-2276st.
2. Balfour-Lynn IM, Primhak RA, Shaw BNJ. Home oxygen for children: who, how and when? Thorax. 2005;60:76. https://doi.org/10.1136/thx.2004.031211.
3. Balfour-Lynn IM, Field DJ, Gringras P, Hicks B, Jardine E, Jones RC, et al. BTS guidelines for home oxygen in children. Thorax. 2009;64:ii1. https://doi.org/10.1136/thx.2009.116020.

4. Collins J-A, Rudenski A, Gibson J, Howard L, O'Driscoll R. Relating oxygen partial pressure, saturation and content: the haemoglobin–oxygen dissociation curve. Breathe. 2015;11:194–201. https://doi.org/10.1183/20734735.001415.
5. Khemani RG, Patel NR, Bart RD, Newth CJL. Comparison of the pulse oximetric saturation/fraction of inspired oxygen ratio and the PaO_2/fraction of inspired oxygen ratio in children. Chest. 2009;135(662):668. https://doi.org/10.1378/chest.08-2239.
6. World Health Organization. Oxygen therapy for children: a manual for health workers. 2016.
7. Gozal E, Gozal D. Respiratory plasticity following intermittent hypoxia: developmental interactions. J Appl Physiol 1985. 2001;90:1995–9. https://doi.org/10.1152/jappl.2001.90.5.1995.
8. Benatar A, Clarke J, Silverman M. Pulmonary hypertension in infants with chronic lung disease: non-invasive evaluation and short term effect of oxygen treatment. Arch Dis Child Fetal Neonatal Ed. 1995;72:F14. https://doi.org/10.1136/fn.72.1.f14.
9. Fraser KL, Tullis DE, Sasson Z, Hyland RH, Thornley KS, Hanly PJ. Pulmonary hypertension and cardiac function in adult cystic fibrosis: role of hypoxemia. Chest. 1999;115:1321–8. https://doi.org/10.1378/chest.115.5.1321.
10. Onyekwere OC, Campbell A, Teshome M, Onyeagoro S, Sylvan C, Akintilo A, et al. Pulmonary hypertension in children and adolescents with sickle cell disease. Pediatr Cardiol. 2008;29:309–12. https://doi.org/10.1007/s00246-007-9018-x.
11. Urschitz MS, Wolff J, Sokollik C, Eggebrecht E, Urschitz-Duprat PM, Schlaud M, et al. Nocturnal arterial oxygen saturation and academic performance in a community sample of children. Pediatrics. 2005;115:e204–9. https://doi.org/10.1542/peds.2004-1256.
12. Bass JL, Corwin M, Gozal D, Moore C, Nishida H, Parker S, et al. The effect of chronic or intermittent hypoxia on cognition in childhood: a review of the evidence. Pediatrics. 2004;114:805–16. https://doi.org/10.1542/peds.2004-0227.
13. Rigatto H, Brady JP. Periodic breathing and apnea in preterm infants. II. Hypoxia as a primary event. Pediatrics. 1972;50:219–28.
14. McCoy RW. Options for home oxygen therapy equipment: storage and metering of oxygen in the home. Respir Care. 2013;58:65–85. https://doi.org/10.4187/respcare.01932.
15. Milési C, Boubal M, Jacquot A, Baleine J, Durand S, Odena MP, et al. High-flow nasal cannula: recommendations for daily practice in pediatrics. Ann Intensive Care. 2014;4:29. https://doi.org/10.1186/s13613-014-0029-5.
16. Dysart K, Miller TL, Wolfson MR, Shaffer TH. Research in high flow therapy: mechanisms of action. Respir Med. 2009;103(1400):1405. https://doi.org/10.1016/j.rmed.2009.04.007.
17. Mikalsen IB, Davis P, Øymar K. High flow nasal cannula in children: a literature review. Scand J Trauma Resusc Emerg Medicine. 2016;24:93. https://doi.org/10.1186/s13049-016-0278-4.
18. Kotecha SJ, Vick D, Delgado-Thompson M, West J, Edwards MO. Establishing paediatric ward high-flow nasal cannula usage for infants with bronchiolitis. Acta Paediatr. 2022;111:638–9. https://doi.org/10.1111/apa.15527.
19. Ejiofor BD, Carroll RW, Bortcosh W, Kacmarek RM. PEEP generated by high-flow nasal cannula in a pediatric model. Respir Care. 2019;64:1240–9. https://doi.org/10.4187/respcare.06470.
20. Liew Z, Fenton AC, Harigopal S, Gopalakaje S, Brodlie M, O'Brien CJ. Physiological effects of high-flow nasal cannula therapy in preterm infants. Arch Dis Child Fetal Neonatal Ed. 2020;105:87. https://doi.org/10.1136/archdischild-2018-316773.
21. Sivieri EM, Gerdes JS, Abbasi S. Effect of HFNC flow rate, cannula size, and nares diameter on generated airway pressures: an in vitro study. Pediatr Pulm. 2013;48:506–14. https://doi.org/10.1002/ppul.22636.
22. Nolasco S, Manti S, Leonardi S, Vancheri C, Spicuzza L. High-flow nasal cannula oxygen therapy: physiological mechanisms and clinical applications in children. Front Med. 2022;9:920549. https://doi.org/10.3389/fmed.2022.920549.
23. Steindor M, Wagner CE, Kavvalou A, Bock C, Olivier M, Stehling F. Indications and outcome of home high-flow nasal therapy in children, a single-center experience. Pediatr Pulm. 2022;57(9):2048–52. https://doi.org/10.1002/ppul.25974.

24. Kawaguchi A, Garros D, Joffe A, DeCaen A, Thomas NJ, Schibler A, et al. Variation in practice related to the use of high flow nasal cannula in critically ill children. Pediatr Crit Care Med. 2020;21:e228–35. https://doi.org/10.1097/pcc.0000000000002258.
25. Peterson RJ, Hassumani DO, Hole AJ, Slaven JE, Tori AJ, Abu-Sultaneh S. Implementation of a high flow nasal cannula management protocol in the pediatric ICU. Respir Care. 2020;66:respcare.08284. https://doi.org/10.4187/respcare.08284.
26. Hawkins S, Huston S, Campbell K, Halbower A. High-flow, heated, humidified air via nasal cannula treats CPAP-intolerant children with obstructive sleep apnea. J Clin Sleep Med. 2017;13:981–9. https://doi.org/10.5664/jcsm.6700.
27. Joseph L, Goldberg S, Shitrit M, Picard E. High-flow nasal cannula therapy for obstructive sleep apnea in children. J Clin Sleep Med. 2015;11:1007–10. https://doi.org/10.5664/jcsm.5014.
28. McGinley B, Halbower A, Schwartz AR, Smith PL, Patil SP, Schneider H. Effect of a high-flow open nasal cannula system on obstructive sleep apnea in children. Pediatrics. 2009;124:179–88. https://doi.org/10.1542/peds.2008-2824.
29. Amaddeo A, Khirani S, Frapin A, Teng T, Griffon L, Fauroux B. High-flow nasal cannula for children not compliant with continuous positive airway pressure. Sleep Med. 2019;63:24–8. https://doi.org/10.1016/j.sleep.2019.05.012.
30. Muneuchi J, Sugitani Y, Watanabe M. The safety of home high-flow nasal cannula therapy in children with congenital heart disease and miscellaneous respiratory problems. Pediatr Cardiol. 2022;43:930. https://doi.org/10.1007/s00246-022-02893-1.
31. Israëls J, Nagelkerke AF, Markhorst DG, van Heerde M. Fitness to fly in the paediatric population, how to assess and advice. Eur J Pediatr. 2018;177:633–9. https://doi.org/10.1007/s00431-018-3119-9.
32. Lee AP, Yamatoto LG, Relles NL. Commercial airline travel decreases oxygen saturation in children. Pediatr Emerg Care. 2002;18:78–80. https://doi.org/10.1097/00006565-200204000-00004.
33. Lang M, Société canadienne de pédiatrie, Comité de la pédiatrie communautaire. Les voyages en avion et la santé des enfants. Paediatr Child Healt. 2007;12:53–9. https://doi.org/10.1093/pch/12.1.53.
34. Ahmedzai S, Balfour-Lynn IM, Bewick T, Buchdahl R, Coker RK, Cummin AR, et al. Managing passengers with stable respiratory disease planning air travel: British Thoracic Society recommendations. Thorax. 2011;66:i1. https://doi.org/10.1136/thoraxjnl-2011-200295.
35. Fischer R, Wanka ER, Einhaeupl F, Voll K, Schiffl H, Lang SM, et al. Comparison of portable oxygen concentrators in a simulated airplane environment. Respir Med. 2013;107:147–9. https://doi.org/10.1016/j.rmed.2012.10.001.

Noninvasive MV of PMVed Children

María Ángeles García-Teresa and Marti Pons Odena

1 Introduction

Noninvasive mechanical ventilation (NIMV) provides ventilatory support through an interface attached to the nostrils and/or mouth (outside the airway), avoiding tracheostomy or endotracheal tube [1–4]. Use of prolonged home NIV is growing exponentially worldwide, more in higher developing countries, but also in countries with lower income economies, in all-aged children with chronic respiratory failure (CRF) and sleep-disordered breathing [5–23]. Several factors contribute to this fact. Survival of children with CRF and complex medical conditions has increased due to development and optimization of pharmacological therapy, intensive care, rehabilitation, and surgical techniques, as well as broadening of ethical criteria for their implementation [24]. In addition, detection of sleep-disordered breathing and CRF in children at risk for severe obstructive sleep apnea (OSA) and neuromuscular patients has focused, due to their harmful consequences, on quality of life, behavior, and physical and neurodevelopment. Simultaneously, various favorable technological, financial, and socio-sanitary conditions have been developed for using NIV at home: relatively simple technique with simple and portable ventilation devices and a broad interface availability, funding, moving health care from hospital to home, and family engagement.

Clinical trial-based evidence is sparse to support the use of NIV in pediatrics, but not the evidence based on clinical practice, which reflects improved quality of life, growth, neurocognitive aspects, behavioral features, and neurodevelopment;

M. Á. García-Teresa (✉)
Pediatric Intensive Care Unit, Pediatric Home Ventilation Unit, Niño Jesús University Children's Hospital, Madrid, Spain

M. Pons Odena
University Hospital Sant Joan de Déu Barcelona, Esplugues de Llobregat, Spain

Home Mechanical Ventilation Program, Barcelona, Spain
e-mail: marti.pons@sjd.es

A. Kawaguchi et al. (eds.), *Prolonged and Long-Term Mechanical Ventilation in Children*, https://doi.org/10.1007/978-981-97-8903-0_5

avoidance of exacerbations; preservation of lung function; and increased survival [3, 6, 25]. Prolonged NIV is mainly used as an elective therapy in patients with sleep-disordered breathing and/or CRF, but is also used as a challenging life support therapy in highly selected children without or with sparse respiratory autonomy and alternatively to tracheostomy [26–31].

There are two predominant forms of NIV, continuous positive airway pressure (CPAP) and bilevel positive airway pressure (BLPAP) or pressure support (PS). CPAP is mainly indicated for airway obstruction (OSA). BLPAP is indicated in muscle weakness disorders, chest wall deformity, lung diseases, and abnormal central drive if optimal respiratory rate is assured [32, 33].

Children on prolonged NIV should be comprehensively managed through a home ventilation program, including expertise in pediatric NIV technical skills and sleep and home care education, in addition to other multidisciplinary specialists [34–37]. Family is the key for successful long-term home ventilation, demanding of chronic specialized care that can be exhausting, thus requiring ongoing institutional support. Follow-up goals should include weaning from ventilation if appropriate and transition to adult care if lifelong therapy, in addition to respiratory status stability, side effect minimizing, quality of life, growth, and neurodevelopment [38–40].

This chapter focuses on the indication, technical issues, and outcomes of long-term NIV while avoiding the discharge organizational aspects, post-discharge follow-up, and home care [41–44], which are covered in other chapters.

2 Indication

Normal respiratory function involves a balanced equilibrium between the load on the respiratory system (airway, lung, and chest wall) and the respiratory work capacity (respiratory drive and neuromuscular system). When the load exceeds the work capacity (due to respiratory system, respiratory drive, or neuromuscular disorders), respiratory failure occurs, leading to alveolar hypoventilation [33, 45]. NIV can correct the disequilibrium in the respiratory balance by replacing or supporting the central drive or respiratory muscles, maintaining a stable airway and improving lung compliance [32]. Some pediatric disorders that might benefit from NIV are listed in Table 1 [3, 4, 6, 25, 32, 46–50].

Criteria to be considered in patients who are eligible for home NIV are shown in Tables 2, 3, 4, and 5 [32]. Depending on the patient's characteristics, chronic NIV can be initiated at PICU as a life support therapy or electively, following a sleep study [16, 17, 51].

(a) Clinical and physiological criteria for chronic respiratory failure (Table 2); prolonged NIV should be started if other treatments are ineffective or not available, taking into account age, diagnosis, and prognosis [32, 45, 46, 52].
(b) Global clinical criteria of medical stability required for discharge are shown in Table 3, although each patient should be assessed individually [32, 52].

Table 1 Diseases in pediatric population suitable for prolonged noninvasive mechanical ventilation

Central nervous system (CNS) disorders
• Congenital and acquired disorders affecting the control of the respiratory center
- Congenital central hypoventilation syndrome, ROHHAD
- Central hypoventilation secondary to a metabolic disease (carnitine, pyruvate kinase deficiencies), syndrome (Leigh, Moebius, Prader-Willi), tumor, trauma, stroke, asphyxia, or infection
• Myelomeningocele and Arnold-Chiari malformation
• Spinal muscular atrophy
• Spinal cord injury
Neuromuscular disorders
• Congenital hypotonia
• Myasthenia gravis and congenital myasthenic syndromes
• Phrenic and diaphragmatic palsy
• Myopathies
• Muscular dystrophy
• Guillain-Barré syndrome
• Botulism
• Charcot-Marie-Tooth disease
• Diaphragmatic hernia
Skeletal disorders
• Kyphoscoliosis
• Thoracic wall deformities
Congenital and acquired cardiopathies
Respiratory disorders
Upper airway obstruction
• Sleep-related respiratory disorders: hypoventilation and obesity syndrome, obstructive sleep apnea (OSA)
• Down syndrome
• Craniofacial syndromes (Pierre Robin, Treacher Collins)
• Laryngotracheomalacia
• Tracheoesophageal fistula
• Subglottic stenosis
• Arnold-Chiari malformation
• Vocal cord paralysis
Bronchopulmonary disorders
• Bronchopulmonary dysplasia
• Cystic fibrosis
• Pulmonary hypoplasia
• Ciliary dyskinesia
• Bronchiolitis obliterans
• Complications from infectious or chemical pneumonias

(continued)

Table 1 (continued)

• Sequelae of pediatric acute respiratory distress syndrome
• Pulmonary fibrosis
Other metabolic disorders
• Glycogenoses
• Mucopolysaccharidoses
• Palliative care

Table 2 Criteria of chronic respiratory failure

Cardiopulmonary disorders	Central nervous system, neuromuscular and skeletal disorders
• Clinical criteria: - Decreased air entry detected during auscultation. - Sternal retraction, use of accessory muscles. - Diminished activity. - Poor weight gain. • Physiological criteria: - $PaCO_2 > 45$ mmHg. - $PaO_2 < 65$ mmHg. - $SatO_2 < 95\%$ on room air.	• Clinical criteria: - Weak cough. - Accumulation of secretions in the airway. - Use of accessory muscles. - Inability to swallow. - Weak or absent cough reflex. - Diminished activity. - Paradoxical breathing. • Physiological criteria: - Vital capacity <15 ml/kg (older children). - $PaCO_2 > 45$ mmHg. - $PaO_2 < 70$ mmHg. - $SatO_2 < 95\%$ on room air.

Table 3 Clinical criteria of stability required for discharge

• Patient should be free of repeated episodes of infection or fever.
• Adequate oxygenation, with consistent ventilator settings.
• Stable airway: NIV with minimal risk of aspiration.
• Spontaneous or assisted clearance of secretions.
- Absence of continuous moderate dyspnea and episodic severe dyspnea or tachypnea.
• Absence of life-threatening cardiac disease or dysrhythmias.
- Stable renal function.

(c) Clinical criteria for initiating NIV electively in adults with stable or slow-progression CRF have been described and used as a general guideline (Table 4) [53, 54]. Also initiating criteria of elective long-term NIV in children are used (Table 4) [3, 46, 47], although not validated and more flexible than adult ones [3, 33]. Criteria are mainly based on nocturnal hypoventilation and sleep disturbance detection and also end-organ morbidity assessment associated with CRF (growth; neurocognitive, behavioral, and neurodevelopment dysfunction; repetitive infections). Screening with at least an overnight Sat O_2 and transcutaneous (tc) PCO_2 recording and if possible polysomnographic should be performed in children with upper airway obstruction, neuromuscular disease, or lung disease that might be associated with nocturnal hypoventilation [33, 51,

Table 4 Criteria to prescribe elective home mechanical ventilation in adults and children (stable or slowly progressive chronic respiratory failure)

Adults
Neuromuscular and chest wall diseases
- Repeated hospital admissions due to respiratory exacerbations.
- Symptomatic hypoventilation or sleep disorders: Morning headache, restless sleep, nightmares, daytimesleepiness, cognitive or behavior disorders, malnourishment, recurrent respiratory infections, cor pulmonale (late manifestation).
- $PaCO_2$ > 45–50 mmHg while awake.
- Nocturnal hypoventilation with sustained O_2 desaturation (SpO_2 < 88% for >5 consecutive minutes) and symptoms (e.g., morning headache, hypersomnolence).
- FVC <50% of the theoretical value.
- Maximum inspiratory pressure below −60 cm H_2O (i.e., less negative than −60 cm H_2O; e.g., −50 cm H_2O).
- Maximum expiratory pressure < 40 cm H_2O.
- Sniff-nasal inspiratory force <40 cm H_2O.
- Vital capacity <15 to 20 mL/kg, <60% predicted, <1 liter, or decrease >30 to 50% compared with baseline.
Chronic obstructive lung diseases
- Hypoxia and hypercapnia despite adequate physiotherapy, bronchodilators, antibiotics, and nutritional support.
- Advanced disease with $PaCO_2 \geq$ 55 mmHg or $PaCO_2$ 50–54 mmHg and nocturnal hypoxemia despite oxygen therapy at ≥2 L/min or $PaCO_2$ 50–54 mmHg and more than two hospitalizations for hypercapnic respiratory failure in the previous year or after a life-threatening episode of acute on chronic respiratory failure.
- Specific CF criteria: Prevent or treat severe respiratory exacerbations; patient's desire to relieve dyspnea; rapid deterioration of lung function; end-stage palliative care; pre- and postoperative pulmonary transplantation; optimization of physiotherapy.
Children
- Repeated hospital admissions due to respiratory exacerbations.
- After a PICU admission due to acute respiratory failure or anesthetic procedure and unsuccessful weaning from ventilation.
- Prior to elective arthrodesis.
- Symptomatic hypoventilation or sleep disorders: Paradoxical breathing, morning headache, restless sleep, nightmares, insomnia, daytime sleepiness, fatigue or hyperactivity, cognitive or behavior disorders, malnourishment, recurrent respiratory infections, nocturnal enuresis, cor pulmonale (late manifestation).
- $PaCO_2$ > 45–50 mmHg while awake or $PaCO_2$ > −50 mmHg nocturnal.
- Tc $PCO_2 \geq$ 50 mmHg during ≥2% of recording time.
- Sat <90% during ≥2% of recording time.
- FVC <50% of the theoretical value, vital capacity <15 mL/kg.
- Pulmonary hypertension, right cardiac failure on echocardiogram.
- All patients*: Absence of contraindications for NIV: Significant upper airway/bulbar dysfunction, inability to clear secretions, severely weakened cough, uncooperative patient/family after an adequate period for adaptation, uncontrolled gastroesophageal reflux, severe aerophagia.

Table 5 Clinical, polysomnographic, and respiratory support criteria in pediatric OSA

Clinical criteria
- Sleep disorders: Heavy snoring, observed apneas, restlessness during sleep, excessive sweating, mouth breathing, nocturnal enuresis
- Daytime involvement: Excessive sleepiness, inattention/hyperactivity, cognitive deficits and learning difficulties, behavioral disorder
- Failure to thrive, systemic arterial hypertension, pulmonary hypertension, cor pulmonale
Polysomnographic criteria
- Apnea-hypopnea index (AHI): >1–4.9, mild OSA; 5–9.9, moderate OSA; >10, severe OSA.
- End tidal or transcutaneous $CO_2 > 50$ mmHg for >25% total sleep time (obstructive hypoventilation).
Treatment
- Depending on child's age, clinical symptoms, comorbidities, risk factors, and polysomnographic result if performed
- Important to consider:
- AHI >5 or AHI >1 and comorbidity.
- End tidal or transcutaneous $CO_2 > 50$ mmHg for >25% total sleep time (obstructive hypoventilation).
- Ventilation strategy (CPAP, BPAP):
- It will be discussed after considering adeno-tonsillectomy/weight loss/nasal corticosteroid therapy/antileukotriene treatment/orthodontics.
- It may be necessary before adeno-tonsillectomy if severe symptoms and hypoxemia are present.

$PaCO_2$ partial pressure of arterial carbon dioxide, *PaO_2* partial pressure of arterial oxygen, *SpO_2* oxygen saturation measured by pulse oximetry, *FVC* forced vital capacity, *OSA* obstructive sleep apnea, *AHI* Apnea-Hypopnea Index, *CPAP* continuous positive airway pressure, *BPAP* bilevel positive airway pressure, *CO_2* carbon dioxide, *CF* cystic fibrosis. *See text

55]. Chronically stable patients are typically hospitalized to initiate elective NIV for 2 or 3 days, but may also be set up at regular outpatient visits or more rarely at home in selected patients, with good outcomes on efficacy and compliance [16, 17, 36, 51]. Progressive adaptation is carried out at home.

(d) Specific clinical, polysomnographic, and respiratory support criteria for patients with obstructive sleep apnea (OSA) in children are shown in Table 5 [56].

(e) Family criteria: the family should be informed of the diagnosis and prognosis of disease and of the advantages, disadvantages, and risks of home NIV in order to assume dedication and responsibility for home care. Caregivers and patient training are essential. The absence of tracheostomy usually significantly facilitates home care [26]. However, infants and children on life support NIV require high vigilance during sleep to detect and treat early interface displacement and life-threatening hypoventilation. Very long home mechanical ventilation becomes a way of life for the child and family.

Contraindications for NIV have been listed: significant upper airway/bulbar dysfunction, inability to clear secretions, severely weakened cough, uncooperative patient/family after an adequate period for adaptation, uncontrolled gastroesophageal reflux (GER), and severe aerophagia. However, several collaborative strategies between patient/family and health team have been described to promote NIV in these challenging patients: manual and mechanical assisted cough; treatment of hypersalivation; use of mouthpiece during meals; a trial of NIV with nasal if uncontrolled GER; and family and child intensive support to improve adherence [4]. Other relative contraindications, as a facial abnormality and complications related to an interface, may be overcome with special, customized, or cloth masks. Also, selected patients without or with sparse respiratory autonomy (e.g., neuromuscular teenagers with ventilation for >16 h a day or infants with nocturnal life support therapy) are treated with NIV, alternatively to tracheostomy.

Ethical Considerations The technical capacity to extend life by mechanical ventilation makes the current approach more "what should be done" than "what can be done." Patients and parents play an essential role in shared decision-making, assessing all positive and negative aspects of the patient's current life condition with psychological support. The medical team is responsible for providing complete and accurate information on disease prognosis, technique, and possible alternatives, including tracheostomy, and on expected outcomes in terms of quality of life and expected life span. Palliative care is an emergent indication of NIV; however, the balance between relieving symptoms and prolonging suffering can be challenging [24].

3 Technical Issues on NIV

3.1 Ventilation Setup

3.1.1 Modes [32, 57, 58]

Pressure mode, volume mode (with or without pressure support), or hybrid mode, pressure with guarantee volume mode (available in new ventilators), can be used. Pressure mode is the most often used in NIV, due to its ability to compensate for leaks and to generate constant pressures when compared with volume ventilation. In this section, we will highlight hybrid modes, since the others (pressure or volume) have been previously explained in the invasive ventilation chapter.

Pressure-control mode with adaptive control scheme, also known as volume-targeted pressure ventilation (VTPV) or volume-assured pressure ventilation (VAPV), is characterized by a decelerated inspiratory flow curve, providing a variable pressure (between a minimum and maximum pressure set values) that automatically adapts to changes in airway resistance and lung compliance, to target a predetermined minimum expiratory volume. This hybrid mode aims to combine advantages of both pressure and volume modes, ensuring ventilation with more physiological inspiratory flow. The mode can be used with both PC (VAPC, volume-assured pressure control) and PS (VAPS, volume-assured pressure support).

However, it should be used with caution if closed circuits are used, where non-intentional leaks may be erroneously compensated by the software, leading to hyperventilation (in double-limb circuit systems) or hypoventilation (in single-limb circuit with exhalation valve) [59, 60]. A minimum pressure which guarantees adequate ventilation should be set in order to minimize the risk of hypoventilation, if closed circuits are used. Ventilators on VTPV using controlled-leak single-limb circuits compensate for non-intentional leaks correctly, thus mitigating misinterpretation leaks.

Depending on the BLPAP device, different intelligent algorithms and setting variables are used to provide the minimum assured volume, resulting in different NIV VTPV brands, such as AVAPS® (Average Volume Assured Pressure Support, from Philips-Respironics), iVAPS® (intelligent Volume Assured Pressure Support, from ResMed), or Target Volume® (from Breas). In AVAPS® and Target Volume® modes, a minimum target tidal volume is set, while in iVAPs® mode, a minimum target minute alveolar volume is fixed. The minimum tidal volume delivered by a given device may be too high for younger infants and therefore may limit the use of these hybrid modes in such children. Currently, usage of new hybrid modes is growing [61]. Despite their theoretical benefits, several adults' clinical trials have shown no differences in ventilation or sleep quality between PS and volume-assured modes. There is currently very little data in the literature on the use of these ventilation modes in children [62, 63]. Such devices were more effective than conventional BLPAP in reducing hypercarbia [64], in improving stability of transcutaneous carbon dioxide profile in different sleep states in congenital central hypoventilation syndrome (CCHS) [65–68], and in improving adherence in children with neuromuscular diseases [69, 70]. However, evidence of long-term outcomes in children is lacking.

3.1.2 Modes and Level of Respiratory Support [32]

Continuous mandatory ventilation (CMV), intermittent mandatory ventilation (IMV), or continuous spontaneous ventilation (PC-CSV) modes can be used according to the autonomy of the patient's own breathing and pathology. As a policy, greater patient participation in ventilation should be encouraged in order to optimize synchrony.

Continuous Mandatory Ventilation *Volume-control, pressure-control, and pressure-control modes with adaptive targeting scheme.* Volume-controlled, pressure-controlled, T mode (timed) in ventilators with bilevel positive airway pressure or "BLPAP" and assisted/controlled (A/C) modes are included. The ventilator will deliver the set breath (tidal volume or pressure) without any intervention from the patient or only his/her triggering inspiration. The ventilator always terminates every breath; either ventilator or patient can initiate it. The ventilator dictates inspiratory time duration. Controlled ventilation modes should be used whenever the ventilator cannot detect any respiratory effort from the patient, meaning those patients with disturbances of the respiratory center, children without respiratory effort (bulbomedullous lesions), or children who are unable to trigger the ventilator.

Intermittent Mandatory Ventilation (IMV) Volume- or pressure-controlled intermittent mandatory ventilation with set-point targeting scheme. Every respiratory cycle is divided into mandatory and spontaneous periods of time with a sensitivity window during the mandatory period. If the patient initiates the breath within this window, the ventilator will provide a mandatory ventilation (equal to assisted ventilation), and if the patient triggers after the window, a spontaneous pressure-supported breathing will be delivered.

S/T Mode (Spontaneous/Timed) PS with a backup rate. These modes are included in the self-regulating modes. They are an IMV in which variable mandatory breaths (T) are delivered only if spontaneous respiratory rate falls below a programmed backup respiratory rate (RR). If the patient stops breathing, or the ventilator does not detect the patient's breaths, or the patient breathes at a lower frequency than the programmed rescue rate, the device then provides a number of mandatory breaths in order to complete the patient's respiratory rate until backup rate. The ventilator supports all spontaneous breaths (S) with a pressure support (PS), which are added to EPAP, resulting in IPAP (see below).

S/T mode is probably the most widely used mode in NIV, because it is designed for all patients, regardless of their level of participation. However, patients with poor, irregular, or no involvement (those with weakness, shortness of breath, or apnea) are at risk of hypoventilation when backup rate triggers and some parameters are improperly adjusted. For example, (a) the set IPAP may be insufficient or (b) the set minimum inspiratory time (min Ti) may be short. a) Insufficient IPAP: The same pressure is fixed for both programmed and spontaneous breaths in home devices. This IPAP, enough to achieve an adequate tidal volume in spontaneous breathing, becomes insufficient in rescue ventilations, since the patient's effort disappears. Therefore, if controlled ventilation is kept over time, hypoventilation will appear if set pressure is not increased. b) Short minimum inspiratory time (min Ti): Usually, a brief minimum inspiratory time of spontaneous breaths is set in order to avoid asynchronies. Stable neuromuscular patients will perform an adequate spontaneous inspiratory time. However, they may produce a very short sigh (less than set min Ti) during decompensation/illness, which triggers the set min Ti, leading to low tidal volume and hypoventilation. On the other hand, sometimes the min Ti value also sets the Ti for backup breaths; if short for the patient's age, it will cause hypoventilation when rescue breaths are triggered. Therefore, all parameters (IPAP, RR, Ti, min Ti) should be properly set if S/T mode is used in patients with inconstant participation (central hypoventilation), and also, they should be modified during decompensations in neuromuscular patients.

Continuous Spontaneous Ventilation (PC-CSV) Pressure support mode in home ventilators and S mode (spontaneous) in BLPAP ventilators. Respiratory rate is decided by the patient and, ideally, also the inspiratory time. The ventilator detects the patient's effort and supports it with a pressure, until expiratory trigger is activated. The ventilator cycles between EPAP and IPAP (or between EPAP and PIP) according to the patient's breathing pattern and effort. The ventilator provides a constant expiratory pressure (EPAP or PEEP), and, whenever the patient initiates a breath, the ventilator will pressurize and will deliver a pressure support ventilation (PS = IPAP or PIP—EPAP). The ventilator will keep the inspiratory flow, until the patient activates the expiratory trigger (inspiratory cycle off) when the inspiratory flow finishes and so the inspiratory time. The duration of the inspiratory time will depend on the patient's inspiratory effort, leakages, programmed cycling flow rate percentage—expiratory trigger—and minimum and maximum inspiratory times set. Pressure support must be set up in order to achieve an adequate ventilation (assess chest rise or VT 6–10 mL/kg).

Pressure support improves the patient's comfort and patient-ventilator synchrony in the absence of leaks. This mode will be used electively when the patient's respiratory center works properly and whenever the patient is capable of triggering the system.

CPAP The ventilator delivers a constant pressure throughout the respiratory cycle. It is the simplest, cheapest, and more comfortable mode of NIV, where synchrony is full assured. As ST mode, it is also a widely utilized mode, with its main indication being obstructive sleep apnea (OSA).

3.1.3 Ventilator Setting

Monitoring Tools Ventilator settings should be adjusted individually and according to pathology and age of the patient. Several monitoring tools such as comfort, chest movement, patient's breathing mechanics, snoring, blood gas, or overnight pulse oximetry (SpO_2) and $tcPCO_2$ will be useful to set up the optimal ventilator settings in clinical practice [51]. Some of them can also be used at home, saving incomes. Ideally, polysomnography can get better settings, but is an expensive and sparse resource. Other sophisticated and invasive approaches have been used in lab conditions, albeit unwarranted in most of the patients [71].

Targets Normocapnia should be the target in patients with central drive disorders, regardless of age; neonates and infants with central hypoventilation have healthy lungs and should not be ventilated according to the protective pulmonary strategy for preterm babies. Also, normocapnia will be attempted in children and adolescents with neuromuscular or chest diseases. Mild/moderate hypercapnia can be tolerated in children with any lung disease. Adequate transcutaneous oxygen saturation should be achieved in all ($SpO_2 > 95\%$ in children without any cyanotic cardiac defect), and patients with bronchopulmonary diseases can need adding oxygen to the ventilator. However, hypoxemia in a patient without pulmonary pathology or shunt means hypoventilation; then, setting should be adjusted instead of O_2 adding [27]. In addition to optimal gas exchange, comfort and synchrony should be achieved to optimize tolerance and adherence to NIV, considering the proper mask fit and avoiding leaks.

Parameter Setting (Table 6)

Volume control: •Tidal volume: 10–30 mL/kg, upper range for ventilation with leaks through mask. Expiratory tidal volume can guide ventilation in patients without expiratory leaks, targeting 6–10 mL/Kg. There are very few home devices capable of delivering and monitoring less than 50 mL.

Table 6 Parameter settings; see text to set up O_2 therapy and alarms

Parameter	Value	Comments
Tidal volume (TV)	10–30 mL/kg	Upper range if leaks Target: 6–10 mL/kg expiratory TV if no expiratory leaks
Inspiratory pressure (IPAP)	Variable for adequate chest rise -Young NM: Lower -scoliosis, obesity: Higher -control mode or central drive disorders: Higher -CF: Higher (mean 16 cmH_2O)	Depends on patient's condition, respiratory effort, compliance, resistance, and underlying disease - targets: 6–10 mL/kg expiratory TV if no expiratory leaks. Desired TC CO_2
Expiratory pressure (EPAP)	- Normal lungs: 4–5 cmH_2O -airway obstruction: Higher -lung disease: Higher -Young CF: 0 -adult CF: 4 cmH_2O	
Respiratory rate (RR)	Control mode: Full RR ST mode: Lower	According to patient's condition and age ST mode: Full RR and Ti if: - irregular breathing pattern - unable to trigger the ventilator
Inspiratory time (Ti)	- 0.4-1.5 seconds –1:2 I:E	Control mode, ST mode: According to age
Minimum Ti (min Ti) Maximum Ti (max Ti)		PS mode, ST mode: For synchrony Min Ti: According to age if weakness, shallow or no breathing Max Ti: To avoid an excessively long Ti due to leaks
Inspiratory trigger	-scale	Sensitive, but avoiding auto-triggering For synchrony
Expiratory trigger sensitivity (ETS) or Inspiratory cycle off	–25–35% -higher with leaks* and airway obstruction -automatic in some brands	For synchrony
Inspiratory rise time	- 0.05–0.4 seconds - 1-5 (increasing scale)	As short as the patient can tolerate For comfort and synchrony
Ramp time	5, 10, 15, 20 min	Adjustable by the patient for better adaptation
CPAP	5–15 cmH_2O (mean 8 cmH_2O)	CPAP titration CPAP mode

Abbreviations: *CPAP* continuous positive airway pressure, *CF* cystic fibrosis, *NM* neuromuscular, *ST* spontaneous timed, *TC* CO_2 transcutaneous carbon dioxide. *See Fig. 1

Pressure control: •Inspiratory pressure. Peak pressure (PIP, IPAP) and pressure support (PS) are the required pressures to achieve an adequate chest rise (and therefore adequate tidal volume of around 6–10 mL/kg or more depending on the uncontrolled leaks and the interface's dead space) and to obtain the desired PCO_2. Ventilation volume is obtained by the set pressure, the patient's respiratory effort, and the compliance and resistance of the patient's respiratory system. Respiratory mechanics vary in accordance with the severity and underlying disease (healthy airway and lungs or pulmonary disease) and with physiological changes during sleep in central drive, lung compliance, and airway resistance. Thus, optimal inspiratory pressure should be set according to these factors. Young neuromuscular patients require low inspiratory pressure, but adjustments will be necessary in older children and in those with scoliosis or obesity. Patients with central drive disorders need higher pressures because of lack of patient's respiratory effort. Children with cystic fibrosis need higher inspiratory pressure (optimum at a mean of IPAP 16 $cmHO_2$) and no EPAP, according to some physiological studies [72].

- Expiratory pressure (PEEP, EPAP): Usually, a physiological pressure of 4–5 cmH_2O is enough in the absence of airway obstruction (e.g., central drive and neuromuscular disorders). A high level of expiratory pressure may be necessary in order to overcome intrinsic PEEP in some lung diseases (bronchiolitis obliterans, bronchopulmonary dysplasia) [73]. As shown above, usually, young people with cystic fibrosis do not have intrinsic PEEP, and then EPAP is not recommended for them trying to avoid overdistension produced by EPAP (extrinsic PEEP) [72]. On the other hand, moderate EPAP is usually set in adults with CF.
- Respiratory rate (programmed or guaranteed): Optimal ventilation has to be achieved. Therefore, a full RR and inspiratory time (Ti) appropriate to the age of each patient have to be set for those patients with a lack of adequate breathing pattern (as central hypoventilation syndrome, Arnold-Chiari, spinal cord injury) or in those unable to trigger the ventilator. In those patients capable of maintaining an adequate respiratory rate, this parameter can be set up just as a backup rate (S/T mode).
- Inspiratory time: It can be set as a value on seconds (Ti: 0.4–1.5 seconds, depending on the age of the patient) or as an inspiratory:expiratory ratio (I:E): 1:2.

Minimum and maximum inspiratory time can be set in some ventilators in pressure support mode in order to improve comfort and synchrony. Minimum Ti should be set according to age, in order to avoid hypoventilation in patients with weakness and shallow or no breathing (see above). Maximum Ti should be set to avoid an excessively long Ti due to leaks.

In addition to the pressures (IPAP, EPAP) or the TV, and the RR with inspiratory time, other comfort parameters such as inspiratory ramp (or rise) time, inspiratory trigger, and expiratory cycle off sensitivity can be set or are automatically fixed. These parameters influence the patient-ventilator synchrony [74]:

- Inspiratory trigger. It regulates the ventilator's sensitivity to the patient's effort to initiate spontaneous inspiration. Set as sensitive as possible but avoid auto-triggering. Usually flow trigger is used. When pressure trigger and PEEP are used simultaneously, the trigger level has to be set up 1 cmH_2O lower than the PEEP level to avoid excessive patient effort.
- Expiratory trigger sensitivity (ETS) or inspiratory cycle off (Fig. 1): It will decide inspiratory time during spontaneous breathing on pressure support mode. Usually 25–35%, but will be higher in case of leaks or airway obstruction [72]. ETS is very important for the patient-ventilator synchrony. Sometimes, both "triggers" are automatically set. Some brands have special algorithms for automatic adaptation to the patient's flow, looking for better comfort and synchrony (Autotrack®, Respironics; Vsync®, ResMed).

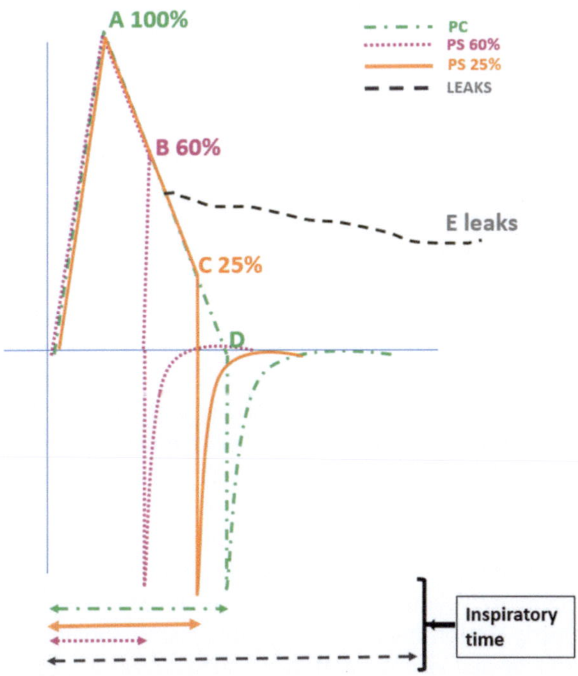

Fig. 1 Expiratory trigger sensitivity (ETS) or inspiratory cycle off. It decides inspiratory time (Ti) during spontaneous breathing on pressure support (PS) mode. Inspiration time ends when the decreasing inspiratory flow reaches a preset percentage of the maximum inspiratory flow. Point A: maximum inspiratory flow. Point B: ETS is set on 60%. Point C: ETS is set on 25%. Point D: End of inspiratory time on pressure control (PC) mode. Ti is shorter in B than in C (the higher the percentage, the lower the Ti). Usually a 25–35% ETS is set up. In case of leaks (E), the inspiratory flow will remain high in an attempt to compensate for them. In that case, if the ETS is low (C), the patient will never reach it: the inspiratory flow will not decrease to that percentage setup (C), and the inspiratory time will be too long (E). So, in case of leaks, a high ETS (B) or a maximum Ti should be set up

- Inspiratory rise time: It is the time taken during the inspiratory phase to achieve the set peak pressure (0.05–0.4 seconds). Indirectly, it regulates the velocity of the air going into the child (the higher inspiratory rise time, the lower flow) and will also affect the patient's comfort and synchrony. It is not always available. Rise time should be set as short as the patient can tolerate to optimize delivered volume. Rise time can be set up as absolute time (in seconds) or using an increasing scale from 1 to 5.
- Ramp time: Ramp means the time (5, 10, 15, 20 min) the ventilator takes to reach the set pressure (IPAP or CPAP). Pressure increases progressively, so the chronic patients will adapt better while asleep or during every new connection to the ventilator after a period without NIV. It can be adjusted by the patient himself/herself in many home ventilators.
- CPAP: CPAP titration should be performed individually, ideally, during polysomnography (PSG) in a pediatric sleep laboratory, starting at 4 cmH_2O, and progressively increasing until snoring and airflow obstruction resolve [56]. Optimal CPAP ranges between 5 and 15 cmH_2O, depending on the severity of the obstruction, although a mean pressure level of 8 cmH_2O has been reported [75]. In infants with severe obstruction, pressure should be set, at least 2 cmH_2O more than titrated CPAP, because this value underestimates optimum CPAP [72]. CPAP autotitration is possible in some devices (auto-CPAPs), and more information is shown below.
- Oxygen can be delivered through the ventilator (if it has an oxygen blender) or via the inspiratory limb at the edge of the ventilator or through the interface. Later options may offer lower FiO_2 and may generate different levels of asynchrony, depending upon the type of ventilator used. Older home ventilators usually do not have air-oxygen blender or oxygen meter, so they cannot supply high oxygen concentration. Therefore, patients with high O_2 requirements should be hospitalized at PICU for switching to ventilator with blender. Patients with central drive and neuromuscular disorders will not require oxygen in a stable condition if hypoventilation has been addressed with properly set NIV parameters.
- Alarms: They must be properly set for the patient's safety. Inappropriate and frequent activation causes discomfort and should be avoided. Disconnection and power failure alarms are essential and preset by the manufacturer. Low pressure and high inspiratory volume alarms also ensure disconnection warning, so they must be properly set for this purpose. Volume alarms should be set in pressure control ventilation and vice versa. If unintentional leaks are known and not corrected, expiratory volume alarms should be overridden.

Change in Parameters Ventilator settings (mainly volume, RR, and Ti) may need to be adjusted periodically during post-discharge follow-up. The younger the patient is, the more frequent the adjustment should be (every 1 or 2 months in infants and young children) to accommodate patient growth. Also, during weaning from the ventilator, the patients will require frequent control. Ventilator settings can be modified in hospitals during a nap or at night or at regular outpatient visit after home recordings. Acute respiratory infection often leads to increased ventilatory time, some parameters (RR, min Ti, IPAP, EPAP), humidification, and physiotherapy intensity. A preset "illness" configuration (available on the new devices) allows caregivers to easily elevate parameters at home during respiratory infection. Respiratory muscle weakness, weak cough, and increased secretions facilitate the formation of atelectasis and rapid progression to acute respiratory failure (ARF) with high O_2 requirement. In this scenario, switching to a hospital noninvasive device with O_2 blender or admission in PICU and intubation may be required.

3.2 Equipment

Required equipment for home discharge are shown in Table 7.

3.2.1 Devices [32, 57, 76, 77]

Currently, home available devices are CPAP devices, BLPAP devices, home ventilators, and high-flow devices. CPAP and BLPAP devices are the most used for long-term NIV.

CPAP devices They supply just a CPAP set pressure through an easy turbine system, and OSA is its main indication. To enhance comfort when falling asleep, the patient can usually adjust the "ramp," progressively increase the time of the pressure

Table 7 Equipment required for home mechanical ventilation (individualized for each patient)

Specific ventilator for home ventilation (2 units if round-the-clock ventilation or life support therapy).
- Heated humidifier.
- Interface (various models).
- Stethoscope.
- Complete ventilator circuits.
Depending on the patient:
- Pulse oximeter.
- External battery for ventilator.
- Respiratory physiotherapy device: IPPD (Alpha 200®), I-EM (Cough Assist®).
- Suction pump machine.
- Manual resuscitation bag and face mask.
- Oxygen source, O_2 extension sets, nasal cannula, face masks.
- Medication nebulizer.
- Feeding pump, silicone nasogastric tube, gastrostomy connection, 50 and 10 ml syringes.
- Wheelchair, external battery.

IPPD Intermittent Positive Pressure Device, *I-EM* Mechanical Insufflation and Exsufflation
Arrangements with health insurance should be made for ensuring devices and regular supply of interfaces and other consumables

(e.g., 5, 10, 15, or 20 min), and regulate the humidifier, if present. Usually mask disconnection and power failure alarms are available on CPAP devices, but not internal battery. CPAPs use a single-limb circuit, with exhalation port on distal end or on interface.

Autotitrated CPAP devices automatically adjust CPAP pressure between a set range, based on the analysis of patient flow curve and airway resistance by the software. Auto-CPAP is effective, well tolerated, and widely used in adult patients, but it has not been shown to be superior to constant CPAP in improving adherence, apnea/hypopnea index, and sleep quality. It is more expensive, so not first-line treatment. However, auto-CPAPs allow significantly reduced costs by CPAP pressure titration performance at home, instead of at a sleep lab. Smaller self-titrated than polysomnographic titrated pressure level has been reported in children [77]. Pressure relief technology (C-Flex®, Respironics) provides a slight decrease of pressure during the onset of expiration to facilitate air release and comfort. Scarce data have been shown from using these novel CPAPs in children; therefore they should not generally be recommended. Manufacturers recommend at least a 10 kg or 30 kg weight for using.

Bilevel PAP, or BLPAP, Devices It is also known as BiPAP for the ventilatory mode it provides. System operates with a turbine, capable of generating high gas flows and easily compensating for all leaks (intentional—exhalation holes—or unintentional—through the interface or mouth). It delivers a desired pressure support by matching to the patient's effort through inspiratory and expiratory flow triggers, whose sensitivity is automatically or manually programmed, depending on devices. BLPAPs can provide the described pressure support ventilation modes (S, ST, T) and CPAP with their related settings, depending on devices (BLPAP-S or BLPAP-ST). Variable pressure support with a minimum assured volume is available in several brands and referred to by different terms, as described above. Several models allow programming ramp time to improve patient adaptation. Mask disconnection, power supply, and high/low-pressure alarms are available on most modern designs. Some can be connected to an external battery (BiPAP Synchrony®), but few include an internal battery (Vivo 3®, by Breas). Disconnection alarm and battery can be required for safety at night on highly ventilator-dependent patients or during transport if acute exacerbation.

BLPAPs take room air and generally do not have an O_2 high-pressure connection. O_2 can be added through a low-pressure oxygen inlet port. In older models, O_2 should be added on inspiratory limb or on mask hole, reaching no more than 50% O_2 concentration, which limits the use of older BLPAP in very hypoxemic patients. Some devices have a built-in humidification-heater system. BLPAPs operate with a single-limb circuits and exhalation port (controlled leak), located close to the patient, usually on the interface, or less frequently on the limb distal end. BLPAPs are designed for mask ventilation; however, they are utilized for invasive ventilation in developing countries where more expensive and sophisticated ventilators are not available.

Home Ventilators They are more sophisticated and expensive than BLPAPs, and currently many of them offer the features of ICU ventilators with lightweight and portable design, easily adaptable to the baby stroller or wheelchair. As BLPAP, almost all operate with a turbine. Only one, PLV 100®, operates with a pneumatic compressor. Usually, they have CMV, IMV, and CSV on pressure and volume control, and guaranteed volume modes, with both invasive and noninvasive modes. Quite a few models have the option of mouthpiece ventilation and allow sigh setting, both useful for NIV 24-h MV dependence patients. The delivered minimum tidal volume ranges from 30 ml to 100 ml, depending on the brand, and the appropriate device should be chosen for a neonate or an infant. They have a wide range of alarms (volume, pressure, frequency, apnea, disconnection, low battery) and monitoring screens with parameters, curves, and trend graphs. Although they are mains powered, they integrate an internal battery and can be connected to an external battery or car battery. They take room air and have a low-pressure oxygen inlet port with optional connection to high-pressure O_2 and FiO_2 measurement. Most devices do not integrate humidification systems and must be provided with a heated humidifier or a heat and moisture exchanger (HME). New ventilators allow various scenarios to be preset (e.g., "day," "night," "illness") that caregivers can easily choose according to the patient status. Home ventilators are indicated in children with NIV and life support therapy during sleep or more than 16-h ventilation or with tracheostomy.

Some new devices (BLPAP and home ventilators) have a built-in input port for TC capnography and/or pulse oximetry monitoring and also a software for manual downloaded or remote monitored data transmission (such as adherence, leakage, ventilation parameter, AHI, and cycling). Built-in monitoring is particularly useful for centers which have a limited access to sleep studies. However, there is not yet a commercially available pediatric specific built-in software or validated data [41, 42, 78, 79].

High-Flow Devices Recently incorporated to home therapy, high-flow (HF) nasal cannula may be an alternative for OSA children not compliant with CPAP, although portable devices provide a minimum 15 Lpm flow and are not approved for below 30 kg [80]. However, a few new ventilators offer optional high flow if the patient requires to alternate NIV support and rest periods on HF.

3.2.2 Interfaces [81, 82]

Widespread NIV use favors the availability of different sizes of interfaces, suitable for children, including neonates and infants. Variability and alternating designs and seal materials (plastic, silicone, gel, even cloth) attempt to improve comfort, adherence, and efficacy, minimizing leaks and side effects. There are mainly five interface types used for chronic NIV.

Nasal Interface **Nasal masks** fit over the nostrils between the upper lip and the nose bridge. Sizes are available for infants with design preventing pressure sores on nasal bridge. **Nasal prongs**, inserted inside the nostrils, avoid pressure sores on nasal bridge although they can produce nostril irritation. Nasal prongs are widely used for newborn and infants on acute CPAP, but not available for them in chronic setting. Alternatively, RAM and high-flow nasal cannulas have been successfully used in small children intolerant to commercial interfaces [83, 84].

Oronasal masks cover the nose and mouth. They should be provided with an anti-rebreathing valve to prevent asphyxiation due to a power cut or ventilator failure, allowing breathing the room air, and with a quick-release strap to prevent aspiration in case of vomiting. Large adult nasal masks can be used as oronasal masks in young children, as a very limited infant-sized availability.

Full-face masks cover the entire face, including eyes; easy fitting, good tolerance, preventing nasal bridge pressure sores, avoiding chronic facial deformity, and availability of all sizes may make them a first-choice interface in young children with life support ventilation.

Mouthpiece is used during daytime ventilation in cooperating awake neuromuscular chronic patients, alternating with another night interface. Mouthpiece is held close to the patient's mouth, who seals his/her lips around it to receive a requested breath. There are angled mouthpieces and straw mouthpieces. Some ventilators have a specific ventilation mode for use of a mouthpiece interface. Of note, interface may produce increased salivation, orthodontic problems, gastric distension, and nose leaks. Oral masks are also available [30].

Helmet has been exceptionally used at home in patients with facial deformities with severe OSAs unable to adapt to common commercial interfaces.

In addition, masks can be custom-made with silicone, and current 3D technology appears to be a promising option for designing and fabricating the most appropriate mask for selected patient [85]. Facial growth will require periodic replacement. Interfaces may or may not have intentional leaks, with the former being called "vented" and the latter "non-vented." Vented interfaces are the most used on NIV. Vented interfaces are used with single-limb circuit. Non-vented mask must be used with double-limb circuit or with a single-limb circuit plus exhalatory valve.

Last but not least, **headgear** is also an important, adequate fitting that should uniformly distribute a suitable pressure in order to avoid facial injuries and excessive air leaks.

Selection of the Interface

Several factors determine interface choice, including availability, effectiveness, preferences of patient or family, age and weight, cranial anatomy, nasal patency, mouth breathing, hours of ventilation, expected duration of therapy, and pros and cons.

At home, nasal mask is the most commonly used, followed by oronasal mask, although alternating with a full-face mask is preferred for infants and young children for preventing face deformity. Nasal interface is comfortable, less claustrophobic, and better tolerated, as the child can talk, cry, expectorate, and eat (although eating with a mask is not recommended for preventing aspiration). However, it can offer greater resistance, and mouth leaks can cause discomfort and worsen ventilation; chin straps or a pacifier attempts to correct this problem. Care should be taken to avoid nares obstruction due to nasal interface malposition or secretions, especially in young children. Infection and nasal congestion can be a challenge in patients with nasal NIV and life-sustaining therapy (e.g., central hypoventilation). In addition to increased humidification, local medications (antibiotics, anti-inflammatory, and vasoconstrictors) and/or temporary change to an oronasal mask may be necessary.

Oronasal and full-face mask can also cause upper airway obstruction, as both can displace soft palate and tongue backward [86]. Risk of aspiration during vomiting may occur if patients are not able to remove their oronasal or full-face mask, due to short age, muscle weakness, or mental retardation.

Dead space (full-face mask > oronasal mask > nasal mask) can take part on ventilation, although, in full-face masks, it has been shown that dynamic or actual dead space (device on) is much lower than static dead space (device off). Facial deformity due to chronic pressure is an unpleasant side effect, being more dangerous in younger children with a highly moldable and growing bone structure. Maxillary deformity and midfacial hypoplasia have been described with nasal mask usage, and less with oronasal mask, and are avoided by full-face mask.

Careful interface selection, a well-fitting headgear, and also a mask desensitization and adaptation procedure are critical to the success of NIV, avoiding leaks, discomfort, and side effects. Motivating the child with stories and mask games and fitting the mask without headgear or air can help tolerance and adaptation [82]. Optimal adherence can be a challenge, especially in young children at the beginning because of intolerance to technique or unavailability of a proper interface. Early close follow-up at home (telephone and home visits) constitutes a major factor of the success of a home NIV program; regular screening for NIV side effects (leaks, pain, bedsores), respiratory symptoms, and sleep quality can detect and resolve issues early, promoting compliance. Mask changing, custom-made interface, optimal ventilatory setting titration, and warm humidifier adding can also optimize adherence [87–90].

3.2.3 Limb Circuits and Expiratory Systems

There are two expiratory systems for the tubing used on NIV, the "exhalation port" and the "exhalatory valve." The "exhalation port" is a full respiratory cycle open hole, placed on the interface (most often and preferred location) or at the end of the single circuit limb. The "exhalatory valve" opens only during expiration, being inserted at the end of the single-limb circuit or built-in ventilator attached to the expiratory limb of the double-limb circuits.

CPAP devices and BLPAP devices use single-limb circuits + vented mask. Home ventilators can use (i) single-limb circuit + vented mask (most common option in NIV); (ii) single-limb circuit + "expiratory valve" + non-vented mask; and (iii)

Double-limb circuit + non-vented mask. When single-limb circuits are used, the expiratory system should be as close as possible to the nose/mouth or cannula (if invasive ventilation), as the circuit in between the nose/mouth and the expiratory system will behave as dead space. This can be particularly significant in younger children.

3.2.4 Other Devices

Pulse Oximeter It should be simple; reliable, with acoustic alarms if nocturnal monitoring; battery operated; and easily transportable devices.

Suction Pump Machine Mandatory for tracheostomized patients, may be recommendable for selected children on NIV and a poor management of pharyngeal secretions. It can be powered by mains, battery, or manually. It should be light, portable, easy to handle, and with adjustable suction pressure.

Humidification The natural humidification and warming system (the nostrils) is preserved during NIV, but may be insufficient due to high gas flow rates. Humidification improves NIV adherence [75, 76]. Two artificial humidification methods (passive humidification—heat and moisture exchanger (HME)—and active humidification—heated humidifier) are available. Only the latter can be used on one single-limb circuit NIV, where the tiny HME cannot contact exhaled air, a prerequisite to function as designed. In-line HMEs are used in children with tracheostomy. Heated humidifier efficiently warms and humidifies the air to a desired temperature, used for either tracheostomy ventilation or NIV. The heater and sterile water reservoirs are electrically powered and inserted into the inspiratory limb or built-in BPAP devices. Sophisticated and expensive servo-control systems are used in the hospital, and simpler ones at home. The latter may require condensation water traps adding to the inspiratory circuit.

Respiratory Physiotherapy Device Intermittent positive-pressure devices (IPPDs), such as the Alpha 200®, and mechanical insufflation and exsufflation (I-EM) devices, such as the Cough Assist®. Both can be used with a mask or tracheostomy. The Alpha 200® can be used to achieve air stacking and improve the cough mechanism. I-EM involves passive lung expansion using positive-pressure insufflation, followed by rapid negative-pressure exsufflation to generate a sufficiently high expiratory flow rate to clear secretions. The Vest® and Percussionaire® devices can also help for airway clearance. Cough assistance should be considered mandatory in children with weakness and impaired spontaneous cough. When cough devices are not available, family training in manual cough assistance is crucial.

Home Oxygen Therapy [91]
It is delivered through BLPAP device in case of input port, inspiratory limb, interface, nasal cannulas, or tracheostomy. As shown above, the BLPAP device cannot

deliver a high concentration of oxygen, which limits its use on severe hypoxemic patient.

Indications include the following: (i) $PaO_2 < 60$ mmHg on room air; (ii) pulse oximetry during sleep with desaturations below 90% despite optimized ventilation setting; and (iii) Pulmonary hypertension and/or right ventricular hypertrophy and/or polycythemia, due to chronic hypoxemia.

Home Oxygen Sources

- Compressed oxygen: The gas is stored in the classic bullet or cylinder; some sizes are available, but even the small one is still heavy for mobility.
- Liquid oxygen: O_2 is stored in a reservoir ("nurse") at −183 °C in a liquid state from where, with a simple maneuver, it is transferred to a small refillable and easily portable backpack. Two sizes of backpacks are available; the classic one can supply 8 h on 1–2 L/min O_2 flow rate; the modern and lighter one (Heliox plus®, 1.6 kg weight) can supply 22 h on 2 L/min O_2 flow rate with on-demand delivery. Liquid O_2, although expensive, provides great autonomy and mobility, which makes it preferable for children. However, caregiver should be aware that stored gas evaporates and is consumed even if not used, so O_2 content should be monitored frequently and the tank replaced periodically.
- Oxygen concentrator: It does not need refilling because it takes room air for O_2 concentrating. Therefore, O_2 does not run out. Device provides a maximum of 4–6 L/min O_2 flow rate, only suitable if low O_2 requirements. Two types of O_2 concentrators are available: one is inexpensive, noisy, large, and heavy (16–23 kg), with mains plugged, and is widely used for nocturnal therapy; another is portable, lighter (2.3–8 kg), small, and battery-powered (internal battery—lasts up to 3 h—or external battery—lasts up to 10 h), although expensive and with limited availability. The portable concentrator is the only source of O_2 authorized by airlines for traveling.

Home oxygen devices can provide continuous flow during inspiration and expiration or only during the patient's inspiration by a demand valve; the latter spends less gas, so devices can weigh less and enable mobility; however, they cannot be used with a ventilator. Demand valve can be available on liquid O_2 backpacks and O_2 concentrators.

4 Outcomes

Benefits of home versus hospital care for children on chronic life support NIV [6, 25, 48, 49, 92, 93]: (i) extends life; (ii) provides an environment that will enhance individual potential; (iii) Reduces morbidity (avoids prolonged hospitalization side effects: nosocomial infections, iatrogenic effect, affective deprivation, sleep disturbance, lack of positive stimuli, hostile environment, no or inadequate family, social, and school life); (iv) promotes the child's physical, psychological, intellectual, and social development; (v) facilitates family life; (vi) enhances the quality of life; and vii. Offers cost-effectiveness (increases hospital bed availability, reduces cost).

Benefits of prolonged NIV [4, 6, 25, 26, 94, 95]: improvement in survival, quality of life, sleep, growth, behavior, and neurocognitive development; decrease in respiratory symptoms (airway obstruction, hypoventilation, postoperative complications) and respiratory exacerbations; avoidance of tracheostomy; allowing decannulation; prevention of chest deformity; and preservation of lung function.

Disadvantages for the family [96–100]: The acquired commitment may lead to stress, fear, and overwhelming, initial feelings that can improve and be exchanged for comfort and security over time. However, fatigue, refusal, and pessimism can appear if it is very-long-term ventilation. Family demands increase; mothers usually take on the role of the main caregiver, quitting her out-of-home job. Surveillance and noisy devices cause sleep disturbance. Changes in family and social life routines occur, and family conflicts and inattention to siblings may arise. Privacy is reduced when a personal care assistant works at home. Home NIV generates additional expenses. Institutional financial and healthcare support is often insufficient.

Adverse Events

Inadvertent ventilator disconnection/failure can lead to death or severe neurological sequelae, if absent or sparse respiratory autonomy; pulse oximeter monitoring allows early detection.

Children with chronic NIV may develop facial deformity (midface hypoplasia, class III malocclusion) due to interface and headgear long-term pressure, which can be prevented by alternating various interfaces [101–105]. However, orthodontic periodical consultation is recommended. Also, dental deformity due to mouthpiece should be followed.

Other side effects are generally mild, but they can lead to poor adherence or, if severe, withdrawal of NIV for a time. Adequate interface choice and an effective minimum pressure setting are essential for preventing these unintentional outcomes/complications. The following have been described: (i) Skin pressure sores, mostly on nasal bridge, are the most frequent complication, and temporary NIV discontinuation may be necessary, until the lesion heals, or transition to an alternative mask (to nasal prongs, total face, custom-molded, or cloth mask). Skin protection with hydrocolloid dressings and proper headgear pressure fitting are preventing and healing procedures [106]. (ii) Contact dermatitis, due to allergy to mask materials, requires mask change and topical corticosteroids. (iii) Ocular irritation or trauma (conjunctivitis, abrasion, corneal ulcer), due to leaks or pressure on the conjunctiva, is avoided by adjusting and choosing adequate interface size and pressure setting. (iv) Chronic nasal discomfort (congestion, irritation, dry mucus, sinusitis, epistaxis, rhinorrhea) can be prevented with suitable humidification. (v) Gastric distension is prevented or corrected by lower value pressure setting, avoiding vomiting and aspiration. (vii) Discomfort, agitation, claustrophobia, poor adherence, and rejection are more frequent at the beginning and can improve after a period of adaptation. As discussed above, careful interface selection, a well-fitting headgear, and mask desensitization are recommended for adaptation [82]. Early detection of NIV side effects (leaks, pain, bedsores) by a close follow-up, mask changing, custom-made interface, optimal ventilatory setting titration, and warm humidifier adding can also optimize adherence [87–90].

5 Conclusion

A home ventilation program will optimize the management of long-term NIV children, including expert health workers, education, and family support, as they are often primary caregivers. Follow-up goals should include weaning from ventilation if appropriate and transition to adult care if lifelong therapy, in addition to respiratory status stability, side effect minimizing, quality of life, growth, and neurodevelopment. Continuous positive airway pressure (CPAP) for airway obstruction diseases, pressure support for neuromuscular disorders, and pressure control for central drive disturbances are the predominant forms of home NIV. The interface is a fundamental conditioning factor for the safety, efficacy, and quality of NIV.

References

1. Sullivan CE, McNamara F, Waters KA, et al. Nasal CPAP: use in the management of infantile apnea. Sleep. 1993;16(8 Suppl):S108e13.
2. Guilleminault C, Pelayo R, Clerk A, et al. Home nasal continuous positive airway pressure in infants with sleep-disordered breathing. J Pediatr. 1995;127:905–12.
3. Fauroux B, Abel F, Amaddeo A, et al. ERS statement on paediatric long-term noninvasive respiratory support. Eur Respir J. 2022;59:2101404. https://doi.org/10.1183/13993003.01404 2021.
4. Praud JP. Long-term non-invasive ventilation in children: current use, indications and contraindications. Front Pediatr. 2020;8:584334. https://doi.org/10.3389/fped.2020.584334.
5. Amos L, Afolabi-Brown O, Gault D, et al. Age and weight considerations for the use of continuous positive airway pressure therapy in pediatric populations: an American Academy of sleep medicine position statement. J Clin Sleep Med. 2022;18(8):2041–3.
6. Castro Codesal ML, Dehaan K, Featherstone R, et al. Long-term non-invasive ventilation therapies in children: a scoping review. Sleep Med Rev. 2018;37:148–58. https://doi.org/10.1016/j.smrv.2017.02.005.
7. Nathan AM, Loo HY, de Bruyne JA, et al. Thirteen years of invasive and noninvasive home ventilation for children in a developing country: a retrospective study. Pediatr Pulmonol. 2017;52:500–7.
8. Leske V, Guerdile MJ, Gonzalez A, et al. Feasibility of a pediatric long-term home ventilation program in Argentina: 11 years' experience. Pediatr Pulmonol. 2020;55:780–7.
9. Chatwin M, Tan HL, Bush A, Rosenthal M, Simonds AK. Long term noninvasive ventilation in children: impact on survival and transition to adult care. PLoS One. 2015;10(5):e0125839.
10. McDougall CM, Adderley RJ, Wensley DF, Seear MD. Long-term ventilation in children: longitudinal trends and outcomes. Arch Dis Child. 2013;98(9):660e5.
11. Sovtic A, Minic P, Vukcevic M, et al. Home mechanical ventilation in children is feasible in developing countries. Pediatr Int. 2012;54(5):676e81.
12. Francisco Prado A, Pamela SF. At-home non-invasive ventilatory assistance for children: initial impact of a national program in Chile [asistencia ventilatoria no invasiva domi-

ciliaria en ninos: Impacto inicial de un programa nacional en Chile]. Rev Chil Pediatr. 2011;82(4):289e99.
13. Wallis C, Paton JY, Beaton S, Jardine E. Children on long-term ventilatory support: 10 years of progress. Arch Dis Child. 2011;96(11):998e1002.
14. Edwards EA, Hsiao K, Nixon GM. Paediatric home ventilatory support: the Auckland experience. J Paediatr Child Health. 2005;41(12):652e8.
15. Kamm M, Burger R, Rimenzsberger P, et al. Survey of children supported by long-term mechanical ventilation in Switzerland. Swiss Med Wkly. 2001;131(19e20):261e6.
16. Amin R, Sayal P, Syed F, et al. Pediatric long-term home mechanical ventilation: twenty years of follow-up from one Canadian center. Pediatr Pulmonol. 2014;49:816–24.
17. Chau SK, Yung AW, Lee SL. Long-term management for ventilator-assisted children in Hong Kong: 2 decades' experience. Respir Care. 2017;62:54–64.
18. Fauroux B, Boffa C, Desguerre I. Long-term noninvasive mechanical ventilation for children at home: a national survey. Pediatr Pulmonol. 2003;35:119–25.
19. Gonzalez Cortes R, Bustinza Arriortua A, Pons Odena M, García Teresa MA, Cols Roig M, Gaboli M, et al. Domiciliary mechanical ventilation in children: a Spanish multicentre study. An Pediatr. 2013;78:227–33.
20. Racca F, Berta G, Sequi M, et al. LTV Paediatric Italian network. Long-term home ventilation of children in Italy: a national survey. Pediatr Pulmonol. 2011;46:566–72.
21. Bertrand P, Fehlmann E, Lizama M, et al. Home ventilatory assistance in Chilean children: 12 years' experience. Arch Bronconeumol. 2006;42:165–70.
22. Hsia SH, Lin JJ, Huang IA, Wu CT. Outcome of long-term mechanical ventilation support in children. Pediatr Neonatol. 2012;53:304–80. https://doi.org/10.1016/j.pedneo.2012.07.005.
23. Povitz M, Rose L, Shariff SZ, et al. Home mechanical ventilation: a 12-year population-based retrospective cohort study. Respir Care. 2018;63(4):380–7.
24. Krivec U, Caggiano S. Noninvasive ventilation in palliative care and ethical dilemma. Front Pediatr. 2020;8:483. https://doi.org/10.3389/fped.2020.00483etica).
25. Bedi PK, Castro-Codesal ML, Featherstone R, AlBalawi MM, Alkhaledi B, et al. Long-term non-invasive ventilation in infants: a systematic review and meta-analysis. Front Pediatr. 2018;6:13. https://doi.org/10.3389/fped.2018.00013.
26. García Teresa MA, Porto Abal R, Rodríguez Torres S, et al. Spanish patients with central hypoventilation syndrome included in the European Registry. The 2015 data. An Pediatr. 2017;86:255–63. https://doi.org/10.1016/j.anpedi.2016.05.008.
27. Trang H, Samuels M, Ceccherini I, et al. Guidelines for diagnosis and management of congenital central hypoventilation syndrome. Orphanet J Rare Dis. 2020;15:252.
28. Paglietti MG, Porcaro F, Sovtic A, et al. Decannulation in children affected by congenital central hypoventilation syndrome: a proposal of an algorithm from two European centers. Pediatr Pulmonol. 2019;54:1663–9. https://doi.org/10.1002/ppul.24448.
29. Lloyd-Owen SJ, Donaldson GC, Ambrosino N, et al. Patterns of home mechanical ventilation use in Europe: results from the Eurovent survey. Eur Respir J. 2005;25:1025–31. https://doi.org/10.1183/09031936.05.00066704.
30. Bach JR. Noninvasive respiratory management of patients with neuromuscular disease. Ann Rehabil Med. 2017;41:519–38.
31. Gonçalves MR, Bach JR, Ishikawa Y, et al. International study group on Continuous Noninvasive Ventilatory Support in Neuromuscular Disease (CNVSND). Continuous non-invasive ventilatory support outcomes for patients with neuromuscular disease: a multicenter data collaboration. Pulmonology. 2021;27:509–17. https://doi.org/10.1016/j.pulmoe.2021.06.007.
32. García-Teresa MA, Pons-Ódena M, De Lama G, et al. Chapter 24: Home mechanical ventilation in paediatrics. In: Medina A, Pilar J, García Cusco M, et al., editors. Handbook of paediatric and neonatal mechanical ventilation. 2nd ed. Las Palmas de Gran Canaria: Tesela ediciones; 2021.
33. Amaddeo A, Frapin A, Brigitte F. Long-term non-invasive ventilation in children. Lancet Respir Med. 2016;4:999–1008.

34. Amin R, MacLusky I, Zielinski D, el al. Pediatric home mechanical ventilation: a Canadian thoracic society clinical practice guideline executive summary. Can J Respir Crit care. Sleep Med. 2017;1:7–36. https://doi.org/10.1080/24745332.2017.1300463.
35. Windisch W, Geiseler J, Simon K, et al. German National Guideline for treating chronic respiratory failure with invasive and non-invasive ventilation - revised edition 2017: part 2. Respiration. 2018;96:171–203. https://doi.org/10.1159/000488667.
36. Castro-Codesal ML, Dehaan K, Bedi PK, et al. Longitudinal changes in clinical characteristics and outcomes for children using long-term non-invasive ventilation. PLoS One. 2018;13:e0192111. https://doi.org/10.1371/journal.pone.0192111.
37. Chatwin M, Heather S, Hanak A, et al. Analysis of home support and ventilator malfunction in 1,211 ventilator-dependent patients. Eur Respir J. 2010;35:310–6. https://doi.org/10.1183/09031936.00073409.
38. Mastouri M, Amaddeo A, Griffon L, et al. Weaning from long term continuous positive airway pressure or noninvasive ventilation in children. Pediatr Pulmonol. 2017;52(10):1349–54. https://doi.org/10.1002/ppul.23767.
39. Onofri A, Broomfield A, Tan H-l. Transition to adult Care in Children on long-term ventilation. Front Pediatr. 2020;8:548839. https://doi.org/10.3389/fped.2020.548839.
40. Dale CM, Carbone S, Amin R, et al. A transition program to adult health services for teenagers receiving long-term home mechanical ventilation: a longitudinal qualitative study. Pediatr Pulmonol. 2020;55:771–9. https://doi.org/10.1002/ppul.24657.
41. Khirani S, Amaddeo A, Griffon L, et al. Follow-up and monitoring of children needing long term home ventilation. Front Pediatr. 2020;8:330. https://doi.org/10.3389/fped.2020.00330.
42. Côté A. On behalf of the CTS pediatric home ventilation guidelines panel. Section 4: home monitoring and follow-up of home ventilated children. Can J Respir Crit Care Sleep Med. 2018;2:23–31. https://doi.org/10.1080/24745332.2018.1494978.
43. Muñoz-Bonet JI, López-Prats JL, Flor-Macián EM, et al. Usefulness of telemedicine for home ventilator-dependent children. J Telemed Telecare. 2020;26:207–15. https://doi.org/10.1177/1357633X18811751.
44. Trucco F, Pedemonte M, Racca F, et al. Tele-monitoring in paediatric and young home-ventilated neuromuscular patients: a multicenter case-control trial. J Telemed Telecare. 2019;25:414–24. https://doi.org/10.1177/1357633X18778479.
45. Pilmer SL. Prolonged mechanical ventilation in children. Pediatr Clin N Am. 1994;41:473–512.
46. Bach JR, Turcios NL, Wang L. Respiratory complications of Paediatric neuromuscular diseases. Pediatr Clin N Am. 2021;68:177–91.
47. Fauroux B, Khirani S, Griffon L, et al. Non-invasive ventilation in children with neuromuscular disease. Front Pediatr. 2020;8:482. https://doi.org/10.3389/fped.2020.00482.
48. AlBalawi MM, Castro-Codesal M, Featherstone R, et al. Outcomes of long-term noninvasive ventilation use in children with neuromuscular disease. Systematic review and meta-analysis. Ann Am Thorac Soc. 2022;19:109–19. https://doi.org/10.1513/AnnalsATS.202009-1089OC.
49. Hudson S, Abusido T, Sebastianski M, et al. Long-term non-invasive ventilation in children with down syndrome: a systematic review. Front Pediatr. 2022;10:886727. https://doi.org/10.3389/fped.2022.886727.
50. Verhulst S. Long term continuous positive airway pressure and non-invasive ventilation in obstructive sleep apnea in children with obesity and down syndrome. Front Pediatr. 2020;8:534. https://doi.org/10.3389/fped.2020.00534.
51. Amaddeo A, Frapin A, Touil S, et al. Outpatient initiation of long-term continuous positive airway pressure in children. Pediatr Pulmonol. 2018;53:1422–8.
52. Panitch HB, Downes JJ, Kennedy JS. Guidelines for home care of children with chronic respiratory insufficiency. Pediatr Pulmonol. 1996;21:52–6.
53. Ergan B, Oczkowski S, Rochwerg B, et al. European Respiratory Society guidelines on long-term home non-invasive ventilation for management of COPD. Eur Respir J. 2019;54:1901003. https://doi.org/10.1183/13993003.01003-2019.
54. Macrea M, Oczkowski S, Rochwerg B, et al. Long-term noninvasive ventilation in chronic stable hypercapnic chronic obstructive pulmonary disease. An official American Thoracic

Society clinical practice guideline. Am J Respir Crit Care Med. 2020;202(4):e74–87. https://doi.org/10.1164/rccm.202006-2382ST.
55. Amaddeo A, Moreau J, Frapin A, et al. Long term continuous positive airway pressure (CPAP) and noninvasive ventilation (NIV) in children: initiation criteria in real life. Pediatr Pulmonol. 2016;51:968–74.
56. Kaditis AG, Alonso Alvarez ML, Boudewyns A, et al. Obstructive sleep disordered breathing in 2- to 18-year-old children: diagnosis and management. Eur Respir J. 2016;47:69–94.
57. Pavone M, Verrillo E, Onofri A, et al. Ventilators and ventilatory modalities. Front. Pediatr. 2020;8:500. https://doi.org/10.3389/fped.2020.00500.
58. Rabec C, Rodenstein D, Leger P, et al. Ventilator modes and settings during non-invasive ventilation: effects on respiratory events and implications for their identification. Thorax. 2011;66:170–8. https://doi.org/10.1136/thx.2010.142661.
59. Carlucci A, Schreiber A, Mattei A, et al. The configuration of bi-level ventilator circuits may affect compensation for non-intentional leaks during volume-targeted ventilation. Intensive Care Med. 2013;39:59–65.
60. Khirani S, Louis B, Leroux K, Delord V, Fauroux B, Lofaso F. Harms of unintentional leaks during volume targeted pressure support ventilation. Respir Med. 2013;107:1021–9.
61. Lofaso F, Prigent H, Tiffreau V, et al. Association Française Contre les myopathies research group. Long-term mechanical ventilation equipment for neuromuscular patients: meeting the expectations of patients and prescribers. Respir Care. 2014;59:97–106. https://doi.org/10.4187/respcare.02229.
62. Saddi V, Thambipillay G, Martin B, et al. Front Pediatr. 2022;10:868625. https://doi.org/10.3389/fped.2022.868625.
63. Diaz-Abad M, Isaiah A, Rogers VE, et al. Use of noninvasive ventilation with volume-assured pressure support to avoid tracheostomy in severe obstructive sleep apnea. Case Rep Pediatr. 2018;2018:4701736. https://doi.org/10.1155/2018/4701736.
64. Saddi V, Thambipillay G, Pithers S, et al. Average volume-assured pressure support vs. conventional bilevel pressure support in pediatric nocturnal hypoventilation: a case series. J Clin Sleep Med. 2021;17:925–30. https://doi.org/10.5664/jcsm.9084.
65. Saddi V, Teng A, Thambipillay G, Allen H, Pithers S, Sullivan C. Nasal mask average volume-assured pressure support in an infant with congenital central hypoventilation syndrome. Respir Case Rep. 2019;7:e00448. https://doi.org/10.1002/rcr2.448.
66. Veeravigrom M, Desudchit T. Prevalence of sleep disorders in Thai children. Indian J Pediatr. 2016;83:1237–41. https://doi.org/10.1007/s12098-016-2148-5.
67. Vagiakis E, Koutsourelakis I, Perraki E, et al. Average volume-assured pressure support in a 16-year-old girl with congenital central hypoventilation syndrome. J Clin Sleep Med. 2010;6:609–12. https://doi.org/10.5664/jcsm.27997.
68. Khayat A, Medin D, Syed F, et al. Intelligent volume-assured pressured support. (iVAPS) for the treatment of congenital central hypoventilation syndrome. Sleep Breath. 2017;21:513–9. https://doi.org/10.1007/s11325-017-1478-5.
69. Sunkonkit K, Al-Saleh S, Chiang J, Hamilton A, Medin D, Syed F, et al. Volume-assured pressure support mode for noninvasive ventilation: can it improve overnight adherence in children with neuromuscular disease? Sleep Breath. 2021;21:1. https://doi.org/10.1007/s11325-021-02288-1.
70. Gentin N, Williamson B, Thambipillay G, et al. Nocturnal respiratory failure in a child with congenital myopathy - management using average volume-assured pressure support (AVAPS). Respir Case Rep. 2015;3:115–7. https://doi.org/10.1002/rcr2.117.
71. Khirani S, Ramírez A, Aloui S, et al. Continuous positive airway pressure titration in infants with severe upper airway obstruction or bronchopulmonary dysplasia. Crit Care. 2013;17:R167. https://doi.org/10.1186/cc12846.
72. Fauroux B, Nicot F, Essouri S, et al. Setting of noninvasive pressure support in young patients with cystic fibrosis. Eur Respir J. 2004;24:624–30.
73. Gibbs K, Jensen EA, Alexiou S, et al. Ventilation strategies in severe Bronchopulmonary dysplasia. NeoReviews. 2020;21:e226. https://doi.org/10.1542/neo.21-4-e226.

74. Subirà C, de Haro C, Magrans R, et al. Minimizing asynchronies in mechanical ventilation: current and future trends. Respir Care. 2018;63:464–78. https://doi.org/10.4187/respcare.05949.
75. Marcus CL, Ward SL, Mallory GB, et al. Use of nasal continuous positive airway pressure as treatment of childhood obstructive sleep apnea. J Pediatr. 1995;127:88–94. https://doi.org/10.1016/s0022-3476(95)70262-8.
76. Fauroux B, Leroux K, Desmarais G. Performance of ventilators for noninvasive positive-pressure ventilation in children. Eur Respir J. 2008;31:1300–7.
77. Mihai R, Vandeleur M, Pecoraro S, et al. Autotitrating CPAP as a tool for CPAP initiation for children. J Clin Sleep Med. 2017;13:713.
78. Perrem L, Mehta K, Syed F, Baker A, Amin R. How to use non-invasive positive airway pressure device data reports to guide clinical care. Pediatr Pulmonol. 2020;55:58–67. https://doi.org/10.1002/ppul.24555.
79. Khirani S, Delord V, Olmo Arroyo J, et al. Can the analysis of built-in software of CPAP devices replace polygraphy in children? Sleep Med. 2017;37:46–53. https://doi.org/10.1016/j.sleep.2017.05.019.
80. Amaddeo A, Khirani S, Frapin A, et al. High-flow nasal cannula for children not compliant with continuous positive airway pressure. Sleep Med. 2019;63:24.
81. Ferreira R. Interfaces, circuits and humidifiers. Front Pediatr. 2020;8:557301. https://doi.org/10.3389/fped.2020.557301.
82. Castro-Codesal ML, Olmstead DL, MacLean JE. Mask interfaces for home non-invasive ventilation in infants and children. Pediatr Respir Rev. 2019;32:66–72.
83. Overbergh C, Installe S, Boudewyns A, et al. The Optiflow™ interface for chronic CPAP use in children. Sleep Med. 2018;44:1–3.
84. De Jesus RW, Samuels CL, Gonzales TR, et al. Use of nasal non-invasive ventilation with a RAM cannula in the outpatient home setting. Open Respir Med J. 2017;11:41–6.
85. Willox M, Metherall P, Jeays-Ward K, et al. Custom-made 3D printed masks for children using noninvasive ventilation: a feasibility study of production method and testing of outcomes in adult volunteers. J Med Eng Technol. 2020;44:213–23. https://doi.org/10.1080/03091902.2020.1769759.
86. Teo M, Amis T, Lee S, Falland K, Lambert S, Wheatley J. Equivalence of nasal and oronasal masks during initial CPAP titration for obstructive sleep apnea syndrome. Sleep. 2011;34:951–5. https://doi.org/10.5665/SLEEP.1134.
87. Tuggey JM, Delmastro M, Elliott MW. The effect of mouth leak and humidification during nasal non-invasive ventilation. Respir Med. 2007;101:1874–9. https://doi.org/10.1016/j.rmed.2007.05.005.
88. Nilius G, Franke KJ, Domanski U, Schroeder M, Ruhle KH. Effect of APAP and heated humidification with a heated breathing tube on adherence, quality of life, and nasopharyngeal complaints. Sleep Breath. 2016;20(1):43–9.
89. Koontz KL, Slifer KJ, Cataldo MD, et al. Improving pediatric compliance with positive airway pressure therapy: the impact of behavioral intervention. Sleep. 2003;26:1010–5.
90. Watach AJ, Xanthopoulos MS, Afolabi-Brown O, et al. Positive airway pressure adherence in pediatric obstructive sleep apnea: a systematic scoping review. Sleep Med Rev. 2020;51:101273.
91. Brian K, Walsh BK. Smallwood CD pediatric oxygen therapy: a review and update. Respir Care. 2017;62:645–61. https://doi.org/10.4187/respcare.05245.
92. Make BJ, Hill NS, Goldberg AI. Mechanical ventilation beyond the intensive care unit. Report of a consensus conference of American College of Chest Physicians. Chest. 1998;113:289S–344.
93. Paulides FM, Plötz FB, Verweij-van den Oudenrijn LP. Thirty years of home mechanical ventilation in children: escalating need for pediatric intensive care beds. Intensive Care Med. 2012;38:847–52.
94. Young HKA, Lowe A, Fitzgerald DA. Outcome of noninvasive ventilation in children with neuromuscular disease. Neurology. 2007;68:198–201.

95. Bach JR, Niranjan V. Spinal muscular atrophy type I: a non-invasive respiratory management approach. Chest. 2000;117:1100–5. https://doi.org/10.1378/chest.117.4.1100.
96. Yotani N, Ishiguro A, Sakai H, Ohfuji S, Fukushima W, Hirota Y. Factor-associated caregiver burden in medically complex patients with special healthcare needs. Pediatr Int. 2014;56(5):742e7.
97. González R, Bustinza A, Fernandez SN, García M, Rodriguez S, García-Teresa MÁ, Gaboli M, et al. Quality of life in home-ventilated children and their families. Eur J Pediatr. 2017;176:1307–17. https://doi.org/10.1007/s00431-017-2983-z.
98. Mattson J, Lunnelie J, Löfholm T, et al. Quality of life in children with home mechanical ventilation - a scoping review. SAGE Open Nurs. 2022;8:23779608221094522. https://doi.org/10.1177/23779608221094522.
99. Bjerregaard Alrø A, Klitnaes C, Dahl Rossau C, Dreyer P. Living as a family with a child on home mechanical ventilation and personal care assistants-A burdensome impact on family life. Nurs Open. 2021;8:3340–8. https://doi.org/10.1002/nop2.879.
100. Nonoyama ML, Katz SL, Amin R, et al. Healthcare utilization and costs of pediatric home mechanical ventilation in Canada. Pediatr Pulmonol. 2020;55:2368–76. https://doi.org/10.1002/ppul.24923.
101. Roberts SD, Kapadia H, Greenlee G, et al. Midfacial and dental changes associated with nasal positive airway pressure in children with obstructive sleep apnea and craniofacial conditions. J Clin Sleep Med. 2016;12:469–75. https://doi.org/10.5664/jcsm.5668.
102. Bariani RCB, Guimarães TM, Cappellette M Jr, et al. The impact of positive airway pressure on midface growth: a literature review. Braz J Otorhinolaryngol. 2020;S1808–8694(20):30068–9. https://doi.org/10.1016/j.bjorl.2020.05.010.
103. KK, Riley RW, Guilleminault C. An unreported risk in the use of home nasal continuous positive airway pressure and home nasal ventilation in children: mid-face hypoplasia. Chest. 2000;117:916–8.
104. Fauroux B, Lavis JF, Nicot F, et al. Facial side effects during noninvasive positive pressure ventilation in children. Intensive Care Med. 2005;31:965–9.
105. Villa MP, Pagani J, Ambrosio R, Ronchetti R, Bernkopf E. Mid-face hypoplasia after long-term nasal ventilation. Am J Respir Crit Care Med. 2002;166:1142–3.
106. Visscher MO, White CC, Jones JM, Cahill T, Jones DC, Pan BS. Face masks for noninvasive ventilation: fit, excess skin hydration, and pressure ulcers. Respir Care. 2015;60:1536–47. https://doi.org/10.4187/respcare.04036.

Invasive MV of PMVed Children

Fabrizio Chiusolo and Giorgio Picardo

Abbreviations

APRV	Airway pressure release ventilation
ARDS	Acute respiratory distress syndrome
CDC	Centers for Disease Control
CO_2	Carbon dioxide
ECMO	Extracorporeal membrane oxygenation
EAdi	Electrical activity of the diaphragm
ETT	Endotracheal tube
FiO_2	Fraction of inspired oxygen
HME	Heat and moisture exchanger
ICU	Intensive care unit
IMV	Invasive mechanical ventilation
MAP	Mean airways pressure
MV	Mechanical ventilation
NAVA	Neurally adjusted ventilatory assisted
NNIS	National Nosocomial Infections Surveillance System
$PaCO_2$	Arterial blood carbon dioxide pressure
PACV	Assist-controlled pressure ventilation
PARDS	Pediatric acute respiratory distress syndrome
PAV	Proportional assist ventilation

F. Chiusolo (✉)
Anesthesia and Critical Care Medicine, ARCO Rome, Bambino Gesù Children's Hospital Rome, Rome, Italy
e-mail: fabrizio.chiusolo@opbg.net

G. Picardo
Department of Biomedical Sciences, Humanitas University, Milan, Italy
e-mail: giorgio.picardo@hunimed.eu

A. Kawaguchi et al. (eds.), *Prolonged and Long-Term Mechanical Ventilation in Children*, https://doi.org/10.1007/978-981-97-8903-0_6

PCV	Pressure controlled ventilation
PEEP	Positive end expiratory pressure
PICU	Pediatric intensive care unit
PIP	Peak inspiratory pressure
PMV	Prolonged mechanical ventilation
PRVC	Pressure regulated volume control
PSV	Pressure support ventilation
RCT	Randomized controlled trial
SIMV	Synchronized intermittent mandatory ventilation
SpO_2	Peripheral oxygen saturation
TIAEs	Tracheal intubation-associated adverse events
VACV	Volume assist-control ventilation
VAEs	Ventilation-associated events
VAP	Ventilator-associated pneumoniae
VILI	Ventilator induced lung injury
VT	Tidal volume
WOB	Work of breathing

1 Introduction

The improvement in critical care has led to better clinical outcomes such as mortality, but at the same time, a prolonged hospital stay leads to an increase in morbidity [1], which in many cases results in prolonged mechanical ventilation (PMV) [2, 3].

Respiratory indications for admission influence the length of stay of infants in the pediatric intensive care unit (PICU) and also increase the likelihood of readmission to PICUs [4].

After resolution of the acute clinical and respiratory phase, a strategy should be structured that aims for respiratory stabilization over time and potential weaning from MV, adjusting for factors such as age, comorbidities, and disability. This would lead to faster patient recovery and discharge by reducing complications related to the care pathway and optimizing the available resources. It is considered a must that the focus on mechanical ventilation (MV) in the acute phase is also accompanied by long-term ventilatory management (when applied) planning to facilitate a transition to a subacute setting or discharge. Special attention should be paid to the transition between different ventilatory modes, and between endotracheal tube and tracheotomy, and to changing ventilator (home ventilator).

Morbidity and mortality increase as the duration of invasive mechanical ventilation (IMV) increases: post-extubation atelectasis and upper airway obstruction are complications of PMV. Morbidity also increases if there is associated nutritional or neurological impairment [5–7].

The function of MV is to improve respiratory exchange and minimize respiratory work [8]. New ventilator generations allow the use of different ventilatory modes, but not all modes are tested with clinical outcomes such as mortality, length of stay

Table 1 Main invasive ventilation modes used in PMV and their application

Ventilation modes		Application
Controlled		
	Pressure-controlled ventilation and pressure assist-controlled ventilation	Clinical
	Volume-controlled ventilation and volume assist-controlled ventilation	Clinical
	Pressure-regulated volume control	Clinical
	Synchronized mandatory intermittent ventilation	Clinical
	Airway pressure release ventilation	Clinical/research
Assisted		
	Pressure support ventilation	Clinical
	Neurally adjusted ventilatory assist	Clinical
	Proportional assist ventilation	Research

Clinical: if a ventilation mode was based on studies with clinical outcomes
Research: if a ventilation mode is based on case series, case report, and physiological studies without clinical outcomes

in PICU, and complications (Table 1). Invasive ventilation is indicated when a patient's spontaneous breathing is not adequate to guarantee normal oxygenation. The choice of interfaces enables a stable connection between the patient and the ventilator. Depending on the contribution given by the patient, IMV can be divided into two modes which can be full support, if the patient's work of breathing (WOB) is totally absent, and partial support, if the respiratory activity is partially preserved. When ventilatory support is total, sedation and, if necessary, muscle relaxants should be administered [9], and reduction and thinning of the diaphragm muscle may occur if applied for long periods [10]. In partial-support ventilation, the minimization of WOB depends on patient-ventilator interaction. IMV must assume a monitoring system with alarms of patient responses to ventilator settings.

2 Indications

Tracheal intubation is performed when noninvasive ventilation is insufficient to maintain respiratory gas exchange or in the context of other pathophysiology where consistency in breathing or secretion clearance is essential, such as severe alteration of consciousness or cardiovascular instability. Pathological conditions of significant severity of the upper airway (i.e., subglottic stenosis, vocal cord paralysis) or degenerative neurological diseases may necessitate long-term tracheostomy cannula placement. In these cases, the use of IMV techniques is not always necessary. Based on the NAMDRC definition of PMV [11], approximately 2.5–3% of patients admitted to the PICU receive MV for more than 21 days [2, 12–14], and generally, these are patients who require rehabilitation [15], and almost all require invasive ventilation as they have a tracheotomy [16, 17].

Variability in age and size of pediatric patients undergoing MV over the years has led to heterogeneous application of MV with highly variable modalities and indications among centers; this is due to the lack of RCTs in this area [18].

Recently, international scientific societies have extensively reviewed the available pediatric literature and published recommendations with the aim of standardizing and providing indications on the use of MV in different cases of pediatric respiratory failure [19].

During assisted ventilatory modes, it is critical to set ventilation parameters so as to avoid episodes of asynchrony between the patient and the ventilator. With particular caution, one must limit the use of very high ventilation pressures because of the increased risk of developing ventilator-induced lung injury (VILI). It is recommended to maintain a plateau pressure < 28 cm H_2O (to be increased to 30 in the case of diseases with reduced thoracic compliance).

There are no data regarding maximum acceptable values of peak, plateau, or transpulmonary pressures to be observed. In cases of severe pediatric acute respiratory failure, it is important to maintain a tidal volume (VT) of no more than 8 ml per kg of ideal weight. A different cutoff should be considered in ventilated children with nonparenchymal lung disease. Indeed, high-compliance lungs benefit from higher VTs, so VT should be cut off according to the severity of lung damage [20, 21].

A combination of factors should be evaluated in patients undergoing PMV. Clinical studies have considered a mean airway pressure (MAP) higher than 13 cm H_2O as a risk factor for prolonged ventilation in the pediatric population [12]. In a multicenter study of ex-preterm bronchodysplasic infants, settings for prolonged invasive ventilation varied significantly between clusters and centers, with peak inspiratory pressure (PIP) values ranging in 25–55 cm H_2O, PEEP 8–12 cm H_2O, inspiratory time 0.5–0.7 seconds, and MAP 12–18 cm H_2O [22].

Ventilation adjustment requires repeated daily multiparametric assessments that take into account the presence/absence of spontaneous ventilatory activity (WOB), peripheral oxygenation, capnography, and metabolic pattern.

First, determine if the patient has spontaneous ventilatory activity and if sedation or muscle relaxants are needed. If the patient requires assisted/semi-assisted ventilatory support, the flow or electrical trigger should be adjusted to match the patient's inspiratory effort, possibly avoiding auto-trigger or ineffective efforts; poor synchronization of the patient with the ventilator is a common condition and can lead to abnormal WOB [23] and increase the likelihood of PMV [24–27]. PEEP values of 3–5 cm H_2O would be indicated in the management of ventilated patients without pulmonary injury, whereas in respiratory failure, PEEP should be set considering the impact on hemodynamics and oxygenation. Setting controlled ventilatory safety breaths helps prevent hypoxia and pulmonary derecruitment when the patient may experience episodes of apnea or bradypnea.

The setting of controlled ventilation should always take into account the sensitivity of the trigger and the interface (whether there are air leaks; endotracheal tubes, or tracheostomy cannulas cuffed or not) and leak compensation. In the case of non-cuffed endotracheal tubes and tracheostomy cannulae, choosing a pressurometric setting would allow monitoring of adequate exhaled VT ensuring lung expansion; choosing a volumetric mode, air leak could expose the patient to hypoventilation and subsequent atelectasis due to circuit leakage or hyperventilation with high VT and risk of VILI.

In a retrospective study conducted in PARDS patients, PEEP values lower than the FiO_2/PEEP table of ARDSNet of adults are associated with higher mortality [28]. There is no evidence regarding the use of recruitment maneuvers. The use of active humidifiers is very important, although the superiority of active methods over passive ones has not been demonstrated.

During a ventilator setting, one must consider the detrimental effects caused by high oxygen concentrations that may reduce vital capacity (from uptake atelectasis) and retinopathy of prematurity [29].

Although there is no evidence regarding the threshold level of oxygen toxicity [30], it is common practice among pediatric intensivists not to exceed a FiO_2 threshold of 50–60% during the management of PMV, and to accept a value lower than expected for paO_2 [31].

The use of heat and moisture exchanger (HME) filters should be considered according to the increased dead space and increased WOB. In the PICU, HME should be used for patients for whom a short period of MV is expected.

The drafting of protocols targeting ICU release on Pain Assessment, Spontaneous Awakening and Breathing Tests, Choice of Sedation, Monitoring/Management of Delirium, Early Exercise/Mobility, and Family Involvement/Entertainment (ABCDEF) in the adult population has resulted in improved outcomes including survival [32–34]. In the pediatric setting, there is a strong awareness of the issue. In a survey of 161 PICUs worldwide regarding the application of the ABCDEF bundle, only 1/3 of centers have a ventilator weaning protocol, as well as only half apply spontaneous breath testing protocols [35]. Application of the ABCDEF bundle in a human resource-limited PICU in 88 patients (compared with 137) is associated with a significant reduction in sedative and opioid medication use and reduced MV duration and PICU length of stay [36].

3 Interfaces

The endotracheal tube allows IMV, management of airway secretions, and administration of pharmacological agents. Correct placement of the endotracheal tube (ETT) avoids complications concerning pulmonary atelectasis (partial and total) and vocal cords by facilitating the process of liberation from MV. The utility of low-pressure cuffs (with minimal occlusion volumes) allows the reduction of complications related to the ETT itself. In high-volume, low-pressure, cuffed tubes, the cuff pressure must be kept below 20 cm H_2O [37, 38]. The use of non-cuffed tubes, except for the neonatal period, has been decreasing in children with prolonged ventilation [39]. Newth et al. demonstrated that the use of cuffed tubes in pediatric intensive care did not expose patients to post-extubation stridor [37]. Autocycling of ventilators occurs mainly in the presence of gas leak respiratory system, especially when using uncuffed tubes [40].

In the adult population, the orotracheal intubation is preferred because of the lower rate of pneumonia associated with ventilation [41]. The oral route has been shown to be easier and faster, especially in emergencies [42, 43]. Given the shorter duration of the procedure, oral tracheal intubation would be preferable when rapid sequence induction is planned for fast intubation. In a multicenter study conducted in 121 US PICUs, 12,088 tracheal intubations were performed, of which only 5.6% were nasotracheal [44]. Because of its infrequency and prolonged procedure, nasotracheal intubation should be performed by skilled healthcare providers [41, 45–50], although there is no difference in complications related to the nasal and tracheal intubation procedure (e.g., number of attempts, change in SpO_2 from baseline, adverse TIAEs) [43, 51–53].

The nasotracheal tube has advantages such as safer fixation of the tube itself; less trauma to the lips, tongue, and larynx; lower rate of unplanned extubation; lower rate of post-extubation airway obstruction; and higher patient tolerance of the ETT [44, 54–56]. The presence of the nasal tube may allow for diagnostic tests such as transesophageal echocardiography because the oral cavity and oropharynx are unobstructed [44]. The stability of the nasotracheal tube position allows greater safety during maneuvers to change the patient's position, and especially in the prone position. Nasal intubation allows greater tolerance of the tube, especially during weaning from the ventilator, when deep sedation and myoresolution are not necessary, and spontaneous ventilatory activity should be stimulated.

Nasal skin lesions and bleeding are more commonly associated with nasotracheal intubation. The use of a skin dressing helps reduce pressure-induced skin breakdown. When comparing the two routes (oral and nasal) of intubation, there are fewer unplanned extubations in nasotracheal tube patients and no differences in post-extubation obstruction and sinusitis [44, 51].

The transition from the oral to the nasal route should be made when early extubation is not expected (within the first few days after intubation) and when the patient is expected to require prolonged periods of IMV (due to cardiorespiratory instability, surgical reinterventions, planned surgical and nonsurgical procedures, evolving and to-be-determined neurological status, anticipated difficult weaning from MV, timing of tracheotomy). The most frequent indications for which a patient may need tracheotomy are airway anomalies and the need for PMV due to chronic lung disease or neurologic disease [57–59]. Tracheotomy demonstrates advantages in terms of less need for analgosedation and shorter weaning from MV [60, 61].

A more detailed description of the indications and management of tracheostomy is provided in the following section, "Tracheostomy Management and Strategy."

4 Ventilators

Positive-pressure ventilation is based on the application of a higher than atmospheric pressure at the upper respiratory tract. The pressure gradient obtained between the upper airways and the alveoli allows gas to pass through the airways to the alveoli. Positive-pressure ventilators were invented in the 1950s. Since the 1970s, there has been a revolution in the design of mechanical ventilators, and this was due to the introduction of electronics in ventilator technology and the progressive application of positive end expiratory pressure in clinical practice. Chatburn first classified ventilators based on input power, power conversion and transmission, control scheme, output variables, and alarm systems [62].

The purpose of MV is to ensure adequate alveolar ventilation without causing lung damage, hemodynamic changes, and changes in comfort. It is necessary to clarify that the variable controlled by the ventilator is called the independent variable. It is easily recognized on the monitor because it usually takes a square geometric shape and depends solely on its setting. Conversely, the variable that is patient related is called the dependent variable and is related to the mechanical characteristics of the respiratory system and any spontaneous respiratory activity. To define a ventilatory mode, one must identify the primary control variable (pressure, volume, or flow), the type of breath, and the mode of control the operator will exert over the controlled variable. To distinguish two similar ventilatory modes, we also need to define the second classification variable. For the detailed description of a ventilatory mode, all three variables must be specified. In all ventilatory modes, only one variable can be controlled at a time (pressure, volume, or flow) so that pressure-controlled, volume-controlled, and flow-controlled modes can be distinguished. Knowing that volume and flow are inverse functions (flow is the derivative of volume over time, and volume is the integral area standing under the flow curve), we can directly classify pressure- and volume-controlled ventilatory modes. During pressure-controlled ventilation, the independent variable is the pressure that is set, while volume and flow are derived variables that are dependent on the pressure and properties of the respiratory system. Conversely, in volume-controlled ventilation, volume and flow are constant, while pressure is the dependent variable.

All ventilatory modes can be described according to phase variables. Each breath during positive-pressure ventilation can be divided into four key phases:

1. Breath onset or trigger.
2. Limit.
3. Cycle.
4. Baseline.

4.1 Initiating Breath or Trigger

The mechanical ventilator takes into account multiple variables (time, flow, pressure, volume, or diaphragmatic electrical activity), and when the expiratory phase ends, the inspiratory phase begins as soon as one of these variables reaches a set threshold value. Flow or electrical triggers are considered the most sensitive triggers and are applied in special cases to improve synchronization between the ventilator and the patient and cases where patients demonstrate weak muscular respiratory effort [63–65].

4.2 Limit

The ventilator delivers gas flow to the patient until a threshold value is reached. During the inspiratory phase, pressure and flow in the airway are taken into account by the ventilator and are considered control variables. During a ventilation mode, the ventilator will assume only one of these two variables by considering it as an independent variable, while the other is considered as a dependent variable. When pressure-controlled ventilation is applied to a patient, the pressure variable is independent, while the flow (and volume) depends on the respiratory system (compliance and resistance). Conversely, if the flow (and volume) is considered an independent variable, the pressure generated by the flow depends on the characteristics of the respiratory system.

4.3 Cycle

The cycle variable describes the process that determines the end of the inspiratory phase and allows the transition to the expiratory phase. Pressure, volume, flow, and diaphragmatic electrical activity are the cycle variables. In a ventilatory mode, if the cycle variable is time, the operator sets the respiratory rate (per minute) and the duration of a single respiratory act considering the time of inspiration and exhalation. If the cycle variable is flow, exhalation starts when a certain percentage value of inspiratory flow from the initial peak is reached; this percentage value can be adjusted to improve synchrony between patient and ventilator. If the cycle variable is diaphragmatic electrical activity, then exhalation starts when a 70% percentage value of the maximum Edi peak is reached.

4.4 Exhalation

Generally, the transition from the inspiratory phase to the expiratory phase is determined by time (defined as the duration of the inspiratory phase) during controlled ventilation or flow (defined as the percentage reduction in maximal inspiratory flow of 75–80%) during assisted ventilation. During almost all invasive ventilation modes, most part of exhalation is passive. When the inspiratory phase is in the end, the ventilator expiratory valve opens, and the elastic recoil of the lungs and chest wall (due to alveolar surface tension and tissue elasticity) consents to exhale gas from lungs. The volume exhaled depends on the relationship between lung compliance and airway resistance, defined as time constant. The expiratory time constant is the total time that the lung needs to exhale the 63% inspired VT [66]. Increased airway resistance or lung compliance results in increased constant time.

4.5 Type of Breath

Each of the inspiratory variables can be controlled by the patient or the ventilator. Therefore, two types of breathing are identified: spontaneous breaths (which also include assisted breaths) and controlled breaths (which include assisted-controlled cycles).

During spontaneous breathing, the patient controls all phases of breathing from beginning to end. In assisted spontaneous breathing, the ventilator performs part of the breathing cycle. For example, in pressure support ventilation, the single breath is assisted because the inspiratory pressure increases until the set pressure level is reached, but it is also considered a spontaneous breath because the patient controls both the initial phase of inspiration and the transition from inspiration to exhalation.

Conversely, if during the respiratory cycle the patient does not control the inspiratory phase or expiratory phase, it is called controlled ventilation. If the patient controls only either the inspiratory phase or the expiratory phase, it is called assist-controlled ventilation.

Three respiratory sequences are thus distinguished:

1. Fully controlled ventilation: each breath is controlled only by the ventilator.
2. Totally spontaneous ventilation: the patient controls every breath in all phases of breathing.
3. Intermittently controlled ventilation: some spontaneous breaths are allowed during controlled ventilatory cycles.

Considering the control variables (flow/volume and pressure) and the three possible ventilatory sequences (controlled, spontaneous, and intermittently controlled), we can distinguish the following conventional ventilatory modes:

1. Flow/volume-controlled and assisted-controlled ventilation.
2. Pressure-controlled and assisted-controlled ventilation.
3. Spontaneous pressurometric ventilation.
4. Intermittently controlled volumetric or pressurometric ventilation.

5 Conventional Invasive Ventilation

5.1 *Volume-Controlled and Volume Assist-Control Ventilation*

The goal of this mode is to deliver a set VT at a constant rate (constant inspiratory flow), over a given period of time, and at a preset respiratory rate [67].

Variables to be set:

- FiO_2.
- Respiratory rate.
- VT.
- PEEP.
- I:E or inspiratory time.
- Slope of the pressure rise curve.
- Inspiratory pause time.
- Safe limit pressure.
- Trigger: if the patient is passive, it will not be operative, but during assisted/controlled ventilation, it is important to set it correctly.

The operator sets the VT, respiratory rate, inspiratory time or inspiration/exhalation ratio, and PEEP. In this ventilatory mode, flow and volume are controlled by the ventilator; each breath is initiated by the ventilator and terminated according to a prefixed time.

In this mode, the limit variable is volume or flow, and the cycle variable is a set volume or time, depending on whether there is an inspiratory pause. In some cases, the limit variable may be pressure if a maximum airway pressure limit has been set.

Generally, in the flow graph, the wave is square (at constant flow), although some ventilators allow a choice of wave shapes. It is possible to set a flow or pressure trigger level that allows the patient to be able to trigger inspiration (volume assist-control ventilation, VACV).

During VACV, the ventilator always delivers the same preset VT regardless of whether there is patient inspiratory effort or a change in airway pressure/flow. The inspiratory phase can be triggered by patient effort (as the ventilator senses through the trigger sensor the inspiratory effort generated by the respiratory muscles) or initiated by the ventilator itself at a predetermined volume and frequency (in case the patient does not produce inspiratory effort).

In this ventilatory mode, the patient has his own respiratory rate, but also a set "safe" respiratory rate. Frequently, the ventilator does not control volume, but rather flow through inspiratory valves operated by microprocessors, and they then calculate volume through transducers internal to the ventilator circuit. Similarly, exhalation is controlled by expiratory valves that also allow for the ability to maintain a desired PEEP.

In recent years, the goals of controlled ventilation in acute respiratory failure have changed: there is a tendency to maintain a VT of 5–8 ml/kg (predicted body weight) while also tolerating increases in carbon dioxide [19]. Differently in acute brain damage with normal respiratory function, carbon dioxide must be monitored to avoid consequences on cerebral hemodynamics. For patients undergoing controlled invasive ventilation, it is recommended to maintain a plateau pressure at values below 28 cm H_2O so as to limit damage to normally ventilated lung areas. Plateau pressure depends on VT, PEEP, and respiratory system compliance; usually, the plateau pressure value corresponds to the end inspiratory alveolar pressure. In patients with increased chest wall stiffness (e.g., obese patients), plateau pressure may overestimate alveolar pressure [68]. This can be achieved by decreasing respiratory rate and VT and increasing expiratory time and gas flows; this allows for improved alveolar distribution of inspired gas. When patients have minimal spontaneous ventilatory activity, setting PEEP to values similar or just above intrinsic PEEP allows for a reduction in respiratory work.

If the patient is ventilated in the assist-control mode and activates the inspiratory trigger, the total respiratory rate will be higher than the set rate; consequently, the respiratory cycle duration will be shorter. In this condition, as the duration of the inspiratory phase is set, the expiratory phase will be reduced exposing the patient to the risk of dynamic hyperinflation, altering the synchrony between the patient and the ventilator and causing ineffective inspiratory efforts [69, 70]. It is important to set the inspiratory flow to ensure proper alveolar gas distribution while minimizing the WOB.

Reducing inspiratory flow results in increasing the patient's WOB, leading to a deformation of the pressure-time curve with an upward concave appearance [71]. Analysis of the pressure-volume curve allows the inspiratory flow to be set to achieve the best possible comfort for the patient.

The volume-controlled mode is indicated in cases of impaired respiratory exchanges and in cases where respiratory work increases the risk of cardiac arrest [67]. One advantage is the reduction of the patient's respiratory work. In addition, the volume delivered is constant. If patients are paralyzed, it is possible to calculate ventilatory parameters such as lung compliance, airway resistances, and time constant. If the patient has minimal ventilatory activity, it is possible that the patient may not adapt to this ventilatory mode (leading to periods of over-assistance and periods of under-assistance), and this may be a limitation of this mode. In fact, as soon as the level of analgosedation/myoresolution is reduced and respiratory exchanges have improved, it would be better to switch to an assisted mode such as pressure support ventilation.

Moreover, the longer the muscle inactivity lasts, the more the patient is exposed to the risk of muscle atrophy (especially of the diaphragm and respiratory muscles) making the weaning phase from MV more complex [10, 72–78].

5.2 *Pressure-Controlled and Pressure-Controlled Assist-Control Ventilation*

During pressure-controlled ventilation (PCV), the ventilator is able to do 100% of WOB; the independent variable is airway pressure (which takes a square form on the pressure/time diagram), while volume is a dependent variable. The limit variable is pressure, and the cycle variable is time [67]. Use of this ventilatory mode has developed more because of the increased attention to VILI and the risks of high inspiratory pressures [79, 80].

The goal of this mode is to apply a constant pressure, for a given period of time and at a preset frequency.

Variables to be set:

- FiO_2.
- Respiratory rate.
- Pressure controlled over PEEP.
- PEEP.
- I:E or inspiratory time.
- Slope of the pressure rise curve.
- Safe limit pressure.
- Trigger.

The ventilator can initiate breaths (PCV), while in the assisted-controlled mode, the patient's inspiratory effort can trigger ventilator action (pressure assist-control ventilation, PACV). When the ventilator generates pressure, a pressure difference is created between the ventilator and the alveoli determining the direction of airflow. The pressure though does not guarantee the volume delivered. This depends on how much flow the pressure difference can generate, and the impedance of the respiratory system. Each increase in the impedance of the respiratory system corresponds to a reduction in the VT delivered.

When the set inspiratory phase is short, the balance between delivered pressure and alveolar pressure is not achieved, and the latter will be less than delivered pressure. The slope of the pressure rise can be set. The delivered pressure is the sum of PEEP and the set pressure [67].

In PCV or PACV, the VT depends on the pressure setting above PEEP, duration of the inspiratory phase, and respiratory mechanics (respiratory system compliance and airway resistances). The presence of intrinsic PEEP reduces the difference between set and alveolar pressure leading to a reduction in VT [67]. Similarly, if the pressure and the inspiration/exhalation ratio remain constant and the respiratory rate increases, this results in an increase in intrinsic PEEP and consequent reduction in VT. This phenomenon is especially exacerbated in patients with restrictive lung disease where lung compliance is greatly reduced.

In obstructive lung disease, the increase in respiratory rate results in reduced inspiratory time producing a decrease in VT for dead-space ventilation and consequently an increase in $PaCO_2$ [81].

The ventilator can change the pressurization rise time and consequently the initial flow rate. A faster rise time results in a higher peak flow rate with more rapid reaching of the pressure limit and subsequent termination of the inspiratory act. This effect can cause asynchronies between the ventilator and the patient.

Conversely, if the ramp is very slow, the flow rate may decelerate to a value of zero before the expiratory phase begins. This would allow for better distribution of gases at the alveolar level and elimination of CO_2. In special cases of increased oxygen demand (such as fever), this phenomenon could trigger the patient's increased inspiratory effort [82–84].

The indications are similar to the volumetric controlled or assisted-controlled mode.

The basic goal is to reduce alveolar overdistension and barotrauma, although it is known that lung damage from MV is due to increased transpulmonary pressure (airway pressure minus pleural pressure) [85].

Therefore, the pressure limit is not always a protective factor since it may be enough for excessive patient effort to result in a more negative pleural pressure (with consequent increase in transpulmonary pressure); in these cases, the risk of lung damage can be reduced by giving the patient analgosedation and myoresolution.

VT is variable so that in cases of respiratory instability, there would be a risk of hypoventilation [85].

Unlike VACV, PACV controls inspiratory time and not flow which is affected by the patient's respiratory mechanics and effort intensity.

Asynchronies can also occur in this method, such as when the patient starts exhalation during the final inspiratory phase of the ventilator; this results in increased airway pressure or, more frequently, a reduction in VT.

5.3 *Pressure Support Ventilation*

It is a ventilatory mode in which a constant pressure is applied to the airway during the inspiratory phase only if the patient initiates his or her own inspiratory activity, that is, each breath is spontaneous and is assisted by the ventilator. This ventilatory mode provides synchronization of the mechanical ventilator with the patient's spontaneous respiratory activity. The setting includes:

- FiO_2.
- PEEP.
- Supportive pressure (above PEEP).
- Rise time.
- Inspiratory trigger (pressure or flow).
- Expiratory trigger.
- Limit safety pressure.

This ventilatory mode is spontaneous because it depends on the patient's inspiratory effort. The ventilator controls the pressure to be applied each time the patient triggers an inspiratory act by keeping the pressure limit [67, 86, 87] as the control variable.

Inspiratory triggering depends on the patient's inspiratory effort and on reaching a threshold value of inspiratory phase activation (inspiratory trigger). The inspiratory trigger can be of pressure when in the respiratory circuit with valves (inspiratory and expiratory) closed and at the end of the expiratory phase, a pressure drop is generated due to the patient's effort reaching an established threshold value.

Differently in the flow trigger, the inspiratory phase begins when at circuit with open valves, a subtraction of flow is determined (reaching a set threshold value) due to the patient's inspiratory effort. Studies have shown that with the flow trigger, the patient makes less inspiratory effort than with the pressure trigger [88].

During the inspiratory phase, airway pressure reaches the set value while flow is decreasing. The transition from the inspiratory to expiratory phase occurs when the inspiratory flow decreases to a certain threshold value called the expiratory trigger. This threshold value corresponds to the value of flow such that the inspiratory muscle relaxation phase begins and the expiratory phase can start.

The expiratory trigger value can be expressed as an absolute value or percentage value of the peak inspiratory flow (and is settable).

Since controlled respiratory acts are not delivered, when the patient's apnea occurs, the ventilator can trigger "apnea ventilation" by delivering controlled breaths.

The WOB changes according to the pressure support ventilation (PSV) setting. The respiratory pattern decreases proportionally to the level of care set [89]. The patient will be over-assisted when the level of pressure assistance is higher than the patient's individual limit. Reducing the level of pressure assistance has been shown to be accompanied by decrease of TV and increases in respiratory rate, whereas an increase in assisted pressure is associated with an increase in VT [89–91].

Assist level can also be assessed by respiratory rate: a high respiratory rate leads to increased muscle work [67, 92, 93]. Conversely, an increased level of assist is associated with hyperinflation, respiratory alkalosis, reduced respiratory rate to apnea pauses [40, 48], and asynchronies between patient and ventilator [24, 94, 95]. A velocity that is too slow to reach the target pressure value can cause increased WOB, especially in patients with high airway resistance [82–84, 96, 97]. Conversely, a high pressurization velocity may result in early termination of the inspiratory phase [96].

Thus, the possibility of modifying the expiratory trigger allows the inspiratory and expiratory phases and VT to be better matched to the patient's condition by reducing asynchronies.

With the reduction of sedation, the prevention of diaphragm muscle atrophy due to its reduced use is allowed [72, 98]. PSV is used in the resolution phases of PARDS as a weaning mode [99]. There are ventilators with closed-loop modes that allow varying the pressure level in each breath while maintaining a target VT, respiratory rate, and end-tidal CO_2 [100–104].

A failure to synchronize can occur if the patient makes ineffective respiratory efforts, for example, when the patient is ventilated with high VT and supportive pressure (over-assistance). Conversely, self-triggering results in pressure delivery when the patient has not initiated inspiratory effort: this depends on circuit issues (humidity, leakage, patient's cardiac oscillations). Asynchronies can occur when the inspiratory ramp (and thus the flow rate) is inappropriately set or when multiple cycles occur, during auto-triggering with high pressurization velocity [83, 105] or a too short inspiratory time. In a study on weaning from MV in the pediatric patient, PSV does not result in significant inspiratory efforts compared with PCAC and also does not increase the WOB and discomfort of patients [106].

5.4 Synchronized Mandatory Intermittent Ventilation

Synchronized intermittent mandatory ventilation (SIMV) is a mixed ventilatory mode in which there are mandatory (controlled) breaths and spontaneous or assisted breaths. The variables to be considered for the setting of SIMV are:

- FiO_2.
- Controlled volume or pressure.
- PEEP.
- Rise time.
- Inspiration/exhalation.
- Controlled respiratory rate.
- SIMV cycle duration.
- Expiratory trigger.
- Inspiratory trigger.
- Pressure support.

Controlled cycles can be in volumetric or pressurometric mode and are synchronized with the patient's spontaneous activity. In case the patient does not initiate spontaneous breaths, the ventilator would provide controlled breaths at the preset rate.

Ventilatory support depends on the controlled respiratory rate: the higher the rate, the more the intensity of support increases. If the preset frequency decreases, there will be a greater chance that the patient will perform spontaneous/assisted breaths by reducing respiratory work [107, 108].

The flow trigger is the most widely used because it allows better synchronization to the patient's demand. SIMV is more like an assisted-controlled ventilatory mode (by volume or pressure).

Initially, it was believed that SIMV respiratory effort decreased with increasing controlled acts and that muscle activity became more active during lower controlled respiratory rates (in which spontaneous/assisted ventilatory acts were favored). This concept has been overcome: inspiratory effort then is similar during both controlled and spontaneous/assisted breaths [109–111].

The advantage of a properly set SIMV is the stimulation of spontaneous ventilatory activity, thus weaning from controlled ventilation. SIMV as the final mode of weaning from MV has been shown to be inferior to PSV or spontaneous ventilation with T-tube and is associated with prolongation of MV itself [112, 113].

6 Nonconventional Invasive Ventilation

6.1 Pressure-Regulated Volume Control

In this mode, the ventilator adjusts the pressure applied to the patient in order to achieve a set VT, breath by breath. Pressure-regulated volume control (PRVC) belongs to closed-loop ventilations, in which a feedback signal is used to adjust the output of a system. The difference between set volume and obtained (expired) volume is useful to guide the ventilator to deliver inspiratory pressure such that a set VT is obtained.

The setting includes:

- FiO_2.
- VT.
- Respiratory rate.
- PEEP.
- I:E.
- Rise time.
- Inspiratory trigger.
- Safety pressure limit.

An advantage of this method is that the predetermined VT is achieved with the lowest inspiratory pressure, avoiding the reaching of high airway pressures. In addition, if the patient is able to trigger, the respiratory rate is controlled by the patient.

The principle of operation is similar to PCV (for constant inspiratory pressure and decreasing flow) with the advantage of volume-controlled ventilation, that is, guaranteeing a prefixed VT. PRVC is commonly used in pediatric setting especially in pediatric acute respiratory distress and in postsurgical patients [114–117].

6.2 *Proportional Ventilation*

Assisted ventilatory modes are still based on a closed-loop system. For example, relying on a back-loop system, already in SIMV, there are controlled acts in the midst of which the patient can take spontaneous breaths; same thing happens during PSV where in a closed system, pressor support is delivered to the change in flow or pressure in the loop itself.

Relatively new pressurometric assisted ventilatory modes make it possible to quantify the patient's inspiratory effort and correspond to this with a consensual pressure that varies with the intensity of the inspiratory effort itself. Under these conditions, there is no prefixed VT to be achieved.

Inspiratory effort recognition systems are based on the electrical activity of the diaphragm or calculations based on resistivity and elastance of the patient's respiratory system.

The ultimate goal is to ensure the greatest ventilator-patient synchronization, give the patient greater control of VT, reduce ineffective inspiratory efforts (not recognized by the ventilator), and limit over-suppression.

These new modalities are shown to be physiologically effective, although there is a need for conclusive studies on their clinical efficacy (Table 1).

6.2.1 Neurally Adjusted Ventilatory Assist

Neurally adjusted ventilatory assist (NAVA) is a ventilatory mode based on the synchronization of positive-pressure application with inspiration and electrical activity of the diaphragm (EAdi) [118]. Variables to consider during the setting of NAVA are:

- FiO_2.
- Neural inspiratory flow trigger.
- NAVA level ($cmH_2O/\mu V$).
- PEEP.
- Pmax.
- Backup ventilation.
- Pressure-support ventilation.
- Neural inspiratory trigger (Edi trigger).

The ventilator delivers assisted breaths after receiving the electromyographic signal of the diaphragm detected by electrodes in the nasogastric tube (currently the best signal for estimating respiratory drive). EAdi represents the final neural signal from the breath centers (through the phrenic nerves) to the diaphragm [118]. The cycling between inspiration and exhalation has been established at 70% of the maximal EAdi peak by the manufacturer. The level of assistance is based on the level of EAdi: the pressure support value is set for each 29 microvolt of electromyographic signal from the diaphragm [119, 120].

NAVA is unaffected by intrinsic PEEP and allows for better ventilator-patient synchrony by reducing over-assistance.

A fundamental condition for better synchrony outcome is the integrity of the breath centers, phrenic nerves, and diaphragmatic neuromuscular junctions and that no sedative drugs (that affect EAdi signal integrity and voltage) are administered.

Comparison studies between PSV and NAVA regarding asynchrony index (expressed as numbers of synchronous acts/total number of ventilatory acts) have been conducted in the pediatric setting, confirming the advantages of neural trigger over pneumatic and that in NAVA there is better synchronization and reduced over-assistance [65]. Similar results were obtained when NAVA was compared with CPAP in infants during weaning from invasive ventilation [121].

In a meta-analysis of prospective/retrospective studies in 464 neonates/children, the application of NAVA (compared with conventional methods) resulted in significant improvement in asynchronies, peak inspiratory pressure, and oxygenation indices [122].

Crossover comparison studies in neonates/children with ARDS, multiple organ failure, bronchiolitis, prematurity, congenital heart disease, and in postoperative period confirm lower asynchrony index and peak inspiratory pressure in favor of NAVA, while there is no gain for gas exchange and hemodynamic parameters [123–127].

Two studies demonstrate increased patient comfort during NAVA application compared with conventional modalities [128, 129].

In a pilot study, NAVA compared with PSV during weaning in infants affected by severe ARDS (and treated with high-frequency oscillatory ventilation) was associated with less peak inspiratory pressure and lower $PaCO_2$, heart rate, mean arterial pressure, COMFORT score, and duration of support. In a randomized controlled trial on 161 pediatric patients, NAVA (compared to pressure-controlled ventilation in neonates or pressure-regulated volume control in older) was associated with lower FiO_2 and peak inspiratory pressure, while no differences were found in terms of gas exchange, complications, and duration of invasive ventilation [129]. Trigger delay and asynchrony index are demonstrated to be lower in infants affected by bronchiolitis, ARDS, acute respiratory failure, and multiple organ failure, when ventilated with NAVA [125, 127, 130].

Similarly in the cardiac patient and after cardiac surgery, NAVA is shown to be associated with lower asynchronies and PIP [123, 131, 132]. A retrospective study of patients undergoing ECMO demonstrates better synchronization of patients when undergoing NAVA during weaning from MV [133].

All of these studies have demonstrated the feasibility and benefits of NAVA on some clinical/respiratory parameters, but there are currently no large trials that correlate NAVA with clinical outcomes such as mortality, duration of IMV, length of ICU stay, and failure of extubation when compared with conventional ventilation.

Recently, a review paper focused on bronchopulmonary dysplasia patients showed some relevant clinical advantages of using NAVA and NIV-NAVA for this group, like reduced time on mechanical ventilation, less extubation failure rate, and shorter length of stay in intensive care [134].

6.2.2 Proportional Assist Ventilation (PAV)

When applying proportional assist ventilation (PAV), the pressure delivered varies for each respiratory cycle. While in PSV the pressure delivered to the patient is constant (through inspiratory trigger activation) and decreases when the percentage threshold of peak inspiratory flow is reached for cycling on exhalation [24, 67, 86, 89], during PAV, the pressure delivered changes breath by breath [135], so it depends on the intensity of muscle effort generated and is proportional (based on the desired level of assistance, 0–100%) to the flow, volume, and pressure generated by the muscles themselves. During PAV, it is possible to select the level (as a percentage) of assistance that the ventilator will constantly apply considering the elastance and resistivity of the respiratory system.

This mode initially required manual and periodic measurements of resistivity and elastance and made PAV very investigative in application. The development of software installed in the ventilator that automatically estimates resistivity and elastance every 8–10 breaths (PAV+) has allowed for greater ease of use and dissemination [136–138]; this allows the operator to set only the desired level of care based on the patient's clinical condition. For example, in patients with neuromuscular disease where respiratory work is reduced, the rate of assistance will be increased until optimal VT and gas exchange are achieved.

Current data confirm that PAV+ can be applied to infants with or at risk of bronchopulmonary dysplasia [139].

At present, PAV/PAV+ remains a research tool. As with NAVA, the current challenge is to demonstrate its efficacy on clinical outcomes [140].

6.2.3 Airway Pressure Release Ventilation

APRV is a pressurometric modality characterized by the application of continuous positive pressure with short release phases allowing partial volumes to be released to the patient. It is an inverse ratio control pressure ventilation in which the high (inspiratory)-pressure application phase is longer lasting than the low-pressure phase. The goal is to deliver breaths in the transition from low to high pressure. The patient can take spontaneous breaths both in high-pressure and low-pressure delivery phase.

The longer duration of high pressure allows an increase in airway pressure leading to increased oxygenation through alveolar recruitment by improving the ventilation/perfusion ratio [141].

Currently, apart from case reports, case series, and retrospective and crossover studies demonstrating improvement in oxygenation and CO_2 clearance, there is only one trial regarding the use of APRV in PARDS compared with low VT controlled ventilation, which stopped due to increased mortality in the APRV group [142–145].

7 Ventilator-Associated Pneumonia

Ventilator-associated pneumonia (VAP) represents one of the most common infections in the pediatric and neonatal intensive care units [146]. Mechanically ventilated patients are at risk of developing VAP [147].

VAP results in increases in morbidity and mortality in PICU/neonatal intensive care unit while increasing the length of hospital stay and management costs [148–150]. In addition, VAP exposes patients to prolonged antibiotic therapy (antibiotic overuse and risk of resistance) [151].

The incidence of VAP varies between 2 and 35% of ventilated patients and between 1 and 63 cases per 1000 days of MV [7, 146, 152–157]. This variability among studies may depend on patient characteristics, nutritional status, resource availability of centers, and different diagnostic criteria adopted.

This is due to the lack of a diagnostic gold standard and an accepted definition of VAP-related outcomes (mortality, organ failure, length of stay, and antibiotic resistance) [158]. Clinical, microbiologic, radiologic, and diagnostic criteria can be subjectively interpreted and be applied differently across centers, thus resulting in this variability in rates.

The most recognized and widely used guidelines for the diagnosis of VAP in general, also applied to pediatric settings, are the 2014 CDC/NNIS criteria updated to 2022 [147, 159]. VAP is defined as pneumonia diagnosed in a patient ventilated by tracheal tube or tracheotomy for at least 48 h.

In addition, the CDC has defined ventilator-associated events (VAEs) to better understand ventilation-related complications. VAEs occur in patients who show an increase in MAP or FiO2 after a period of stabilization or improvement [159]. Frequently, VAEs are not correlated with infection. As a result, solutions are being suggested that may not even be directly related to MV and that aim to reduce ventilation itself, length of stay, and mortality [159]. All recommendations are based on varying levels of evidence due to the lack of experience in the pediatric population as opposed to adult studies.

It is recommended that quantitative criteria be used for the diagnosis of VAP to ensure greater reproducibility of results between centers.

Risk factors most associated with the development of VAP are inoculation of non-sterile solutions during aspiration of tracheobronchial secretions, colonization of airway and digestive mucosa, reintubation, enteral nutrition, gastric proton pump inhibitors, patient transfers, and duration of MV.

Some differences for the neonatal and pediatric population such as bronchopulmonary dysplasia, necrotizing enterocolitis, and hyaline membrane disease that may affect the detection of VAP should also be considered [160, 161].

Risk factors in the adult population are overlapped in infants and children, but not all prevention recommendations for VAP events may be applicable to the pediatric population. Prevention recommendations aim to avoid IMV whenever possible by using noninvasive ventilation. Minimizing the duration of IMV through daily assessment for extubation and avoiding reintubation of patients is one of the key aspects [159]. Effective interventions to prevent VAP should include oral hygiene, head elevation, frequent circuit changes, removal of circuit condensation without returning it to the patient, choice of tubing cuffed at a pressure of 20–24 cm H_2O to reduce the risk of air leak and inhalation, probiotics, daily awakening test with discontinuation of sedation, and early tracheotomy [159].

In a recent study, Chongcharoenyanon demonstrated in a pediatric population of 140 children ventilated for more than 14 days how the incidence of VAP increases significantly with increasing duration of MV (up to 98% of patients ventilated for more than 30 days) [162].

Once VAP is diagnosed, antibiotic therapy should be started rapidly. Delay in the setting of antibiotic therapy has an impact on morbidity, mortality, and cost. Especially in late VAP, isolations of multidrug-resistant bacteria are common [159].

The available data do not allow definitive answers regarding diagnosis and prevention of VAP in the pediatric setting. In fact, all strategies should aim not only to reduce incidence rates but also to limit risk factors and related complications such as duration of antibiotic therapy, hospital stay, and mortality.

8 Conclusion

The increased intensity of care has improved the outcome of critically ill pediatric patients and consequently increased their morbidity. The possibility of being able to choose between different ventilatory modes allows a better fitting to individual patient characteristics. Ventilation-related problems such as diaphragmatic dysfunction must be considered. A common definition regarding the timing of tracheotomy is desirable. New ventilatory modalities would allow the improvement of patient-ventilator synchronization, and future efficacy studies with clinical outcomes would allow their clinical application.

References

1. Iwashyna TJ, Hodgson CL, Pilcher D, Bailey M, van Lint A, Chavan S, et al. Timing of onset and burden of persistent critical illness in Australia and New Zealand: a retrospective, population-based, observational study. Lancet Respir Med. 2016;4(7):566–73.
2. Traiber C, Piva JP, Fritsher CC, Garcia PC, Lago PM, Trotta EA, et al. Profile and consequences of children requiring prolonged mechanical ventilation in three Brazilian pediatric intensive care units. Pediatr Crit Care Med. 2009;10(3):375–80.
3. Lone NI, Walsh TS. Prolonged mechanical ventilation in critically ill patients: epidemiology, outcomes and modelling the potential cost consequences of establishing a regional weaning unit. Crit Care. 2011;15(2):R102.
4. Polito A, Combescure C, Levy-Jamet Y, Rimensberger P, Medicine SSoIC. Long-stay patients in pediatric intensive care unit: diagnostic-specific definition and predictors. PLoS One. 2019;14(10):e0223369.

5. Principi T, Fraser DD, Morrison GC, Farsi SA, Carrelas JF, Maurice EA, et al. Complications of mechanical ventilation in the pediatric population. Pediatr Pulmonol. 2011;46(5):452–7.
6. Mutlu GM, Factor P. Complications of mechanical ventilation. Respir Care Clin N Am. 2000;6(2):213–52. v
7. Rivera R, Tibballs J. Complications of endotracheal intubation and mechanical ventilation in infants and children. Crit Care Med. 1992;20(2):193–9.
8. Navalesi P, Costa R. New modes of mechanical ventilation: proportional assist ventilation, neurally adjusted ventilatory assist, and fractal ventilation. Curr Opin Crit Care. 2003;9(1):51–8.
9. Argov Z, Mastaglia FL. Drug therapy: disorders of neuromuscular transmission caused by drugs. N Engl J Med. 1979;301(8):409–13.
10. Levine S, Nguyen T, Taylor N, Friscia ME, Budak MT, Rothenberg P, et al. Rapid disuse atrophy of diaphragm fibers in mechanically ventilated humans. N Engl J Med. 2008;358(13):1327–35.
11. MacIntyre NR, Epstein SK, Carson S, Scheinhorn D, Christopher K, Muldoon S, et al. Management of patients requiring prolonged mechanical ventilation: report of a NAMDRC consensus conference. Chest. 2005;128(6):3937–54.
12. Payen V, Jouvet P, Lacroix J, Ducruet T, Gauvin F. Risk factors associated with increased length of mechanical ventilation in children. Pediatr Crit Care Med. 2012;13(2):152–7.
13. Polito A, Patorno E, Costello JM, Salvin JW, Emani SM, Rajagopal S, et al. Perioperative factors associated with prolonged mechanical ventilation after complex congenital heart surgery. Pediatr Crit Care Med. 2011;12(3):e122–6.
14. Monteverde E, Fernández A, Poterala R, Vidal N, Siaba Serrate A, Castelani P, et al. Characterization of pediatric patients receiving prolonged mechanical ventilation. Pediatr Crit Care Med. 2011;12(6):e287–91.
15. Jubran A, Grant BJ, Duffner LA, Collins EG, Lanuza DM, Hoffman LA, et al. Effect of pressure support vs unassisted breathing through a tracheostomy collar on weaning duration in patients requiring prolonged mechanical ventilation: a randomized trial. JAMA. 2013;309(7):671–7.
16. Overman AE, Liu M, Kurachek SC, Shreve MR, Maynard RC, Mammel MC, et al. Tracheostomy for infants requiring prolonged mechanical ventilation: 10 years' experience. Pediatrics. 2013;131(5):e1491–6.
17. Holloway AJ, Spaeder MC, Basu S. Association of timing of tracheostomy on clinical outcomes in PICU patients. Pediatr Crit Care Med. 2015;16(3):e52–8.
18. Santschi M, Jouvet P, Leclerc F, Gauvin F, Newth CJ, Carroll CL, et al. Acute lung injury in children: therapeutic practice and feasibility of international clinical trials. Pediatr Crit Care Med. 2010;11(6):681–9.
19. Group PALICC. Pediatric acute respiratory distress syndrome: consensus recommendations from the pediatric acute lung injury consensus conference. Pediatr Crit Care Med. 2015;16(5):428–39.
20. Khemani RG, Conti D, Alonzo TA, Bart RD, Newth CJ. Effect of tidal volume in children with acute hypoxemic respiratory failure. Intensive Care Med. 2009;35(8):1428–37.
21. Kneyber MC, Rimensberger PC. The need for and feasibility of a pediatric ventilation trial: reflections on a survey among pediatric intensivists*. Pediatr Crit Care Med. 2012;13(6):632–8.
22. Kielt MJ, Hatch LD, Levin JC, Napolitano N, Abman SH, Baker CD, et al. Classifying multicenter approaches to invasive mechanical ventilation for infants with bronchopulmonary dysplasia using hierarchical clustering analysis. Pediatr Pulmonol. 2023;58(8):2323–32.
23. Kondili E, Prinianakis G, Georgopoulos D. Patient-ventilator interaction. Br J Anaesth. 2003;91(1):106–19.
24. Thille AW, Rodriguez P, Cabello B, Lellouche F, Brochard L. Patient-ventilator asynchrony during assisted mechanical ventilation. Intensive Care Med. 2006;32(10):1515–22.

25. de Wit M, Pedram S, Best AM, Epstein SK. Observational study of patient-ventilator asynchrony and relationship to sedation level. J Crit Care. 2009;24(1):74–80.
26. Chao DC, Scheinhorn DJ, Stearn-Hassenpflug M. Patient-ventilator trigger asynchrony in prolonged mechanical ventilation. Chest. 1997;112(6):1592–9.
27. Blanch L, Villagra A, Sales B, Montanya J, Lucangelo U, Luján M, et al. Asynchronies during mechanical ventilation are associated with mortality. Intensive Care Med. 2015;41(4):633–41.
28. Khemani RG, Parvathaneni K, Yehya N, Bhalla AK, Thomas NJ, Newth CJL. Positive end-expiratory pressure lower than the ARDS network protocol is associated with higher pediatric acute respiratory distress syndrome mortality. Am J Respir Crit Care Med. 2018;198(1):77–89.
29. West JB, Luks AM. Respiratory physiology. The essentials. 10th ed. Wolters Kluwer; 2012.
30. Lodato RF. Oxygen toxicity. In: Tobin MJ, editor. Principles and practice of mechanical ventilation. 3rd ed. McGraw Hill; 2013. p. 3596–621.
31. Peterson-Carmichael S, Cheifetz I, Storme L. Oxygen supplementation, delivery, and physiologic effects. In: Rimensberger PC, editor. Pediatric and neonatal mechanical ventilation from basics to clinical practice. 1st ed. Springer; 2015. p. 129–30.
32. Barnes-Daly MA, Phillips G, Ely EW. Improving hospital survival and reducing brain dysfunction at seven California Community Hospitals: implementing PAD guidelines via the ABCDEF bundle in 6,064 patients. Crit Care Med. 2017;45(2):171–8.
33. Morandi A, Piva S, Ely EW, Myatra SN, Salluh JIF, Amare D, et al. Worldwide survey of the "assessing pain, both spontaneous awakening and breathing trials, choice of drugs, delirium monitoring/management, early exercise/mobility, and family empowerment" (ABCDEF) bundle. Crit Care Med. 2017;45(11):e1111–e22.
34. Pun BT, Balas MC, Barnes-Daly MA, Thompson JL, Aldrich JM, Barr J, et al. Caring for critically ill patients with the ABCDEF bundle: results of the ICU liberation collaborative in over 15,000 adults. Crit Care Med. 2019;47(1):3–14.
35. Ista E, Redivo J, Kananur P, Choong K, Colleti J, Needham DM, et al. ABCDEF bundle practices for critically ill children: an international survey of 161 PICUs in 18 countries. Crit Care Med. 2022;50(1):114–25.
36. Di Nardo M, Boldrini F, Broccati F, Cancani F, Satta T, Stoppa F, et al. The LiberAction project: implementation of a pediatric liberation bundle to screen delirium, reduce benzodiazepine sedation, and provide early mobilization in a human resource-limited pediatric intensive care unit. Front Pediatr. 2021;9:788997.
37. Newth CJ, Rachman B, Patel N, Hammer J. The use of cuffed versus uncuffed endotracheal tubes in pediatric intensive care. J Pediatr. 2004;144(3):333–7.
38. Weiss M, Dullenkopf A, Fischer JE, Keller C, Gerber AC, Group EPEIS. Prospective randomized controlled multi-Centre trial of cuffed or uncuffed endotracheal tubes in small children. Br J Anaesth. 2009;103(6):867–73.
39. Litman RS, Maxwell LG. Cuffed versus uncuffed endotracheal tubes in pediatric anesthesia: the debate should finally end. Anesthesiology. 2013;118(3):500–1.
40. Schwab RJ, Schnader JS. Ventilator autocycling due to an endotracheal tube cuff leak. Chest. 1991;100(4):1172–3.
41. Committee HICPA, (U.S.) CfDCaP. Guidelines for preventing health-care-associated pneumonia, 2003 recommendations of the CDC and the healthcare infection control practices advisory Committee. Respir Care. 2004;49(8):926–39.
42. Holzapfel L. Nasal vs oral intubation. Minerva Anestesiol. 2003;69(5):348–52.
43. Abdelbaser I, Abourezk AR, Magdy M, Elnegerey N, Sabry R, Tharwat M, et al. Comparison of the outcomes of oral versus nasal endotracheal intubation in neonates and infants undergoing cardiac surgery: a randomized controlled study. J Cardiothorac Vasc Anesth. 2023;37(10):2012–9.
44. Christian CE, Thompson NE, Wakeham MK. Use and outcomes of nasotracheal intubation among patients requiring mechanical ventilation across U.S. PICUs. Pediatr Crit Care Med. 2020;21(7):620–4.

45. Nett S, Emeriaud G, Jarvis JD, Montgomery V, Nadkarni VM, Nishisaki A, et al. Site-level variance for adverse tracheal intubation-associated events across 15 North American PICUs: a report from the national emergency airway registry for children*. Pediatr Crit Care Med. 2014;15(4):306–13.
46. Chevron V, Ménard JF, Richard JC, Girault C, Leroy J, Bonmarchand G. Unplanned extubation: risk factors of development and predictive criteria for reintubation. Crit Care Med. 1998;26(6):1049–53.
47. Listello D, Sessler CN. Unplanned extubation. Clinical predictors for reintubation. Chest. 1994;105(5):1496–503.
48. Boulain T. Unplanned extubations in the adult intensive care unit: a prospective multicenter study. Association des Réanimateurs du Centre-Ouest. Am J Respir Crit Care Med. 1998;157(4 Pt 1):1131–7.
49. Piva JP, Amantéa S, Luchese S, Giugno K, Maia TR, Einloft L. Accidental extubation in a pediatric intensive care unit. J Pediatr. 1995;71(2):72–6.
50. Salord F, Gaussorgues P, Marti-Flich J, Sirodot M, Allimant C, Lyonnet D, et al. Nosocomial maxillary sinusitis during mechanical ventilation: a prospective comparison of orotracheal versus the nasotracheal route for intubation. Intensive Care Med. 1990;16(6):390–3.
51. Kumar V, Angurana SK, Baranwal AK, Nallasamy K, Nasotracheal vs. Orotracheal intubation and post-extubation airway obstruction in critically ill children: an open-label randomized controlled trial. Front Pediatr. 2021;9:713516.
52. Orlowski JP, Ellis NG, Amin NP, Crumrine RS. Complications of airway intrusion in 100 consecutive cases in a pediatric ICU. Crit Care Med. 1980;8(6):324–31.
53. Spence K, Barr P. Nasal versus oral intubation for mechanical ventilation of newborn infants. Cochrane Database Syst Rev. 2000;1999(2):CD000948.
54. Kambestad KK, Huack A, Nair S, Chapman R, Chin S, Langga L, et al. The adverse impact of unplanned Extubation in a cohort of critically ill neonates. Respir Care. 2019;64(12):1500–7.
55. Kanthimathinathan HK, Durward A, Nyman A, Murdoch IA, Tibby SM. Unplanned extubation in a paediatric intensive care unit: prospective cohort study. Intensive Care Med. 2015;41(7):1299–306.
56. Roddy DJ, Spaeder MC, Pastor W, Stockwell DC, Klugman D. Unplanned extubations in children: impact on hospital cost and length of stay. Pediatr Crit Care Med. 2015;16(6):572–5.
57. Egbuta C, Easley RB. Update on ventilation management in the pediatric intensive care unit. Paediatr Anaesth. 2022;32(2):354–62.
58. Berry MF, Villamizar-Ortiz NR, Tong BC, Burfeind WR, Harpole DH, D'Amico TA, et al. Pulmonary function tests do not predict pulmonary complications after thoracoscopic lobectomy. Ann Thorac Surg. 2010;89(4):1044–51. discussion 51–2.
59. Mizuno K, Takeuchi M, Kishimoto Y, Kawakami K, Omori K. Indications and outcomes of paediatric tracheotomy: a descriptive study using a Japanese claims database. BMJ Open. 2019;9(12):e031816.
60. Butler EK, Killien EY, Groner JI, Arbabi S, Vavilala MS, Rivara FP. Optimal timing of tracheostomy in injured adolescents. Pediatr Crit Care Med. 2021;22(7):629–41.
61. Lin CY, Ting TT, Hsiao TY, Hsu WC. Pediatric tracheotomy: a comparison of outcomes and lengths of hospitalization between different indications. Int J Pediatr Otorhinolaryngol. 2017;101:75–80.
62. Chatburn RL. A new system for understanding mechanical ventilators. Respir Care. 1991;36(10):1123–55.
63. Stein H, Firestone K, Rimensberger PC. Synchronized mechanical ventilation using electrical activity of the diaphragm in neonates. Clin Perinatol. 2012;39(3):525–42.
64. Murias G, Villagra A, Blanch L. Patient-ventilator dyssynchrony during assisted invasive mechanical ventilation. Minerva Anestesiol. 2013;79(4):434–44.
65. Spinazzola G, Costa R, De Luca D, Chidini G, Ferrone G, Piastra M, et al. Pressure Support Ventilation (PSV) versus Neurally Adjusted Ventilatory Assist (NAVA) in difficult to wean pediatric ARDS patients: a physiologic crossover study. BMC Pediatr. 2020;20(1):334.

66. Rimensberger PC. Pediatric and neonatal mechanical ventilation. From basics to clinical practice. 1st ed. Springer; 2015.
67. Tobin MJ. Principles and practice of mechanical ventilation. 2nd ed. McGraw-Hill; 2006.
68. Grasso S, Terragni P, Birocco A, Urbino R, Del Sorbo L, Filippini C, et al. ECMO criteria for influenza A (H1N1)-associated ARDS: role of transpulmonary pressure. Intensive Care Med. 2012;38(3):395–403.
69. Kondili E, Prinianakis G, Anastasaki M, Georgopoulos D. Acute effects of ventilator settings on respiratory motor output in patients with acute lung injury. Intensive Care Med. 2001;27(7):1147–57.
70. Laghi F. Effect of inspiratory time and flow settings during assist-control ventilation. Curr Opin Crit Care. 2003;9(1):39–44.
71. Ward ME, Corbeil C, Gibbons W, Newman S, Macklem PT. Optimization of respiratory muscle relaxation during mechanical ventilation. Anesthesiology. 1988;69(1):29–35.
72. Sassoon CS. Ventilator-associated diaphragmatic dysfunction. Am J Respir Crit Care Med. 2002;166(8):1017–8.
73. De Jonghe B, Bastuji-Garin S, Sharshar T, Outin H, Brochard L. Does ICU-acquired paresis lengthen weaning from mechanical ventilation? Intensive Care Med. 2004;30(6):1117–21.
74. Knisely AS, Leal SM, Singer DB. Abnormalities of diaphragmatic muscle in neonates with ventilated lungs. J Pediatr. 1988;113(6):1074–7.
75. Glau CL, Conlon TW, Himebauch AS, Yehya N, Weiss SL, Berg RA, et al. Progressive diaphragm atrophy in pediatric acute respiratory failure. Pediatr Crit Care Med. 2018;19(5):406–11.
76. Goligher EC, Dres M, Fan E, Rubenfeld GD, Scales DC, Herridge MS, et al. Mechanical ventilation-induced diaphragm atrophy strongly impacts clinical outcomes. Am J Respir Crit Care Med. 2018;197(2):204–13.
77. Khemani RG, Sekayan T, Hotz J, Flink RC, Rafferty GF, Iyer N, et al. Risk factors for pediatric Extubation failure: the importance of respiratory muscle strength. Crit Care Med. 2017;45(8):e798–805.
78. Crulli B, Kawaguchi A, Praud JP, Petrof BJ, Harrington K, Emeriaud G. Evolution of inspiratory muscle function in children during mechanical ventilation. Crit Care. 2021;25(1):229.
79. Laffey JG, O'Croinin D, McLoughlin P, Kavanagh BP. Permissive hypercapnia—role in protective lung ventilatory strategies. Intensive Care Med. 2004;30(3):347–56.
80. Brower RG, Matthay MA, Morris A, Schoenfeld D, Thompson BT, Wheeler A, et al. Ventilation with lower tidal volumes as compared with traditional tidal volumes for acute lung injury and the acute respiratory distress syndrome. N Engl J Med. 2000;342(18):1301–8.
81. Nahum A, Burke WC, Ravenscraft SA, Marcy TW, Adams AB, Crooke PS, et al. Lung mechanics and gas exchange during pressure-control ventilation in dogs. Augmentation of CO_2 elimination by an intratracheal catheter. Am Rev Respir Dis. 1992;146(4):965–73.
82. Bonmarchand G, Chevron V, Chopin C, Jusserand D, Girault C, Moritz F, et al. Increased initial flow rate reduces inspiratory work of breathing during pressure support ventilation in patients with exacerbation of chronic obstructive pulmonary disease. Intensive Care Med. 1996;22(11):1147–54.
83. Bonmarchand G, Chevron V, Ménard JF, Girault C, Moritz-Berthelot F, Pasquis P, et al. Effects of pressure ramp slope values on the work of breathing during pressure support ventilation in restrictive patients. Crit Care Med. 1999;27(4):715–22.
84. Chiumello D, Pelosi P, Taccone P, Slutsky A, Gattinoni L. Effect of different inspiratory rise time and cycling off criteria during pressure support ventilation in patients recovering from acute lung injury. Crit Care Med. 2003;31(11):2604–10.
85. Dreyfuss D, Soler P, Basset G, Saumon G. High inflation pressure pulmonary edema. Respective effects of high airway pressure, high tidal volume, and positive end-expiratory pressure. Am Rev Respir Dis. 1988;137(5):1159–64.
86. MacIntyre NR. Respiratory function during pressure support ventilation. Chest. 1986;89(5):677–83.

87. Brochard L, Pluskwa F, Lemaire F. Improved efficacy of spontaneous breathing with inspiratory pressure support. Am Rev Respir Dis. 1987;136(2):411–5.
88. Aslanian P, El Atrous S, Isabey D, Valente E, Corsi D, Harf A, et al. Effects of flow triggering on breathing effort during partial ventilatory support. Am J Respir Crit Care Med. 1998;157(1):135–43.
89. Brochard L, Harf A, Lorino H, Lemaire F. Inspiratory pressure support prevents diaphragmatic fatigue during weaning from mechanical ventilation. Am Rev Respir Dis. 1989;139(2):513–21.
90. Tokioka H, Saito S, Kosaka F. Effect of pressure support ventilation on breathing patterns and respiratory work. Intensive Care Med. 1989;15(8):491–4.
91. Van de Graaff WB, Gordey K, Dornseif SE, Dries DJ, Kleinman BS, Kumar P, et al. Pressure support. Changes in ventilatory pattern and components of the work of breathing. Chest. 1991;100(4):1082–9.
92. MacIntyre NR. Weaning from mechanical ventilatory support: volume-assisting intermittent breaths versus pressure-assisting every breath. Respir Care. 1988;33(2):121–5.
93. Jubran A, Van De Graaff WB, Tobin MJ. Variability of patient-ventilator interaction with pressure support ventilation in patients with chronic obstructive pulmonary disease. Am J Respir Crit Care Med. 1995;152(1):129–36.
94. Giannouli E, Webster K, Roberts D, Younes M. Response of ventilator-dependent patients to different levels of pressure support and proportional assist. Am J Respir Crit Care Med. 1999;159(6):1716–25.
95. Leung P, Jubran A, Tobin MJ. Comparison of assisted ventilator modes on triggering, patient effort, and dyspnea. Am J Respir Crit Care Med. 1997;155(6):1940–8.
96. Chiumello D, Pelosi P, Croci M, Bigatello LM, Gattinoni L. The effects of pressurization rate on breathing pattern, work of breathing, gas exchange and patient comfort in pressure support ventilation. Eur Respir J. 2001;18(1):107–14.
97. MacIntyre NR, Ho LI. Effects of initial flow rate and breath termination criteria on pressure support ventilation. Chest. 1991;99(1):134–8.
98. Sassoon CS, Zhu E, Caiozzo VJ. Assist-control mechanical ventilation attenuates ventilator-induced diaphragmatic dysfunction. Am J Respir Crit Care Med. 2004;170(6):626–32.
99. Esteban A, Anzueto A, Frutos F, Alía I, Brochard L, Stewart TE, et al. Characteristics and outcomes in adult patients receiving mechanical ventilation: a 28-day international study. JAMA. 2002;287(3):345–55.
100. Dojat M, Brochard L, Lemaire F, Harf A. A knowledge-based system for assisted ventilation of patients in intensive care units. Int J Clin Monit Comput. 1992;9(4):239–50.
101. Dojat M, Harf A, Touchard D, Laforest M, Lemaire F, Brochard L. Evaluation of a knowledge-based system providing ventilatory management and decision for extubation. Am J Respir Crit Care Med. 1996;153(3):997–1004.
102. Dojat M, Pachet F, Guessoum Z, Touchard D, Harf A, Brochard L. NéoGanesh: a working system for the automated control of assisted ventilation in ICUs. Artif Intell Med. 1997;11(2):97–117.
103. Dojat M, Harf A, Touchard D, Lemaire F, Brochard L. Clinical evaluation of a computer-controlled pressure support mode. Am J Respir Crit Care Med. 2000;161(4 Pt 1):1161–6.
104. Bouadma L, Lellouche F, Cabello B, Taillé S, Mancebo J, Dojat M, et al. Computer-driven management of prolonged mechanical ventilation and weaning: a pilot study. Intensive Care Med. 2005;31(10):1446–50.
105. Jubran A. Inspiratory flow rate: more may not be better. Crit Care Med. 1999;27(4):670–1.
106. van Dijk J, Koopman AA, de Langen LB, Dijkstra S, Burgerhof JGM, Blokpoel RGT, et al. Effect of pediatric ventilation weaning technique on work of breathing. Respir Res. 2022;23(1):184.
107. Sassoon CS, Del Rosario N, Fei R, Rheeman CH, Gruer SE, Mahutte CK. Influence of pressure- and flow-triggered synchronous intermittent mandatory ventilation on inspiratory muscle work. Crit Care Med. 1994;22(12):1933–41.

108. Giuliani R, Mascia L, Recchia F, Caracciolo A, Fiore T, Ranieri VM. Patient-ventilator interaction during synchronized intermittent mandatory ventilation. Effects of flow triggering. Am J Respir Crit Care Med. 1995;151(1):1–9.
109. Marini JJ, Smith TC, Lamb VJ. External work output and force generation during synchronized intermittent mechanical ventilation. Effect of machine assistance on breathing effort. Am Rev Respir Dis. 1988;138(5):1169–79.
110. Imsand C, Feihl F, Perret C, Fitting JW. Regulation of inspiratory neuromuscular output during synchronized intermittent mechanical ventilation. Anesthesiology. 1994;80(1):13–22.
111. Uchiyama A, Imanaka H, Taenaka N, Nakano S, Fujino Y, Yoshiya I. Comparative evaluation of diaphragmatic activity during pressure support ventilation and intermittent mandatory ventilation in animal model. Am J Respir Crit Care Med. 1994;150(6 Pt 1):1564–8.
112. Brochard L, Rauss A, Benito S, Conti G, Mancebo J, Rekik N, et al. Comparison of three methods of gradual withdrawal from ventilatory support during weaning from mechanical ventilation. Am J Respir Crit Care Med. 1994;150(4):896–903.
113. Esteban A, Frutos F, Tobin MJ, Alía I, Solsona JF, Valverdú I, et al. A comparison of four methods of weaning patients from mechanical ventilation. Spanish Lung Failure Collaborative Group. N Engl J Med. 1995;332(6):345–50.
114. Kıhtır HS, Akçay N, Şevketoğlu E. Pressure-regulated volume control and pressure-control ventilation modes in pediatric acute respiratory failure. Turk J Anaesthesiol Reanim. 2022;50(1):18–23.
115. Kocis KC, Dekeon MK, Rosen HK, Bandy KP, Crowley DC, Bove EL, et al. Pressure-regulated volume control vs volume control ventilation in infants after surgery for congenital heart disease. Pediatr Cardiol. 2001;22(3):233–7.
116. Sward KA, Newth CJL, Khemani RG, Page K, Meert KL, Carcillo JA, et al. Potential acceptability of a pediatric ventilator management computer protocol. Pediatr Crit Care Med. 2017;18(11):1027–34.
117. Newth CJL, Sward KA, Khemani RG, Page K, Meert KL, Carcillo JA, et al. Variability in usual care mechanical ventilation for pediatric acute respiratory distress syndrome: time for a decision support protocol? Pediatr Crit Care Med. 2017;18(11):e521–e9.
118. Sinderby C, Navalesi P, Beck J, Skrobik Y, Comtois N, Friberg S, et al. Neural control of mechanical ventilation in respiratory failure. Nat Med. 1999;5(12):1433–6.
119. Sinderby C, Beck J, Spahija J, de Marchie M, Lacroix J, Navalesi P, et al. Inspiratory muscle unloading by neurally adjusted ventilatory assist during maximal inspiratory efforts in healthy subjects. Chest. 2007;131(3):711–7.
120. Sinderby C, Beck J. Proportional assist ventilation and neurally adjusted ventilatory assist—better approaches to patient ventilator synchrony? Clin Chest Med. 2008;29(2):329–42.
121. Xiao S, Huang C, Cheng Y, Xia Z, Li Y, Tang W, et al. Application of neurally adjusted ventilatory assist in ventilator weaning of infants ventilator weaning. Brain Behav. 2021;11(10):e2350.
122. Karikari S, Rausa J, Flores S, Loomba RS. Neurally adjusted ventilatory assist versus conventional ventilation in the pediatric population: are there benefits? Pediatr Pulmonol. 2019;54(9):1374–81.
123. Bengtsson JA, Edberg KE. Neurally adjusted ventilatory assist in children: an observational study. Pediatr Crit Care Med. 2010;11(2):253–7.
124. Breatnach C, Conlon NP, Stack M, Healy M, O'Hare BP. A prospective crossover comparison of neurally adjusted ventilatory assist and pressure-support ventilation in a pediatric and neonatal intensive care unit population. Pediatr Crit Care Med. 2010;11(1):7–11.
125. Bordessoule A, Emeriaud G, Morneau S, Jouvet P, Beck J. Neurally adjusted ventilatory assist improves patient–ventilator interaction in infants as compared with conventional ventilation. Pediatr Res. 2012;72(2):194–202.
126. Alander M, Peltoniemi O, Pokka T, Kontiokari T. Comparison of pressure-, flow-, and NAVA-triggering in pediatric and neonatal ventilatory care. Pediatr Pulmonol. 2012;47(1):76–83.

127. de la Oliva P, Schüffelmann C, Gómez-Zamora A, Villar J, Kacmarek RM. Asynchrony, neural drive, ventilatory variability and COMFORT: NAVA versus pressure support in pediatric patients. A non-randomized cross-over trial. Intensive Care Med. 2012;38(5):838–46.
128. Piastra M, De Luca D, Costa R, Pizza A, De Sanctis R, Marzano L, et al. Neurally adjusted ventilatory assist vs pressure support ventilation in infants recovering from severe acute respiratory distress syndrome: nested study. J Crit Care. 2014;29(2):312.e1–5.
129. Kallio M, Peltoniemi O, Anttila E, Pokka T, Kontiokari T. Neurally adjusted ventilatory assist (NAVA) in pediatric intensive care—a randomized controlled trial. Pediatr Pulmonol. 2015;50(1):55–62.
130. Clement KC, Thurman TL, Holt SJ, Heulitt MJ. Neurally triggered breaths reduce trigger delay and improve ventilator response times in ventilated infants with bronchiolitis. Intensive Care Med. 2011;37(11):1826–32.
131. Crulli B, Khebir M, Toledano B, Vobecky S, Poirier N, Emeriaud G. Neurally adjusted ventilatory assist after pediatric cardiac surgery: clinical experience and impact on ventilation pressures. Respir Care. 2018;63(2):208–14.
132. Baez Hernandez N, Milad A, Li Y, Van Bergen AH. Utilization of Neurally Adjusted Ventilatory Assist (NAVA) mode in infants and children undergoing congenital heart surgery: a retrospective review. Pediatr Cardiol. 2019;40(3):563–9.
133. Assy J, Mauriat P, Tafer N, Soulier S, El Rassi I. Neurally adjusted ventilatory assist for children on veno-venous ECMO. J Artif Organs. 2019;22(2):118–25.
134. Shetty S, Evans K, Cornuaud P, Kulkarni A, Duffy D, Greenough A. Neurally adjusted ventilatory assist in very prematurely born infants with evolving/established bronchopulmonary dysplasia. AJP Rep. 2021;11(4):e127–e31.
135. Ranieri VM, Giuliani R, Mascia L, Grasso S, Petruzzelli V, Puntillo N, et al. Patient-ventilator interaction during acute hypercapnia: pressure-support vs. proportional-assist ventilation. J Appl Physiol (1985). 1996;81(1):426–36.
136. Younes M, Kun J, Masiowski B, Webster K, Roberts D. A method for noninvasive determination of inspiratory resistance during proportional assist ventilation. Am J Respir Crit Care Med. 2001;163(4):829–39.
137. Younes M, Webster K, Kun J, Roberts D, Masiowski B. A method for measuring passive elastance during proportional assist ventilation. Am J Respir Crit Care Med. 2001;164(1):50–60.
138. Kondili E, Prinianakis G, Alexopoulou C, Vakouti E, Klimathianaki M, Georgopoulos D. Respiratory load compensation during mechanical ventilation—proportional assist ventilation with load-adjustable gain factors versus pressure support. Intensive Care Med. 2006;32(5):692–9.
139. Hunt KA, Dassios T, Greenough A. Proportional assist ventilation (PAV) versus Neurally Adjusted Ventilator Assist (NAVA): effect on oxygenation in infants with evolving or established bronchopulmonary dysplasia. Eur J Pediatr. 2020;179(6):901–8.
140. Tirupakuzhi Vijayaraghavan BK, Hamed S, Jain A, Chimunda T, Telias I, Friedrich JO, et al. Evidence supporting clinical use of proportional assist ventilation: a systematic review and meta-analysis of clinical trials. J Intensive Care Med. 2020;35(7):627–35.
141. Marini JJ, Ravenscraft SA. Mean airway pressure: physiologic determinants and clinical importance—Part 2: Clinical implications. Crit Care Med. 1992;20(11):1604–16.
142. Lalgudi Ganesan S. Airway pressure release ventilation in children. Curr Opin Crit Care. 2019;25(1):63–70.
143. Yener N, Üdürgücü M. Airway pressure release ventilation as a rescue therapy in pediatric acute respiratory distress syndrome. Indian J Pediatr. 2020;87(11):905–9.
144. Schultz TR, Costarino ATJRAT, Durning SM, Napoli LA, Schears G, Godinez RI, et al. Airway pressure release ventilation in pediatrics. Pediatr Crit Care Med. 2001;2(3):243–6.
145. Lalgudi Ganesan S, Jayashree M, Chandra Singhi S, Bansal A. Airway pressure release ventilation in pediatric acute respiratory distress syndrome. A randomized controlled trial. Am J Respir Crit Care Med. 2018;198(9):1199–207.

146. Iosifidis E, Pitsava G, Roilides E. Ventilator-associated pneumonia in neonates and children: a systematic analysis of diagnostic methods and prevention. Future Microbiol. 2018;13:1431–46.
147. Klompas M, Branson R, Eichenwald EC, Greene LR, Howell MD, Lee G, et al. Strategies to prevent ventilator-associated pneumonia in acute care hospitals: 2014 update. Infect Control Hosp Epidemiol. 2014;35(Suppl 2):S133–54.
148. Chang I, Schibler A. Ventilator associated pneumonia in children. Paediatr Respir Rev. 2016;20:10–6.
149. Modi AR, Kovacs CS. Hospital-acquired and ventilator-associated pneumonia: diagnosis, management, and prevention. Cleve Clin J Med. 2020;87(10):633–9.
150. Vijay G, Mandal A, Sankar J, Kapil A, Lodha R, Kabra SK. Ventilator associated pneumonia in pediatric intensive care unit: incidence, risk factors and etiological agents. Indian J Pediatr. 2018;85(10):861–6.
151. de Neef M, Bakker L, Dijkstra S, Raymakers-Janssen P, Vileito A, Ista E. Effectiveness of a ventilator care bundle to prevent ventilator-associated pneumonia at the PICU: a systematic review and meta-analysis. Pediatr Crit Care Med. 2019;20(5):474–80.
152. Hatachi T, Tachibana K, Takeuchi M. Incidences and influences of device-associated healthcare-associated infections in a pediatric intensive care unit in Japan: a retrospective surveillance study. J Intensive Care. 2015;3:44.
153. Wójkowska-Mach J, Merritt TA, Borszewska-Kornacka M, Domańska J, Gulczyńska E, Nowiczewski M, et al. Device-associated pneumonia of very low birth weight infants in polish neonatal intensive care units. Adv Med Sci. 2016;61(1):90–5.
154. Safdar N, Crnich CJ, Maki DG. The pathogenesis of ventilator-associated pneumonia: its relevance to developing effective strategies for prevention. Respir Care. 2005;50(6):725–39. discussion 39–41.
155. Almuneef M, Memish ZA, Balkhy HH, Alalem H, Abutaleb A. Ventilator-associated pneumonia in a pediatric intensive care unit in Saudi Arabia: a 30-month prospective surveillance. Infect Control Hosp Epidemiol. 2004;25(9):753–8.
156. Barzilay Z, Mandel M, Keren G, Davidson S. Nosocomial bacterial pneumonia in ventilated children: clinical significance of culture-positive peripheral bronchial aspirates. J Pediatr. 1988;112(3):421–4.
157. Elward AM, Warren DK, Fraser VJ. Ventilator-associated pneumonia in pediatric intensive care unit patients: risk factors and outcomes. Pediatrics. 2002;109(5):758–64.
158. Antalová N, Klučka J, Říhová M, Poláčková S, Pokorná A, Štourač P. Ventilator-associated pneumonia prevention in pediatric patients: narrative review. Children (Basel). 2022;9(10):1540.
159. Klompas M, Branson R, Cawcutt K, Crist M, Eichenwald EC, Greene LR, et al. Strategies to prevent ventilator-associated pneumonia, ventilator-associated events, and nonventilator hospital-acquired pneumonia in acute-care hospitals: 2022 update. Infect Control Hosp Epidemiol. 2022;43(6):687–713.
160. Foglia E, Meier MD, Elward A. Ventilator-associated pneumonia in neonatal and pediatric intensive care unit patients. Clin Microbiol Rev. 2007;20(3):409–25.
161. Iosifidis E, Chochliourou E, Violaki A, Chorafa E, Psachna S, Roumpou A, et al. Evaluation of the new centers for disease control and prevention ventilator-associated event module and criteria in critically ill children in Greece. Infect Control Hosp Epidemiol. 2016;37(10):1162–6.
162. Chongcharoenyanon T, Samransamruajkit R, Sophonphan J. Epidemiology, risk factors and outcomes of prolonged mechanical ventilation with different cut-points in a PICU. Front Pediatr. 2023;11:1167595.

Others (Sedation, Hemodynamics, Nutrition, Infection)

Sin Wee Loh, Chengsi Ong, and Jan Hau Lee

1 Analgesia and Sedation

Analgesia and sedation are integral components of critical care management. In children on prolonged mechanical ventilation (PMV), the goals of sedation shift as they transit from hospital to community-based care. In the acute hospital setting, analgesia and sedation are used to reduce discomfort inflicted by noxious stimuli, facilitate invasive procedures, and reduce metabolic demands in critically ill children. However, the goals of analgesia and sedation are much more varied in the home setting. This section discusses the principles of management of analgesia and sedation for a child on PMV transiting from acute to home setting.

S. W. Loh (✉)
Children's Intensive Care Unit, Department of Pediatric Subspecialties, KK Women's and Children's Hospital, Singapore, Singapore
e-mail: loh.sin.wee@singhealth.com.sg

C. Ong
Department of Nutrition & Dietetics, KK Women's and Children's Hospital, Singapore, Singapore

J. H. Lee
Children's Intensive Care Unit, Department of Pediatric Subspecialties, KK Women's and Children's Hospital, Singapore, Singapore

Duke-NUS Medical School, Singapore, Singapore

A. Kawaguchi et al. (eds.), *Prolonged and Long-Term Mechanical Ventilation in Children*, https://doi.org/10.1007/978-981-97-8903-0_7

1.1 Acute Hospital Setting

Most children on PMV would have had prolonged exposure to analgesics and sedatives in the hospital. This predisposes them to a vicious cycle of tolerance, dependence, iatrogenic withdrawal syndrome, and delirium. Therefore, weaning of analgesics and sedatives should begin as soon as the patient no longer requires them to maintain clinical stability or if oversedation is suspected.

There is no consensus to guide the use of analgesia and sedation in children on PMV. In preparation for home, four important considerations during the weaning phase of analgesia and sedation in this group of patients are as follows:

- Regular pain- and sedation-related monitoring using validated scales: validated scales should be used to evaluate the level of analgesia, sedation, presence of withdrawal symptoms, and delirium on a regular basis. The dose of medications should be titrated or weaned to achieve the target level of analgesia and sedation needed to facilitate clinical activities and rehabilitation.
- Iatrogenic withdrawal syndrome (IWS) and delirium: The risk of IWS and delirium is high in children on PMV.
- Weaning strategy: A weaning strategy for gradual tapering of opioid and/or benzodiazepine is essential to prevent IWS and delirium.
- Non-pharmacological methods: Strategies to optimize environment for patient's comfort and sleep and early mobilization can positively impact patient care and decrease parental stress and anxiety level.

1.1.1 Regular Pain- and Sedation-Related Monitoring Using Validated Scales

In addition to vital signs, age-appropriate validated scales should be used to assess pain and depth of sedation on a daily basis. Pain assessment varies with developmental age, patient's comorbidities, and presence of neurodevelopmental delay. These factors affect the child's ability to express and communicate pain and discomfort. The level of analgesia and sedation required in children on PMV is dependent on the type of respiratory support. A patient on MV via tracheostomy should not require regular analgesia and sedation after the first week of tracheostomy creation compared to a patient on MV via endotracheal tube. Likewise, analgesia and sedation are usually not required in a patient on prolonged noninvasive ventilation. All patients on PMV should be assigned a target depth of analgesia and sedation needed for clinical activities and rehabilitation to allow titration and weaning of medications to take place. Some examples of validated scales for analgesia and sedation are listed below:

Validated scales for analgesia [1]:

- Behavioral/observational scales for noncommunicative patients: Face, Legs Activity, Cry, and Consolability (FLACC) or COMFORT-Behavior (COMFORT-B).
- Self-report scales for patients who are able to communicate: Visual Analog Scale (VAS), Numeric Rating Scale, Oucher Scale, or Wong-Baker Faces Pain Scale.

Validated scales for sedation [1]:

- COMFORT-B Scale or the State Behavioral Scale (SBS).

1.1.2 Iatrogenic Withdrawal Syndrome and Delirium

Iatrogenic Withdrawal Syndrome

IWS is a clinical constellation of symptoms that manifest after discontinuation of analgesics and sedatives. It frequently occurs in children who have received opioids or benzodiazepines for more than 3 days and may take up to 48–72 h to manifest. Signs and symptoms of IWS are often nonspecific. They manifest in a constellation of autonomic dysfunction (tachypnea, tachycardia, hyperpyrexia, and diaphoresis), CNS irritability (agitation, jitteriness, seizures, hallucinations, and delirium), and gastrointestinal dysfunction (vomiting and diarrhea).

Risk factors for the development of IWS from opioids and/or benzodiazepines include duration and cumulative dose, use of multiple opioids and sedatives, less than 6 years of age, preexisting cognitive or functional impairment, and CNS disorders [1]. Many of these risk factors frequently exist in children on PMV, putting them at higher risk of IWS.

Screening tools have been developed and validated for the assessment of IWS in children but are unable to accurately differentiate between opioid and benzodiazepine. The use of screening tools during the weaning phase allows for consistency and standardization of diagnosis. These tools include:

- Withdrawal Assessment Tool version 1 (WAT-1): 12-point numerical scale. Scores $\geq$3 are consistent with IWS [2].
- Sophia Observation withdrawal Symptoms-scale (SOS): 15-item scale. Scores $\geq$4 are consistent with IWS [3].

The pharmacological and non-pharmacological management of IWS will be elaborated in the later sections.

1.1.3 Delirium

Delirium is a syndrome of acute brain dysfunction characterized by features of inattention and unawareness, with possible secondary changes in cognition. It can present in forms of hypoactive, hyperactive, or mixed delirium. Some of the risk factors for delirium in critically ill children include younger age, developmental delay, benzodiazepine exposure, deep sedation, use of physical restraints, patient's immobilization, and requirement for MV [4]. Many of these risk factors frequently exist in children on PMV, which puts them at high risk of delirium.

All patients admitted to PICU should be screened for delirium. Examples of validated screening tools for delirium in critically ill children are the following:

- Cornell Assessment of Pediatric Delirium (CAPD) [5]: Observational tools for 0–21 years of age. In a developmentally normal child, a CAPD score of ≥9 has good sensitivity and specificity for delirium. In a child with developmental delay, CAPD ≥9 and the presence of fluctuating SBS scores of ≥2 points in the last 24 h are suggestive of delirium.
- Pediatric Confusion Assessment Method for the ICU (pCAM-ICU) or Preschool Confusion Assessment Method for the ICU (psCAM-ICU) [6]: These are "point in time" assessments that use observational and interactive components to detect PICU delirium.

The management of ICU delirium is beyond the scope of this chapter. We refer you to excellent review articles on the management of ICU delirium [1, 4].

1.1.4 Weaning Strategies and Management of IWS

There is no universal guideline for weaning of opioid and benzodiazepine in PICU. Although practices vary across institutions, the principles of weaning are similar. Children on PMV are at high risk of IWS and will need to be monitored with appropriate validated tools. Figure 1 shows an example of a weaning strategy based on withdrawal risk and management of IWS [7, 8]. Rate of weaning should be individualised based on the risk of IWS. Once enteral feeds are tolerated, intravenous (IV) analgesia and sedation should be converted to oral agents. Table 1 shows conversion formulas of analgesics and sedatives from parenteral to oral form [7]. As IWS might occur in the later stage of weaning or even at home, it is important that the caregivers be educated on the signs and symptoms of withdrawal.

1.1.5 Non-pharmacological Interventions

The high stress and fast-paced environment of the PICU have many negative influences on patient's management and recovery from critical illness. Family-centered care and optimization of the PICU environment have been shown to be effective in the management of IWS and reduction of delirium. They are also important components of the ICU Liberation Initiative to reduce post-intensive care syndrome in pediatrics [9, 10]. Non-pharmacological measures should be implemented as part of routine care in PICU and should also be used as first-line interventions for IWS and ICU delirium. Some of these measures can be extended into the home setting.

These measures include the following:

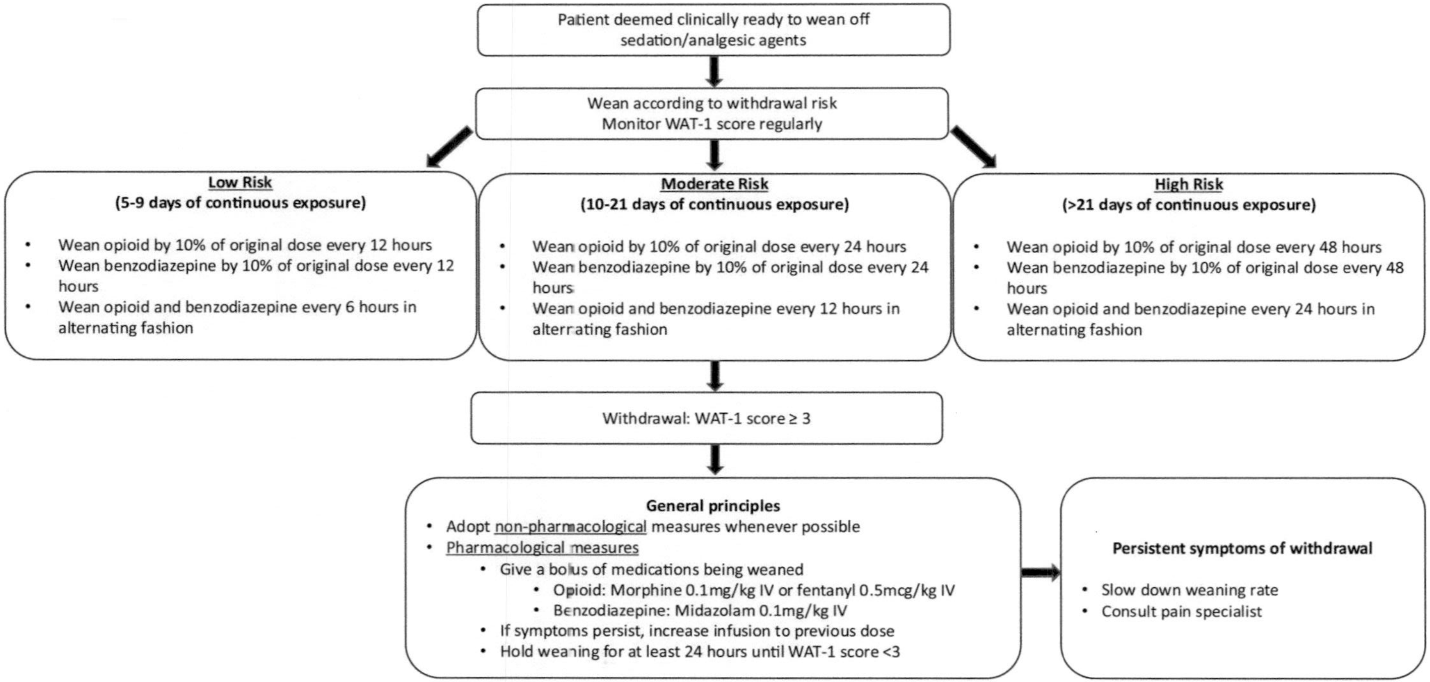

Fig. 1 Weaning strategy and management of IWS [7, 8]

Table 1 Conversion formulas of analgesics and sedatives from parenteral to oral form

Conversion formulas of opioid and benzodiazepine from intravenous (IV) to oral (PO)		
IV agent	**PO agent**	**Formula**
Morphine	Morphine	__mg/24 h IV morphine x 3 = __mg/24 h PO morphine (divide into Q4H dosing)
Fentanyl	Morphine	__mcg/24 h IV fentanyl x 0.1 = __mg/24 h PO morphine (divide into Q4H dosing)
Midazolam	Lorazepam	__mg/24 h IV midazolam x 0.1 = __mg/24 h PO lorazepam (divide into Q6H dosing)

Transitioning of IV to PO opioid/benzodiazepine
Start PO agent at calculated dose.
Wean IV infusion by 50% 30 min after the second PO dose.
Turn IV infusion off 30 min after the third PO dose.

Weaning of PO agent
Continue to wean PO agent as per IV weaning rate (based on the risk of withdrawal).
Once minimum enteral dose is reached, wean frequency of dosing every 24 h:
- Minimum PO morphine dose: 0.1 mg/kg/dose.
  - Q4H > Q6H > Q8H Q12H > Q24H > stop.
- Minimum PO lorazepam dose: 0.02 mg/kg/dose.
  - Q6H > Q8H > Q12H > Q24H > stop.

- Optimize the environment by reducing light, noise, and screen time, especially at night.
- Integration of good sleep hygiene by ensuring wakefulness, promoting physical activity, and minimizing naps during the day.
- Family-centered care by empowering families to be part of the decision-making process for the patient's daily care.
- Early mobilization targeting the highest level of mobility that can be safely achieved.
- Music, play, or distraction therapy.
- Nonnutritive sucking with oral sucrose for neonates and infants.

1.2 Home Setting

Children on PMV often do not require regular analgesia or sedation in the home setting. However, practitioners need to be particularly mindful of two subgroups of patients:

- Patients at risk of IWS who are discharged on weaning doses of oral analgesics and sedatives *(refer to sections on IWS and weaning strategies).*
- Patients with dystonia secondary to central nervous system (CNS) disorders (e.g., cerebral palsy, CNS injury, neuromuscular disorder, neurometabolic conditions).

The use of sedation in children on PMV has to be carefully balanced with its potential adverse effects on respiratory function and upper airway obstruction. This is especially relevant with the increased awareness of sleep disorders in this group of patients (*refer to the section on sleep disorder*).

1.2.1 Dystonia

Children with CNS disorders form a significant proportion of those requiring PMV. Dystonia is characterized by abnormal repetitive movements and/or postures due to intermittent muscle contractions and is prevalent in children with CNS disorders, especially dyskinetic cerebral palsy [11]. Uncontrolled dystonia causes diaphragmatic dysfunction and potentially patient-ventilator desynchrony in a child on PMV [12].

Clonidine is a centrally acting alpha-2 agonist used as one of the second-line medications for dystonia, after trihexyphenidyl (a centrally acting anticholinergic agent) and baclofen (a GABA-agonist). It exhibits sedative effect and, to a lesser extent, also acts as a dose-dependent analgesia. Clonidine has been shown to be an effective treatment for dystonia without major adverse effects [13, 14]. Recommended starting dose is 1 mcg/kg/dose three times per day [14].

2 Nutrition

Nutrition provision in children on PMV can be challenging, due to variability in factors determining nutritional requirements: underlying medical condition, respiratory function, body composition, and physical ability [15, 16]. A singular approach to nutritional provision can result in both under- and overfeeding these children [17]. As such, nutrition provision needs to be individualized to avoid inappropriate growth and weight gain, as well as to optimize respiratory function [18].

2.1 Nutritional Assessment

Nutritional assessment is central to the provision of nutrition in children receiving MV, and a comprehensive baseline nutrition assessment should be conducted upon hospital admission or onset of MV. These constitute basic anthropometry measurements of weight and length. Weights should be paired with length measurements to screen or prevent excessive weight for length status. In hospitalized children, serial measurements should be conducted throughout their stay, although the optimal frequency depends on many factors and should be individualized to the patient's needs [19]. A common frequency of measurement is once a week in hospitalized children [20, 21]. Patients on home MV should also have their weight and length assessed regularly, although the frequency of monitoring is likely to vary depending on the chronicity of the patient and adjustment of feeds.

While weight is the most commonly monitored anthropometrical measurement, it has been regarded as an inaccurate indicator of nutritional status due to confounding by fluid shifts that are common in critical illness [22]. In addition, weight is unable to detect changes in body composition [23]. Inclusion of body composition stores has thus been recommended to complement weight and length measurements [19]. Subjective assessments of body composition include physical examination of muscle and fat stores at various parts of the body including the temple, clavicular, scapular, and limbs [24]. However, small changes in muscle and fat stores can be difficult to detect without objective assessment tools. Bedside objective assessment tools include the mid-upper arm circumference (MUAC) and triceps skinfold (TSF) thickness [19, 25, 26]. MUAC and TSF are most often used together to determine muscle and fat stores of a child, which can be compared to normative values for age to assess baseline nutritional status or be monitored longitudinally to guide nutritional provision [25–27].

2.2 *Nutrition Provision*

2.2.1 Route of Feeding

Children on PMV obtain nutritional intake via several different routes. In a study cohort of 96 children receiving PMV, 50 children (52%) were able to feed orally, although this percentage was significantly lower in those requiring invasive MV compared to those requiring noninvasive MV (28% vs. 61%) [16]. In a smaller group of 20 children enrolled in a home ventilation program, 10% were reported to be feeding orally, 10% were on a combination of oral and tube feeding, while the remainder were on full tube feeding [25]. Concerns for oral feeding in children requiring PMV include swallowing dysfunction and aspiration risk attributed to positive-pressure ventilation, in addition to preexisting dysphagia related to underlying medical conditions (e.g., neurological and neuromuscular conditions) [28]. A feeding assessment should be conducted by a feeding specialist or speech therapist to determine if oral feeding is safe. In addition, the child's oral nutritional intake must be monitored closely by a nutrition professional to determine if they are able to obtain adequate oral intake. Often, caloric dense nutritional supplements and fortification of food are required to achieve this [29].

For those with feeding dysfunction and unable to meet their nutritional requirements orally, nutrition support in the form of nasogastric, nasojejunal, or gastrostomy feeding would be required. Typically, gastric feeding is well tolerated, although the delivery of high positive pressures can increase the risk of gastroesophageal reflux and feeding intolerance [30–32]. In children with persistent feed intolerance, nasojejunal feeds may be required to deliver adequate nutrition.

2.2.2 Macronutrients

One of the goals of energy provision in children with PMV is to maintain appropriate weight for length. As such, appropriate energy provision is important, as even a small degree of daily nutrition provision below or above requirements could accumulate to a large nutritional surplus or deficit over time.

Energy underfeeding can occur due to increased respiratory effort in a child, leading to increase in overall energy requirements. Conversely, energy overfeeding has been observed, particularly in neurologically impaired children requiring PMV. Overfeeding is detrimental as it could result in excess weight without corresponding increases in length [18], making it difficult for caregivers to carry and transfer the child. Overfeeding could also result in excessive carbon dioxide production, thus increasing the oxygen requirements for the child [33].

Most energy requirements have been estimated using energy equations from a child's weight and height. Commonly used equations include the Schofield or the World Health Organization equations [34, 35]. These energy equations should only be used as a starting point, and energy provision should be adjusted based on physical activity, respiratory effort, and other factors, along with longitudinal monitoring of nutritional status. In children with neurological impairment, nutrition provision below their estimated basal metabolic rate may be required to prevent excessive weight gain [36].

While energy estimation equations are widely used in the pediatric population, one criticism is the inaccuracy of estimating requirements. Studies in mechanically ventilated children have shown that energy estimation equations can result in over- or underfeeding of up to 120% depending on the equation used [37–39]. The incidence of over- or underfeeding in children requiring PMV has been reported to be 25% and 44%, respectively. Overfeeding is associated with increased risk of cholestasis and prolonged ventilation, and underfeeding is associated with increased risk of infections and a loss of lean body mass [40, 41]. Both should thus be avoided in children requiring PMV.

Due to the limitations of energy estimation equations, indirect calorimetry is recognized as the gold standard in determining energy requirements. Indirect calorimetry utilizes measurement of inspired oxygen and expired carbon dioxide volumes to calculate energy expenditure based on the modified Weir equation [42]. A study of 16 children requiring home MV demonstrated that an individualized nutrition assessment using indirect calorimetry improved lean body mass [25].

Aside from total energy intake, appropriate protein provision is also important to maintain optimal muscle stores in children requiring PMV. Although the ideal protein provision in these children is unclear, the prior mentioned study demonstrated that protein provision according to recommendations by the American Society for Parenteral And Enteral Nutrition (ASPEN) increased lean body mass in children with PMV [25, 43] (Table 2).

Table 2 Suggested starting macronutrient and fluid requirements in children on PMV

Nutrient	Name	Formula	
Energy	Schofield	0–3 years	Male: (0.167 x W) + (1517.4 x H) – 617.6 Female: (16.252 x W) + (1023.3 x H) – 413.5
		3–10 years	Male: (19.59 x W) + (130.3 x H) + 414.9 Female: (16.97 x W) + (161.8 x H) + 371.2
		10–18 years	Male: (16.25 x W) + (137.2 x H) + 515.5 Female: (8.365 x W) + (465.6 x H) + 200
	WHO	0–3 years	Male: (60.9 x W) – 54 Female: (61 x W) – 51
		3–10 years	Male: (22.7 x W) + 495 Female: (22.5 x W) + 499
		10–18 years	Male: (17.5 x W) + 651 Female: (12.2 x W) + 746
Protein	ASPEN	0–2 years: 2–3 g/kg/day 2–13 years: 1.5–2 g/kg/day 13–18 years: 1.5 g/kg/day	
Fluid	Holliday-Segar	100 ml per kg body weight for the first 10 kg, 50 ml per kg body weight for the next 10 kg, then 20 ml per kg body weight for additional body weight	

W weight in kilograms, *H* height in meters, *ASPEN* American Society for Parenteral and Enteral Nutrition, *WHO* World Health Organization

2.2.3 Micronutrients

There is a paucity of research and limited understanding of micronutrient adequacy in children requiring PMV. While low nutrient levels have been reported in mechanically ventilated children, it is unclear whether additional supplementation improves outcomes, particularly during periods of acute illness [44, 45]. Thus, micronutrient target recommendations in children with PMV are typically similar to target reference values for age, although some considerations exist for certain groups of patients [44]. Children requiring hypocaloric feeds to prevent excessive weight gain may require vitamin and mineral supplementation to meet micronutrient targets if a standard polymeric formula is used [46]. In addition, the prevalence of vitamin D deficiency in neurologically impaired and bed-bound individuals is high, putting them at risk for fractures and osteopenia [47, 48]. These patients may thus require additional vitamin D supplements to maintain serum vitamin D levels within normal levels [48].

2.2.4 Fluids

Early fluid prescriptions in patients on mechanical ventilation (MV) are often conservative, as higher fluid provisions have been associated with worse outcomes, including mortality and longer ventilation requirement [49, 50]. Patients requiring MV are often kept on 80–100% of maintenance fluids, where maintenance fluids are calculated using the Holliday-Segar equation (Table 2) [50–52]. Fluid provision in excess of maintenance fluids has been associated with prolonged mechanical ventilation in PICU children [53]. In patients on PMV in the home setting, fluid provisions typically aim to meet 100% of fluid maintenance, with consideration of additional insensible losses, especially if there are frequent suctioning requirements or insufficient humidification in the ventilator circuit.

3 Hemodynamics

MV can significantly affect a patient's hemodynamics. An understanding of cardiopulmonary interaction is crucial to grasp the impact PMV have on hemodynamics. PMV has direct effects on hemodynamics by altering the preload and pulmonary vascular resistance. The degree of hemodynamic effects is also dependent on baseline lung compliance.

3.1 Cardiopulmonary Interactions in Children on PMV

MV has an unfavorable effect on the right ventricle (RV) by decreasing RV preload and possibly increasing RV afterload [54]. During MV, the intrathoracic pressure throughout the entire respiratory cycle is above atmospheric pressure, which increases right atrial pressure. This results in a decrease in systemic venous return to the right atrium (i.e., RV preload). MV also affects pulmonary vascular resistance (PVR) (i.e., RV afterload) by altering blood pH, alveolar oxygen tension, and lung volumes. For a patient on MV, both lung under- and over-distention increases PVR and hence RV afterload. Ventilating a patient at functional residual capacity is ideal as PVR is lowest at this point.

MV has a more favorable effect on the left ventricle (LV) by decreasing LV afterload, while its effects on LV preload are variable and more complex [54]. MV decreases LV afterload by decreasing transmural pressure, and therefore less gradient is needed to drive blood from the chest to systemic circulation. LV preload is dependent on RV loading conditions and ventricular interdependence. During MV, LV preload is decreased due to decreased RV stroke volume via mechanisms described in the above paragraph. The effect of ventricular interdependence is exaggerated with RV dysfunction. RV dysfunction causes RV diastolic hypertension, deviating the interventricular septum to the left with a net result of decreased LV compliance and LV preload. This phenomenon is known as "diastolic ventricular dependence." A decrease in LV compliance and preload also decreases its assistance to RV ejection, which further impairs LV filling and pressure-generating capabilities in a phenomenon known as "systolic ventricular dependence" [55]. Understanding ventricular dependence is essential in the management of pulmonary arterial hypertension associated with children on PMV.

3.2 *Lung Compliance*

Children on PMV might have heterogeneous lungs secondary to chronic lung disease, atelectasis, or recurrent infections. There is a fine balance in using an optimal positive end-expiratory pressure (PEEP) to allow for better aeration of heterogeneous lung parenchyma to ensure best ventilation/perfusion matching without overdistending the lung, which can lead to decreased stroke volume and cardiac output.

However, lung compliance changes the effects of PEEP on hemodynamics. With poorly compliant lungs, the airway pressure is not as readily transmitted to pulmonary vasculature and hence has a milder effect on hemodynamics. This correlation was seen in both premature infants with respiratory distress syndrome and children with acute respiratory distress syndrome [56, 57].

3.3 *Premature Infants*

Premature infants form the majority of patients needing PMV. This particularly vulnerable patient population is at risk of having comorbidities that will affect their hemodynamic and ventilatory management.

3.3.1 Pulmonary Hypertension

Pulmonary hypertension (PH) is a common complication of premature infants with chronic lung disease (CLD). The pathogenesis of PH is complex and multifactorial. It encompasses both prenatal factors such as impairment in vascular growth resulting in abnormal pulmonary vascular development and postnatal factors such as hypoxia, hyperoxia, and MV-induced baro- and volutrauma [58]. This results in increased RV afterload and varying degree of RV dysfunction due to increased pulmonary vascular resistance. PH can also be associated with congenital heart disease, typically left-to-right shunt defects or left-heart obstructive lesions. Common defects include ventricular septal defect (VSD), atrial septal defect (ASD), and persistent ductus arteriosus (PDA) [59].

Cardiac catheterization is considered the gold standard for assessment of PH. However, echocardiography is more widely utilized for diagnosis due to its noninvasive nature. Echocardiography markers for PH include right ventricular dilatation and hypertrophy, estimated mean pulmonary artery pressure >25 mmHg, right-to-left flow across shunt lesions, and flattening or bowing of septum to the left [60].

In children on PMV with PH, the hemodynamic effects of over-distention (i.e., decreased preload) can be exaggerated and can potentially exacerbate RV dysfunction that is already prevalent in this subgroup of patients. Systemic output can also be compromised due to the effects of ventricular interdependence on LV function and output.

Treatment of PH in children on PMV includes optimizing ventilatory management, targeting factors contributing to lung disease such as hypoxia and chronic aspiration, and addressing pulmonary edema prior to the initiation of vasodilator therapy. Congenital heart diseases such as PDA, VSD, and ASD that contribute to PH should also be surgically treated. Target oxygen saturation in this group of patients should be 92–95% as both hypoxia and hyperoxia can markedly elevate PVR by pulmonary artery vasoconstriction and airway inflammation, respectively [61]. Many pulmonary vasodilators have been utilized, but controlled trials of these agents in BPD are lacking. Sildenafil, a PDE-5 inhibitor that modulates the NO cyclic GMP signaling pathway, has the most evidence of efficacy in this population [62, 63]. Of note in children on PMV with significant lung disease and heterogeneity, sildenafil can potentially worsen V/Q mismatch, as well as increase gastroesophageal reflux symptoms. Other pharmacotherapies are bosentan, inhaled iloprost, intravenous epoprostenol, and milrinone.

3.3.2 Systemic Hypertension

Premature infants with CLD are at increased risk of systemic hypertension which affects LV afterload [64]. Pathogenesis of systemic hypertension in premature infants with CLD is unclear, but plausible causes include umbilical artery thrombosis [65] and reduced clearance of circulating norepinephrine induced by hypoxia disease as shown in animal models [66]. A cohort study (n = 40) reported that premature infants with CLD had increased aortic thickness and systemic vascular resistance compared to healthy control, which might explain higher incidence of systemic hypertension in premature infants with CLD [67]. Systemic hypertension induces LV hypertrophy and affects LV systolic and diastolic function.

Antihypertensive treatment reported to be useful in this cohort includes vasodilators such as hydralazine, angiotensin-converting enzyme inhibitors, calcium channel blockers, alpha- and beta-blockers, and spironolactone-thiazide combination [64, 68]. In children on PMV, beta-blockers should be used with caution as it can exacerbate CLD. In addition to pharmacological therapies, PPV is beneficial for LV afterload reduction for children with sequelae of LV hypertension and cardiac dysfunction.

3.3.3 Left Ventricular Diastolic Dysfunction

LV diastolic dysfunction is an increasingly recognized entity for premature infants with CLD [69]. The pathogenesis remains unclear, but plausible mechanisms include inherent poorly compliant premature myocardium exacerbated by reversible diastolic dysfunction from steroid use and sequelae of systemic hypertension [70]. LV diastolic dysfunction leads to impaired myocardium relaxation, elevated left-sided pressure, and pulmonary venous congestion.

Recognition of LV diastolic dysfunction is important in premature infants with CLD as pulmonary vasodilators used for CLD-associated PH can potentially worsen pulmonary edema and respiratory status. In children on PMV with both CLD and LV diastolic dysfunction, a combination of afterload reduction and diuretics might be needed.

4 Infections

Nosocomial infections are a leading cause of morbidity, mortality, and increased healthcare costs in PICU [71]. In addition to the array of nosocomial infections that a critically ill child is susceptible to, children on PMV are at risk for pneumonia and skin infections compared to those who are not on PMV [72]. This risk amplifies in their home environment where infection control is less stringent. In this subsection, we have focused on preventative strategies of infections in children on PMV.

4.1 Pneumonia

Children on PMV often have retained airway secretions and inadequate cough clearance, predisposing them to pneumonia and atelectasis. Respiratory muscle weakness, from underlying conditions such as neuromuscular disease or critical myopathy from PMV, is an important risk factor for pneumonia in these patients. Children on PMV via tracheostomy are also at increased risk of swallowing dysfunction and aspiration pneumonia from impaired glottic closure and loss of protective laryngeal reflexes [73]. Chronic colonization with highly resistant organisms can occur in children on PMV, especially after prolonged hospitalization [74].

4.1.1 Preventative Strategies for Pneumonia

Most of the preventative strategies for pneumonia benchmark adequate airway clearance as the therapeutic target. Lung volume recruitment (LVR) techniques are commonly used for airway clearance, especially in patients with neuromuscular disorders [75]. They include air stacking, glossopharyngeal breathing, and mechanical insufflation-exsufflation with cough assist devices. Other physiotherapy techniques include percussions and vibrations, which can help mobilize secretions from distal airways. These techniques should be taught to caregivers of children on both noninvasive and invasive PMV as a preventative strategy and intervention for acute respiratory infections [76].

Other methods of enhancing airway clearance include mucolytic agents, increasing mobility, heated humidity, and direct airway suctioning [77, 78]. In children who are ventilated through a tracheostomy, minimally invasive suctioning rather than deep suctioning is recommended as the former has been shown to be equally efficient with fewer adverse effects [79]. Consensus statements suggest that clean, as opposed to sterile, conditions are adequate for home suctioning [78, 80].

4.2 Other Infections

Infection control measures at home should be aligned as much as possible with hospital practices to reduce overall risk of infection. Children on PMV are prone to pressure injuries from respiratory support interfaces and immobility, which predispose them to skin infection [81]. Additional risk factors include low birth weight and gestational age, hemodynamic instability, and nutritional deficiency [81, 82]. Preventative strategies include choosing the right-size NIV mask for the patient's face, adjusting the cords correctly, and keeping skin beneath medical equipment clean and dry [83]. These strategies should be taught to caregivers to be continued in the home environment. More importantly, caregivers should also be taught to recognize early signs of pressure injuries and infections and to seek medical help promptly.

5 Sleep-Disordered Breathing

Sleep plays a vital role in a child's growth and development. Children on PMV are susceptible to sleep disruptions both in the hospital setting and home environment. In the hospital, sleep is often disrupted by acute illnesses, daily routine care and interventions, noise from the ICU environment, and effects of medications [84]. Specific to MV, factors such as alarms, patient-ventilator asynchrony, uncomfortable modes, and inadequate setting with under- or over-assistance can affect sleep quality [85].

There is an increasing interest in sleep-disordered breathing (SDB) in patients needing PMV. SDB encompasses a broad spectrum of ventilatory disorders, such as primary snoring, obstructive sleep apnea syndrome (OSAS), central sleep apnea (CSA), and hypoventilation syndrome (HS) [86]. Children with medical comorbidities form a big proportion of children needing PMV. These children often have alterations in neuromuscular tone, dysfunctions of the central nervous system, and abnormalities in craniofacial structures that predispose them to SDB [87]. SDB has been shown to be up to ten times more prevalent in certain subtypes of children with medical complexities (e.g., neuromuscular disease, cerebral palsy) than in healthy children [88]. The adverse effects of untreated SDB include neurocognitive deficits, growth impairment, cardiovascular complications (e.g., pulmonary hypertension and systemic hypertension), and increased healthcare resource utilization [89]. Under-recognized SDB in children on PMV limits the likelihood of successful weaning from MV and decannulation. Table 3 summarizes definition and risk factors for the different types of SDB [86, 87].

A polysomnography (PSG) is the gold standard for diagnosis of SDB. Children on PMV with risk factors of SDB should be referred to the respiratory physicians

Table 3 Types of sleep-disordered breathing

Sleep-disordered breathing	Definition	At-risk groups
OSAS	Episodes of partial or complete upper airway obstruction (hypopneas, obstructive or mixed apneas) affecting normal oxygenation, ventilation, and sleep patterns	Neuromuscular disorders. Airway abnormalities. Vocal cord dysfunction. Skeletal abnormalities. Central causes. Adenotonsillar hypertrophy. Obesity.
CSA	Prolonged pauses in respiratory effort due to absence in central respiratory drive	Congenital syndromes. Congenital central hypoventilation syndrome. Prader-Willi syndrome. Arnold-Chiari malformation. Neuromuscular disease. Acquired. CNS infection/stroke/space-occupying lesion. Spinal cord trauma. Medications.
HS	Persistent low tidal volume or bradypnea resulting in hypercarbia and hypoxemia Nocturnal HS: Transcutaneous and/or end-tidal carbon dioxide >50 mmHg for >25% total sleep time	Neuromuscular disorders. Skeletal abnormalities. Pulmonary parenchymal disorders. CLD. Cystic fibrosis. Pulmonary hypoplasia.

OSAS obstructive sleep apnea syndrome, *CSA* central sleep apnea, *HS* hypoventilation syndrome, *CNS* central nervous system, *CLD* chronic lung disease for further evaluation to optimize their outcomes. The management of SDB is beyond the scope of this chapter, and we refer the readers to excellent review articles on this topic [86, 90].

6 Conclusion

Children on PMV require optimization of their nutrition and hemodynamic status. They are also at increased risk of iatrogenic withdrawal syndrome, delirium, sepsis, and SDB. Understanding goals of supportive treatment plays an important role in the optimization of outcomes in this group of children, who are increasingly prevalent in our PICU.

References

1. Smith HAB, Besunder JB, Betters KA, Johnson PN, Srinivasan V, Stormorken A, et al. 2022 Society of Critical Care Medicine clinical practice guidelines on prevention and Management of Pain, agitation, neuromuscular blockade, and delirium in critically ill pediatric patients with consideration of the ICU environment and early mobility. Pediatr Crit Care Med. 2022;23(2):e74–e110.
2. Franck LS, Scoppettuolo LA, Wypij D, Curley MAQ. Validity and generalizability of the Withdrawal Assessment Tool-1 (WAT-1) for monitoring iatrogenic withdrawal syndrome in pediatric patients. Pain. 2012;153(1):142–8.
3. Ista E, van Dijk M, de Hoog M, Tibboel D, Duivenvoorden HJ. Construction of the Sophia observation withdrawal symptoms-scale (SOS) for critically ill children. Intensive Care Med. 2009;35(6):1075–81.
4. Smith HA, Brink E, Fuchs DC, Ely EW, Pandharipande PP. Pediatric delirium: monitoring and management in the pediatric intensive care unit. Pediatr Clin N Am. 2013;60(3):741–60.
5. Traube C, Silver G, Kearney J, Patel A, Atkinson TM, Yoon MJ, et al. Cornell assessment of pediatric delirium: a valid, rapid, observational tool for screening delirium in the PICU*. Crit Care Med. 2014;42(3):656–63.
6. Paterson RS, Kenardy JA, De Young AC, Dow BL, Long DA. Delirium in the critically ill child: assessment and Sequelae. Dev Neuropsychol. 2017;42(6):387–403.
7. PICU sedation/analgesia weaning pathway. The Children's Hospital in Philadelphia. 2019.
8. PICU sedation and analgesia weaning guideline. St George's University Hospital. 2016.
9. Manning JC, Pinto NP, Rennick JE, Colville G, Curley MAQ. Conceptualizing post intensive care syndrome in children-the PICS-p framework. Pediatr Crit Care Med. 2018;19(4):298–300.
10. Ely EW. The ABCDEF bundle: science and philosophy of how ICU liberation serves patients and families. Crit Care Med. 2017;45(2):321–30.
11. van Egmond ME, Kuiper A, Eggink H, Sinke RJ, Brouwer OF, Verschuuren-Bemelmans CC, et al. Dystonia in children and adolescents: a systematic review and a new diagnostic algorithm. J Neurol Neurosurg Psychiatry. 2015;86(7):774–81.
12. Fine-Goulden MR, Puppala NK, Durward A. Mechanisms of ventilator dependence in children with neuromuscular and respiratory control disorders identified by monitoring diaphragm electrical activity. Intensive Care Med. 2012;38(12):2072–9.
13. Saini AG, Hassan I, Sharma K, Muralidharan J, Dhawan S, Saini L, et al. Status dystonicus in children: a cross-sectional study and review of literature. J Child Neurol. 2022;37(6):441–50.

14. Sayer C, Lumsden DE, Kaminska M, Lin JP. Clonidine use in the outpatient management of severe secondary dystonia. Eur J Paediatr Neurol. 2017;21(4):621–6.
15. Pavone M, Verrillo E, Onofri A, Caggiano S, Chiarini Testa MB, Cutrera R. Characteristics and outcomes in children on long-term mechanical ventilation: the experience of a pediatric tertiary center in Rome. Ital J Pediatr. 2020;46(1):12.
16. Chau S-K, Yung AW-Y, Lee S-L. Long-term Management for Ventilator-Assisted Children in Hong Kong: 2 Decades' experience. Respir Care. 2017;62(1):54–64.
17. Martinez EE, Smallwood CD, Bechard LJ, Graham RJ, Mehta NM. Metabolic assessment and individualized nutrition in children dependent on mechanical ventilation at home. J Pediatr. 2015;166(2):350–7.
18. Tsuda T, Hehir DA, Thacker D, Lamma A, Tearl D, Gidding SS. Overfeeding and obesity in young children with positive pressure ventilation via tracheostomy following cardiac surgery. Cardiol Young. 2020;30(10):1397–404.
19. Becker P, Carney LN, Corkins MR, Monczka J, Smith E, Smith SE, et al. Consensus statement of the Academy of Nutrition and Dietetics/American Society for Parenteral and Enteral Nutrition. Nutr Clin Pract. 2015;30(1):147–61.
20. Pace A, Zobel A, Gearman L, Seitzer D, Larson-Nath C. Improving the rate of anthropometric measurements in the pediatric intensive care unit. Nutr Clin Pract. 2021;36(6):1276–83.
21. Ahearn MA, Soranno DE, Stidham T, Lusk J, Gist KM. Adherence to daily weights and total fluid orders in the pediatric intensive care unit. Pediatr Qual Saf. 2018;3(5):e110.
22. Ismael S, Savalle M, Trivin C, Gillaizeau F, D'Auzac C, Faisy C. The consequences of sudden fluid shifts on body composition in critically ill patients. Crit Care. 2014;18(2):R49.
23. Reid CL, Murgatroyd PR, Wright A, Menon DK. Quantification of lean and fat tissue repletion following critical illness: a case report. Crit Care. 2008;12(3):R79.
24. Secker DJ, Jeejeebhoy KN. Subjective global nutritional assessment for children. Am J Clin Nutr. 2007;85(4):1083–9.
25. Martinez EE, Bechard LJ, Smallwood CD, Duggan CP, Graham RJ, Mehta NM. Impact of individualized diet intervention on body composition and respiratory variables in children with respiratory insufficiency: a pilot intervention study. Pediatr Crit Care Med. 2015;16(6):e157–e64.
26. Chomtho S, Fewtrell MS, Jaffe A, Williams JE, Wells JCK. Evaluation of arm anthropometry for assessing pediatric body composition: evidence from healthy and sick children. Pediatr Res. 2006;59(6):860–5.
27. Frisancho AR. New norms of upper limb fat and muscle areas for assessment of nutritional status. Am J Clin Nutr. 1981;34(11):2540–5.
28. Amantéa SL, Piva JP, Sanches PR, Palombini BC. Oropharyngeal aspiration in pediatric patients with endotracheal intubation. Pediatr Crit Care Med. 2004;5(2):152–6.
29. Collins PF, Stratton RJ, Elia M. Nutritional support in chronic obstructive pulmonary disease: a systematic review and meta-analysis. Am J Clin Nutr. 2012;95(6):1385–95.
30. Lenihan A, Ramos V, Nemec N, Lukowski J, Lee J, Kendall KM, et al. A retrospective analysis of feeding practices and complications in patients with critical bronchiolitis on non-invasive respiratory support. Children. 2021;8(5):410.
31. Tume LN, Eveleens RD, Mayordomo-Colunga J, López J, Verbruggen S, Fricaudet M, et al. Enteral feeding of children on noninvasive respiratory support: a four-center European study. Pediatr Crit Care Med. 2021;22(3):e192–202.
32. Cantin D, Djeddi D, Carrière V, Samson N, Nault S, Jia WL, et al. Inhibitory effect of nasal intermittent positive pressure ventilation on Gastroesophageal reflux. PLoS One. 2016;11(1):e0146742.
33. Lo HC, Lin CH, Tsai LJ. Effects of hypercaloric feeding on nutrition status and carbon dioxide production in patients with long-term mechanical ventilation. JPEN J Parenter Enteral Nutr. 2005;29(5):380–7.
34. Schofield WN. Predicting basal metabolic rate, new standards and review of previous work. Hum Nutr Clin Nutr. 1985;39(Suppl 1):5–41.

35. No Authors Listed. Energy and protein requirements. Report of a joint FAO/WHO/UNU expert consultation. World Health Organ Tech Rep Ser. 1985;724:1–206.
36. García-Contreras AA, Vásquez-Garibay EM, Romero-Velarde E, Ibarra-Gutierrez AI, Troyo-Sanroman R. Energy expenditure in children with cerebral palsy and moderate/severe malnutrition during nutritional recovery. Nutr Hosp. 2015;31(5):2062–9.
37. Jotterand Chaparro C, Taffé P, Moullet C, Laure Depeyre J, Longchamp D, Perez MH, et al. Performance of predictive equations specifically developed to estimate resting energy expenditure in ventilated critically ill children. J Pediatr. 2017;184:220–6.e5.
38. Dokken M, Rustøen T, Stubhaug A. Indirect calorimetry reveals that better monitoring of nutrition therapy in pediatric intensive care is needed. JPEN J Parenter Enteral Nutr. 2015;39(3):344–52.
39. Mehta NM, Bechard LJ, Dolan M, Ariagno K, Jiang H, Duggan C. Energy imbalance and the risk of overfeeding in critically ill children. Pediatr Crit Care Med. 2011;12(4):398–405.
40. Larsen BMK, Beggs MR, Leong AY, Kang SH, Persad R, Garcia GG. Can energy intake alter clinical and hospital outcomes in PICU? Clin Nutr ESPEN. 2018;24:41–6.
41. Dark DS, Pingleton SK, Kerby GR. Hypercapnia during weaning. A complication of nutritional support. Chest. 1985;88(1):141–3.
42. Weir JBV. New methods for calculating metabolic rate with special reference to protein metabolism. J Physiol. 1949;109(1–2):1–9.
43. Mehta NM, Compher C. A.S.P.E.N. Clinical Guidelines: nutrition support of the critically ill child. JPEN J Parenter Enteral Nutr. 2009;33(3):260–76.
44. Marino LV, Valla FV, Beattie RM, Verbruggen SCAT. Micronutrient status during paediatric critical illness: a scoping review. Clin Nutr. 2020;39(12):3571–93.
45. Cvijanovich NZ, King JC, Flori HR, Gildengorin G, Vinks AA, Wong HR. Safety and dose escalation study of intravenous zinc supplementation in pediatric critical illness. J Parenter Enter Nutr. 2016;40(6):860–8.
46. Duncan B, Barton LL, Lloyd J, Marks-Katz M. Dietary considerations in osteopenia in tube-fed nonambulatory children with cerebral palsy. Clin Pediatr. 1999;38(3):133–7.
47. Narayan O, Dawaishan AA, Sinha A, Wilkinson S, Hughes A, Wright N, et al. Children on long term ventilation are prone to fragility fractures. Eur Respir J. 2020;56(suppl 64):3116.
48. Seth A, Aneja S, Singh R, Majumdar R, Sharma N, Gopinath M. Effect of impaired ambulation and anti-epileptic drug intake on vitamin D status of children with cerebral palsy. Paediatr Int Child Health. 2017;37(3):193–8.
49. Alobaidi R, Morgan C, Basu RK, Stenson E, Featherstone R, Majumdar SR, et al. Association between fluid balance and outcomes in critically ill children: a systematic review and meta-analysis. JAMA Pediatr. 2018;172(3):257–68.
50. Arrahmani I, Ingelse SA, van Woensel JBM, Bem RA, Lemson J. Current practice of fluid maintenance and replacement therapy in mechanically ventilated critically ill children: a European survey. Front Pediatr. 2022;10:828637.
51. Holliday MA, Segar WE. The maintenance need for water in parenteral fluid therapy. Pediatrics. 1957;19(5):823–32.
52. Hassinger AB, Valentine SL. Self-reported management of IV fluids and fluid accumulation in children with acute respiratory failure*. Pediatr Crit Care Med. 2018;19(10):e551–e4.
53. Barhight MF, Nelson D, Chong G, Basu RK, Sanchez-Pinto LN. Non-resuscitation fluid in excess of hydration requirements is associated with higher mortality in critically ill children. Pediatr Res. 2022;91(1):235–40.
54. Bronicki RA, Penny DJ, Anas NG, Fuhrman B. Cardiopulmonary interactions. Pediatr Crit Care Med. 2016;17(8 Suppl 1):S182–93.
55. Santamore WP, Gray L. Significant left ventricular contributions to right ventricular systolic function. Mechanism and clinical implications. Chest. 1995;107(4):1134–45.
56. de Waal K, Evans N, van der Lee J, van Kaam A. Effect of lung recruitment on pulmonary, systemic, and ductal blood flow in preterm infants. J Pediatr. 2009;154(5):651–5.

57. Virk MK, Hotz JC, Wong W, Khemani RG, Newth CJL, Ross PA. Minimal change in cardiac index with increasing PEEP in pediatric acute respiratory distress syndrome. Front Pediatr. 2019;7:9.
58. Baker CD, Abman SH, Mourani PM. Pulmonary hypertension in preterm infants with bronchopulmonary dysplasia. Pediatr Allergy Immunol Pulmonol. 2014;27(1):8–16.
59. Pascall E, Tulloh RM. Pulmonary hypertension in congenital heart disease. Futur Cardiol. 2018;14(4):343–53.
60. Krishnan U, Feinstein JA, Adatia I, Austin ED, Mullen MP, Hopper RK, et al. Evaluation and management of pulmonary hypertension in children with bronchopulmonary dysplasia. J Pediatr. 2017;188:24–34.e1.
61. Mourani PM, Ivy DD, Gao D, Abman SH. Pulmonary vascular effects of inhaled nitric oxide and oxygen tension in bronchopulmonary dysplasia. Am J Respir Crit Care Med. 2004;170(9):1006–13.
62. Mourani PM, Sontag MK, Ivy DD, Abman SH. Effects of long-term sildenafil treatment for pulmonary hypertension in infants with chronic lung disease. J Pediatr. 2009;154(3):379–84, 84.e1–2.
63. Qasim A, Dasgupta S, Aly AM, Jain SK. Sildenafil use in the treatment of bronchopulmonary dysplasia-associated pulmonary hypertension: a case series. AJP Rep. 2018;8(4):e219–e22.
64. Jenkins RD, Aziz JK, Gievers LL, Mooers HM, Fino N, Rozansky DJ. Characteristics of hypertension in premature infants with and without chronic lung disease: a long-term multicenter study. Pediatr Nephrol. 2017;32(11):2115–24.
65. Starr MC, Flynn JT. Neonatal hypertension: cases, causes, and clinical approach. Pediatr Nephrol. 2019;34(5):787–99.
66. Chappell BA, Padbury JF, Habib DM, Martinez AM, Thio SL, Burnell EE, et al. Pulmonary clearance of norepinephrine in lambs. Pediatr Res. 1991;29(1):93–7.
67. Sehgal A, Malikiwi A, Paul E, Tan K, Menahem S. Systemic arterial stiffness in infants with bronchopulmonary dysplasia: potential cause of systemic hypertension. J Perinatol. 2016;36(7):564–9.
68. Blowey DL, Duda PJ, Stokes P, Hall M. Incidence and treatment of hypertension in the neonatal intensive care unit. J Am Soc Hypertens. 2011;5(6):478–83.
69. Sehgal A, Malikiwi A, Paul E, Tan K, Menahem S. A new look at bronchopulmonary dysplasia: postcapillary pathophysiology and cardiac dysfunction. Pulm Circ. 2016;6(4):508–15.
70. Mourani PM, Ivy DD, Rosenberg AA, Fagan TE, Abman SH. Left ventricular diastolic dysfunction in bronchopulmonary dysplasia. J Pediatr. 2008;152(2):291–3.
71. Septimus EJ, Moody J. Prevention of device-related healthcare-associated infections. F1000Res. 2016;5:F1000.
72. Monteverde E, Fernández A, Poterala R, Vidal N, Siaba Serrate A, Castelani P, et al. Characterization of pediatric patients receiving prolonged mechanical ventilation. Pediatr Crit Care Med. 2011;12(6):e287–91.
73. Pullens B, Streppel M. Swallowing problems in children with a tracheostomy. Semin Pediatr Surg. 2021;30(3):151053.
74. Chawla J, Edwards EA, Griffiths AL, Nixon GM, Suresh S, Twiss J, et al. Ventilatory support at home for children: a joint position paper from the Thoracic Society of Australia and New Zealand/Australasian Sleep Association. Respirology. 2021;26(10):920–37.
75. Panitch HB. Airway clearance in children with neuromuscular weakness. Curr Opin Pediatr. 2006;18(3):277–81.
76. Lange DJ, Lechtzin N, Davey C, David W, Heiman-Patterson T, Gelinas D, et al. High-frequency chest wall oscillation in ALS: an exploratory randomized, controlled trial. Neurology. 2006;67(6):991–7.
77. Branson RD. Secretion management in the mechanically ventilated patient. Respir Care. 2007;52(10):1328–42. discussion 42–7.
78. Sherman JM, Davis S, Albamonte-Petrick S, Chatburn RL, Fitton C, Green C, et al. Care of the child with a chronic tracheostomy. This official statement of the American Thoracic

Society was adopted by the ATS Board of Directors, July 1999. Am J Respir Crit Care Med. 2000;161(1):297–308.
79. Van de Leur JP, Zwaveling JH, Loef BG, Van der Schans CP. Endotracheal suctioning versus minimally invasive airway suctioning in intubated patients: a prospective randomised controlled trial. Intensive Care Med. 2003;29(3):426–32.
80. Amin R, MacLusky I, Witmans M, Canadian Thoracic Society, et al. Pediatric home mechanical ventilation: a Canadian Thoracic Society clinical practice guideline executive summary. Can J Respir Crit Care Sleep Med. 2017;1(1):7–36.
81. Nist MD, Rodgers EA, Ruth BM, Bertoni CB, Bartman T, Keller LA, et al. Skin rounds: a quality improvement approach to enhance skin care in the Neonatal Intensive Care Unit. Adv Neonatal Care. 2016;16(Suppl 5S):S33–41.
82. Cooper KL. Evidence-based prevention of pressure ulcers in the intensive care unit. Crit Care Nurse. 2013;33(6):57–66.
83. Cullen GE. Reducing hospital acquired pressure ulcers in intensive care. BMJ Qual Improv Rep. 2015;4(1):u205599.w3015.
84. Bihari S, Doug McEvoy R, Matheson E, Kim S, Woodman RJ, Bersten AD. Factors affecting sleep quality of patients in intensive care unit. J Clin Sleep Med. 2012;8(3):301–7.
85. Rittayamai N, Wilcox E, Drouot X, Mehta S, Goffi A, Brochard L. Positive and negative effects of mechanical ventilation on sleep in the ICU: a review with clinical recommendations. Intensive Care Med. 2016;42(4):531–41.
86. Sateia MJ. International classification of sleep disorders-third edition: highlights and modifications. Chest. 2014;146(5):1387–94.
87. Chiang J, Amin R. Respiratory care considerations for children with medical complexity. Children. 2017;4(5):41.
88. Garcia J, Wical B, Wical W, Schaffer L, Wical T, Wendorf H, et al. Obstructive sleep apnea in children with cerebral palsy and epilepsy. Dev Med Child Neurol. 2016;58(10):1057–62.
89. Marcus CL, Brooks LJ, Draper KA, Gozal D, Halbower AC, Jones J, et al. Diagnosis and management of childhood obstructive sleep apnea syndrome. Pediatrics. 2012;130(3):576–84.
90. Caldarelli V, Porcaro F, Filippo PD, Attanasi M, Fainardi V, Gallucci M, et al. Long-term ventilation in children with medical complexity: a challenging issue. Children. 2022;9(11):1700.

Weaning Strategy of Mechanical Ventilation in Prolonged Mechanical Ventilation in Children

Yolanda M. López-Fernández and Analía Fernández

Abbreviations

ASV	Adaptive support ventilation
ATC	Automatic tube compensation
BiPAP	Bilevel positive airway pressure
CPAP	Continuous positive airway pressure
CPG	Clinical Practice Guidelines
ERT	Extubation readiness testing
ETT	Endotracheal tube
HFNC	High-flow nasal cannula
HMV	Home mechanical ventilation
ICU	Intensive care unit
IMV	Invasive mechanical ventilation
MV	Mechanical ventilation
MMV	Mandatory minute ventilation
PiMax	Maximal inspiratory pressure
PMV	Prolonged mechanical ventilation
NAVA	Neurally adjusted ventilation assist
NRS	Noninvasive respiratory support
NIV	Noninvasive ventilation
PAV	Proportional assist ventilation

Y. M. López-Fernández (✉)
Pediatric Intensive Care Unit, Department of Pediatrics, Cruces University Hospital, BioBizkaia Health Research Institute, Bizkaia, Spain
e-mail: yolandamarg.lopezfernandez@osakidetza.eus

A. Fernández
Pediatric Intensive Care Unit, Hospital General de Agudos "C. Durand", Ciudad Autónoma de Buenos Aires, Argentina

A. Kawaguchi et al. (eds.), *Prolonged and Long-Term Mechanical Ventilation in Children*, https://doi.org/10.1007/978-981-97-8903-0_8

PEEP	Positive end-expiratory pressure
PICU	Pediatric intensive care unit
PS	Pressure support
RCT	Randomized controlled trial
RR	Respiratory rate
SBT	Spontaneous breathing test
SIMV	Synchronized intermittent mandatory ventilation
UAO	Upper airway obstruction
VIDD	Ventilator-induced diaphragmatic dysfunction
VILI	Ventilator-induced lung injury
VS	Volume support
V_T	Tidal volume
WOB	Work of breathing

1 Introduction

There is not yet consensus on a precise operationalized definition of prolonged mechanical ventilation (PMV) in the pediatric and neonatal patients [1, 2]. Reported incidence varies from 2.5% to 4.7% of the population admitted to pediatric intensive care units (PICUs) [3–5] and 10% of all those receiving mechanical ventilation (MV) for more than 12 h [6]. This group of patients consume up to 36.1% of the PICU admission days, with a mortality close to 50% [3–6]. These patients are likely to receive different levels of respiratory support, from invasive mechanical ventilation (IMV) to high-flow nasal cannula (HFNC) oxygen therapy. With additional days expended on MV, the likelihood of related complications (ventilator-induced lung injury, ventilator-induced diaphragmatic dysfunction, ventilator-associated pneumonia, prolonged exposure to sedatives, airway trauma induced by the endotracheal tube (ETT), and subsequent respiratory muscle weakness) increases [7, 8]. The process of liberating a patient from a prolonged course of mechanical ventilation is challenging for the pediatric intensive care team, and the prevalence of children requiring PMV for neurological and neuromuscular diseases, airway abnormalities, or chronic lung diseases is increasing, adding an additional complexity to it [9, 10].

The weaning process is highly related to PMV. Extubation failure (EF) and the need for more than one liberation attempt significantly prolong the duration of MV [11, 13]. On the other side, longer duration of ventilatory support prior to the first separation attempt is associated with higher risk of extubation failure and more days spent on the weaning process [6, 13–16]. Both circumstances are associated with higher healthcare costs and mortality [6, 16]. Children with prolonged invasive ventilation may require noninvasive ventilatory support or a tracheostomy and/or rehabilitation therapies to accurately promote weaning from MV [17]. Persistence of physical deterioration and reduced healthcare-related quality of life in MV survivors has been reported even years after PICU discharge [18, 19].

Pediatric critical care providers should make the effort to improve the management of those patients requiring PMV. With the goal of presenting a review of the literature focused on liberation from prolonged MV in the pediatric patient, this chapter can provide insight into the challenging process of weaning in already complex patients.

2 Weaning Protocols

Patients on PMV might require a simple, difficult, or prolonged process of liberation from MV [21]. In 2007, an International Consensus Conference on weaning from MV proposed a classification based on the number, timing, and results of spontaneous breathing trials and extubation outcomes of adult patients. This classification only considered patients who were ultimately weaned, and as a result, a new definition was proposed: the WIND definition [22]. Briefly, in Group 1—simple or short weaning—the first attempt results in a termination of the weaning process within 1 day; in Group 2—difficult weaning—the weaning is completed after more than 1 day but less than 1 week after the first separation attempt (successful separation or death); and in Group 3—prolonged weaning—weaning is still not terminated at 7th day after the first separation attempt (Group 3a successful, Group 3b without success) [22]. This classification was also evaluated in one pediatric study [15]. Liberation from MV guided by protocols adjusted to these three different groups of patients might be reflected in better weaning outcomes.

The American Thoracic Society (ATS) guidelines (2017) suggest implementing ventilator liberation protocols to manage adults mechanically ventilated for more than 24 h [23]. In patients with PMV, a weaning protocol was associated with better outcomes than standard or non-protocolized clinical practice [24].

In pediatrics, a Cochrane review analyzed three randomized controlled trials (RCTs) comparing the use of a weaning protocol versus standard clinical practice. Two of them were automated protocols in which the pressure level varied according to a computer algorithm. One of the studies showed a decrease in the length of MV, but none of them led to significant improvement of other outcomes (ICU and hospital length of stay, mortality, or ventilator-associated pneumonia) [25, 26]. Three quality improvement studies [27–29] incorporated pre-intervention and intervention comparison using a daily screening test for extubation readiness, which also included an SBT, and other elements related to extubation readiness. The implementation of a protocolized ERT resulted in lower extubation failure rates (absolute risk reduction between 3.3 and 11.7%) [27, 29] and a significant reduction in PICU length of stay (197-h pre-intervention group vs. 177-h intervention group, $p = 0.05$) [29]. However, none of these quasi-randomized studies demonstrated a significant difference with respect to invasive MV duration. An additional concern is the low adherence to protocols. Indeed, compliance with the extubation readiness bundle ranged from 56% [28] to 92% [27, 29], but ongoing training and regular feedback to pediatric critical care practitioners are effective tools to overcome this barrier at implementing a weaning protocol. A pediatric RCT combining targeted sedation protocols and extubation readiness assessments demonstrated a significant reduction in time (2 h) to successful extubation, although the clinical impact of this outcome is debatable despite its statistical significance. Yet, this study has proven the feasibility of a protocolized approach for weaning combined with sedation assessment [30]. Therefore, the Clinical Practice Guidelines (CPG) for Pediatric Ventilator Liberation (2022) also recommend a protocolized approach of weaning in children [31].

Weaning protocols involve objective criteria and algorithms that not only address the reduction of ventilatory support, but also introduce an extubation readiness bundle based on a standardized assessment of the patient's response. Differentiating the concepts of spontaneous breathing trial (SBT) and extubation readiness testing (ERT) is seemingly important. An SBT is a test with minimal predetermined ventilatory support (T-piece, CPAP, ATC, PS) during a variable period (up to 2 h) used to determine the likelihood that the patient will maintain adequate spontaneous ventilation without excessive respiratory effort after extubation. An ERT includes an SBT itself plus other elements such as measures of respiratory muscle strength, assessment of sedation, presence of protective airway reflexes, risk of upper airway obstruction, hemodynamic status, and a plan for post-extubation respiratory support [31]. An ERT is essential for any weaning process, as it enables assessment of the ability of the patient's respiratory system to wean from mechanical ventilation.

Data from RCTs on the efficacy of weaning protocols for patients requiring PMV are limited and lack specific guidance. Still, the liberation procedure should be similar to any general weaning process but considering additional difficulties due to the risks inherent to PMV. Thus, protocolization of weaning in patients with PMV seems even more warranted, and a daily extubation readiness assessment is recommended. However, data from previous pediatric trials should be cautiously extrapolated to patients with PMV, as most studies excluded complex difficult-to-wean patients (i.e., neuromuscular disease or cyanotic congenital heart disease) who oftentimes have prolonged MV courses.

3 Ventilatory Strategies for Weaning

3.1 Simple Weaning

Even when patients on PMV have larger rates of extubation failure, many of them will be successfully weaned after the first attempt of liberation [11–13]. Applying protocolized evaluation according to the Clinical Practice Guidelines for Pediatric Ventilation Liberation might improve outcomes in these patients [31].

According to these protocols, when certain criteria related to respiratory support level, patient's respiratory effort, and overall clinical condition are met, it is time to consider extubation. But this requires that the patient has successfully completed SBT and the other measures that are part of ERT (Fig. 1).

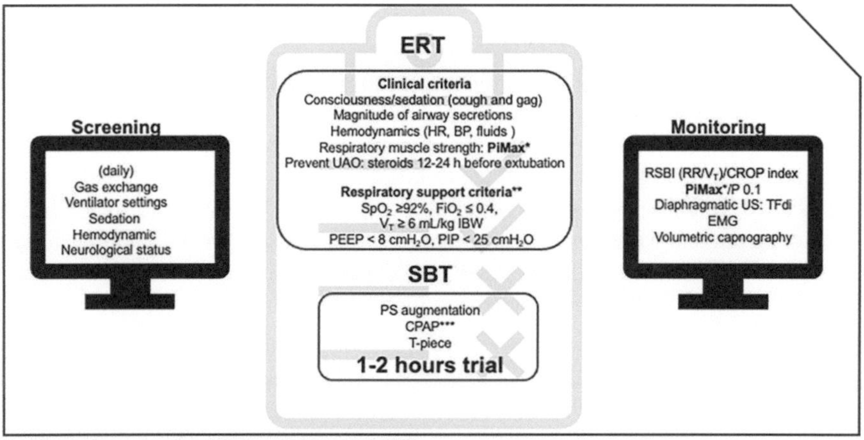

*For children at risk for muscle weakness **PiMax** is suggested as an element of ERT.

****Neuromuscular disease:**SpO_2 ≥94%, FiO_2 0.21, Pre-planned extubation to NIV. Physiotherapy.

***For patients at high risk of extubation failure, **a 60-120 minute SBT** better predicts the post-extubation effort of breathing.

Fig. 1 Extubation phase. The extubation phase includes three steps: (1) screening to determine a favorable clinical status prior to extubation readiness assessment; (2) ERT, which includes an SBT; and (3) monitoring, to consider ERT validated or not. If tests fail, the patient should be placed on pre-ERT ventilator settings and re-examined the next day or as deemed appropriate. *BP* blood pressure, *CPAP* continuous positive airway pressure, *CROP index* compliance, resistance, oxygenation, pressure, *EMG* electromyography, *ERT* extubation readiness testing, *HR* heart rate, *IBW* ideal body weight, *PEEP* positive end-expiratory pressure, *PiMax* maximal inspiratory pressure, *PIP* peak inspiratory pressure, *PS* pressure support, *RR* respiratory rate, *RSBI* rapid shallow breathing index, *SBT* spontaneous breathing trial, *TFdi* diaphragm thickening fraction, *UAO* upper airway obstruction, *US* ultrasound, V_T volume tidal

3.1.1 Screening

Prior to initiation of ERT, a protocolized screening should be performed at regular intervals (usually daily) to identify when a patient has reached pre-specified targets for physiologic parameters (gas exchange), ventilator settings (PEEP, FiO_2, SpO_2, V_T, inspiratory pressure), and sedation (hemodynamic and neurologic status) to safely perform an ERT [31].

3.1.2 Extubation Readiness Test (ERT)

A set of objective measures predictive of the likelihood of a successful extubation. If tests fail, the patient should be placed on pre-ERT ventilator settings and re-examined the next day or as deemed appropriate.

Clinical Criteria

Level of consciousness and/or sedation must be adequate to maintain spontaneous breathing and protective airway reflexes (cough and gag). During weaning, gradual withdrawal of sedatives is required, but oftentimes fluctuations between oversedation and undersedation may contribute to failure of ERT. Additionally, patients are at risk of developing iatrogenic withdrawal syndrome. Hence, valid and reliable sedation, pain, and withdrawal assessment scales with a specific daily target should be used. Use of sedatives that do not suppress their respiratory drive (e.g., dexmedetomidine) may be helpful. In patients with trauma brain injury and severe neurological sequelae, extubation is recommended only when protective airway reflexes are restored, even if the level of consciousness is reduced [30, 32].

Magnitude of airway secretions should be assessed, as an excessive secretion load, especially in a child with an underlying neurological injury or neuromuscular disease, may lead to extubation failure. The patient should be able to manage oropharyngeal secretions or, when failed, use devices such as cough assist. Anticholinergic drugs, such as glycopyrrolate, can be used to decrease the amount of secretions in a certain subset of patients [33].

Hemodynamic condition (heart rate, blood pressure, use of vasoactive drugs) and fluid status should be carefully assessed. Hemodynamic stability is needed for the patient to be able to assume the work of breathing (WOB) induced by the weaning itself. It should also be noted that sedation and analgesia used during MV may contribute to maintaining the vasoactive support, but this requirement will diminish as sedation is gradually reduced while weaning.

Respiratory muscle weakness is a risk factor in difficult weaning. Assessment of respiratory muscle strength is especially important in patients who have been ventilated for a prolonged period and patients with malnutrition or neuromuscular diseases. Maximal inspiratory pressure (PiMax) [34, 35], diaphragmatic ultrasound [36, 37], and respiratory muscle electromyography [38, 39] allow measuring whether there is impairment in respiratory muscle function, although it is PiMax which has been most used for years. Children able to generate a PiMax <20 cmH_2O are at higher risk of failure, whereas those who can generate >50 cmH2O are predicted to be successfully liberated from IMV [31]. In addition, Khemani et al. observed an EF rate of 14% in patients with PiMax $\leq$30 cm H_2O (vs. 5.5%). This rate was increased to 47.5% with the coexistence of UAO. Even when a lower PiMax does not contraindicate extubation in a patient with a successful SBT, it could help to detect patients at risk of EF [34].

Post-extubation upper airway obstruction (UAO): UAO is the most common cause of EF in pediatric critical care. Data on the value of leak pressure measurement in cuffed tubes prior to extubation and peri-extubation corticosteroid administration to prevent EF are not yet conclusive [40, 41]. Still, based on a recent pediatric network meta-analysis, the routine use of peri-extubation corticosteroids cannot be recommended, except in the population of patients considered at high risk for developing UAO, and these include patients with PMV [42]. Consequently, the CPG for Pediatric Ventilator Liberation (2022) suggests that the use of systemic dexamethasone at least 6 (ideally 12–24) hours before the planned extubation attempt may decrease the rate of post-extubation stridor in patients at high risk of post-extubation UAO [31].

Respiratory Support Criteria

The main criteria for a successful ERT are maintaining adequate gas exchange with an $SpO_2 \geq 92\%$ with $FiO_2 \leq 0.4$, $V_T \geq 6$ mL/kg of ideal body weight, PEEP <8 cm H_2O with PIP <25 cm H_2O, and tolerating a period of not less than 30 min on minimal support (SBT). Whether it is anticipated to liberate from IMV to NIV, it may be acceptable to have higher PIP and/or PEEP targets as similar support could be provided with noninvasive respiratory support (NRS) [43]. In patients with neuromuscular disease, it may be cautious to be even more selective and follow a specific weaning protocol. Successful extubation rate of 95% has been reported in patients with SpO2 > 94% at FIO_2 0.21 in combination with NIV and intensive respiratory physiotherapy and cough assistance [44].

3.1.3 Spontaneous Breathing Test (SBT)

Different SBTs can be applied in pediatric patients: inspiratory pressure augmentation (CPAP with PS), CPAP alone, and T-piece. Automatic tube compensation (ATC), not available on all ventilators, provides inspiratory pressure support to overcome the work of breathing imposed by the artificial airway and is an alternative to PS for performing an SBT. Although current adult guidelines recommend the use of 5–8 cm H_2O of PS [43], the reported PS augmentation in pediatric SBTs is highly variable. In some studies, the PS level depends on the size of ETT [45, 46]. PS is set because it is assumed that with a smaller ETT, there is greater WOB imposed due to increased artificial airway resistance, although the fact is that the ETT bypasses natural upper airway resistance. If peak inspiratory flow rates are maintained within age-related limits for a given ETT size, which is the usual situation at the time of extubation, the effects of increased artificial airway resistance are minimal [47, 48]. It has been reported that the use of PS during SBTs underestimates post-extubation WOB, whereas CPAP alone was comparable to post-extubation WOB [48, 49]. The CPG for Pediatric Ventilator Liberation (2022) recommends in patients with PMV who are at higher risk of extubation failure, an SBT with CPAP alone, compared to a PS augmentation SBT, due to a higher degree of accuracy of CPAP-alone SBT in predicting extubation failure [31].

The optimal duration of SBT is an unresolved question yet. In most pediatric studies, a test duration between 10 min and 2 h has been reported [27, 46, 50, 51]. According to the CPG for Pediatric Ventilator Liberation (2022), in patients at high risk of extubation failure, including those with PMV, a 60–120-min SBT better predicts the post-extubation effort of breathing compared to a shorter (30-min) SBT [31].

3.1.4 Assessment of Extubation Failure Predictors

Several indices have been developed to predict success in weaning. Most of them are used in research; these indices have not been routinely implemented in pediatric clinical practice, often due to their complexity or other limitations:

Rapid Shallow Breathing Index (RSBI) or ratio of respiratory rate to tidal volume (RR/V_T): This index, widely used in adult practice as a screening test, includes respiratory rate, and therefore in pediatric ICUs, with different age groups and ranges of normal RR, it has more limited usefulness. RSBI index (normalized to body weight) has been reproduced in children, with good sensibility to predict extubation success with a cut-off point of ≤8 [52] or ≤ 11 breaths/mL/kg [14, 53], but with low specificity to detect extubation failure (AUC 0.51 [0.61–0.70]) [14].

Compliance, Resistance, Oxygenation, Pressure (CROP) Index or dynamic compliance x maximal negative inspiratory pressure x (PaO_2/PAO_2)/RR: This index identifies those patients that decrease their WOB, progressively increasing the negative inspiratory pressure due to low dynamic compliance and lower oxygen requirements, but it is rarely available in routine clinical practice. CROP index was also evaluated in the same pediatric studies, concluding that a CROP value of >0.1 [53] and ≥ 0.15 mL/kg/breaths/min [52] predicted extubation success with good sensibility (83%) but with low specificity (53%).

P 0.1 or the maximum pressure generated by the patient in the airway during the first 100 milliseconds of inspiration when breathing against an occluded tube. P 0.1 is a simple maneuver, although it is not available in all ventilators. More than a measure of WOB, a high P 0.1 value indicates a high respiratory drive needed to maintain adequate alveolar ventilation, and it is associated with EF. However, few data and wide interindividual variability have been reported in the pediatric population, with lower values observed in patients who failed extubation probably due to poorer respiratory drive [54, 55].

Diaphragmatic US: Ultrasound is a promising tool for assessing diaphragmatic function. Diaphragm thickening fraction (TFdi) is used as a measure of contractile activity. TFdi and end inspiratory diaphragm thickness may be useful for predicting extubation outcomes, but more evidence is required regarding the specific value it adds to ERTs [36, 37, 54–57].

Respiratory muscle electromyography (EMG): There is a potential value of EMG of the diaphragm in assessing extubation readiness in pediatric patients, but it requires specific technology not easily implementable or available [38, 39].

Volumetric capnography: The dead space-to-tidal volume ratio (V_D/V_T) has been used as a possible predictor of extubation failure. In a pediatric study (N = 45), $V_D/V_T \leq 0.50$ was found to predict extubation success with 75% sensitivity and 92% specificity, whereas $V_D/V_T > 0.65$ was associated with extubation failure [58]. Volumetric capnography requires specialized exhaled CO_2 monitors, which are not yet available in many PICUs, plus an arterial or capillary blood sample, and posterior studies were not able to reproduce these findings [59, 60].

3.2 *Difficult and Prolonged Weaning*

Extubation should not be delayed in a patient with a successful SBT. However, patients may fail SBT or extubation. The potential for difficult weaning should be anticipated in weaning protocols. These patients have been carefully evaluated before failure; thus, identifying the causes of failure is a real challenge for the PICU team. A predefined list of risk factors for extubation failure could help to recognize them. The actions to address the cause of failure should be promptly performed, and once resolved, a new extubation attempt (ERT) must be performed. If the patient fails two further attempts or cannot be successfully weaned from the ventilator within 1 week, a strategy of prolonged weaning should be followed.

3.2.1 Factors Associated with PMV that Impact the Weaning Process

The underlying disease trajectory and certain clinical factors have been identified as potential barriers to weaning in children with prolonged MV:

Residual airway and lung disease: The ability of the patient's respiratory system to manage the imposed respiratory load will determine the weaning process. Parenchymal lung diseases such as pneumonia, pulmonary edema, interstitial lung disease, and acute respiratory distress syndrome reduce lung compliance and increase WOB. Critical care practitioners should be able to optimize ventilatory settings, avoid further ventilator-induced lung injury (VILI), and monitor lung respiratory compliance to decide the most appropriate time frame to start the liberation process. Inadvertent atelectasis, fluid overload, a new pneumonia, or incomplete resolution of the underlying process might prompt failure.

On the other side, conditions with a predominantly obstructive pattern (severe asthma, viral bronchiolitis, bronchiolitis obliterans, tracheo, and bronchomalacia) increase WOB through airflow obstruction, which in turn can lead to dynamic hyperinflation and auto-PEEP. Optimization of ventilatory settings may help decrease dynamic hyperinflation so that the MV liberation becomes possible in these patients. During SBT excessive levels of PS, inadequate cycling or insufficient PEEP might be responsible of asynchronies and SBT failure [20].

Cardiac dysfunction, pulmonary hypertension, hemodynamic, and fluids: During the weaning process, signs of cardiac failure and hemodynamic instability may appear as mean airway pressures decrease and left ventricular afterload increases. In patients with pulmonary hypertension, as ventilatory support is reduced, pulmonary hypertensive crises may be triggered when pulmonary vascular resistance increases due to atelectasis or other causes of CO_2 retention. Therefore, every attempt should be made to optimize vasoactive support, manage pulmonary hypertension, balance fluid status, and control arrhythmias [20].

Respiratory muscle weakness: Respiratory muscles can develop substantial weakness during long-term MV, and it has been shown to be an independent predictor factor of time to wean from MV. This type of ICU-acquired weakness can be part of critical illness neuromyopathy, a well-known risk factor for PMV in the adult literature, but not so well recognized in pediatric patients. Several factors have been identified as responsible of this multifactorial condition: multiple organ failure, muscle inactivity, neuromuscular blockade, and corticosteroids, among others. These factors should be avoided whenever possible. Of importance is the detection and correction of electrolyte imbalance (especially hypophosphatemia and hyperglycemia) during MV and before SBT.

Ventilator-induced diaphragmatic dysfunction (VIDD) is a rapid form of muscle weakness and has been shown to occur as early as within 12–24 h of MV-imposed diaphragm inactivity and affects primarily infants and small children who have not yet developed effective accessory respiratory muscles. After 48 h of MV, the diaphragmatic fibers begin to show some degree of atrophy. Oxidative stress, protein catabolism, reduced protein synthesis, and apoptosis are considered main causes. A one-third reduction in the force-generating capacity of the diaphragm is observed after 5 days of MV, and the cross-sectional diameter of diaphragmatic fibers is reduced up to 25% after 7 days of MV [61]. Animal studies suggest that continuous mandatory ventilation is directly related with a reduction of diaphragm contractility [57, 62].

Impaired central drive: Sedatives are often used to accomplish ventilator tolerance in the pediatric patient, but simultaneously, these medications often decrease the ability to breathe spontaneously during the weaning process. Conversely, inadequate sedation will increase airway trauma and the risk of post-extubation upper airway obstruction (UAO). Central drive may also be compromised due to damage to neurons controlling respiratory drive in the brainstem following neurocritical diseases or procedures or because of severe metabolic or respiratory alkalosis. Restoration of metabolic balance and reduction of sedatives may enable initiation of the weaning process [20].

Patient-ventilator synchrony: Optimal synchrony requires that every breath initiated by the patient is matched by the ventilator during the respiratory cycle. A mismatch between the patient's ventilatory requirements and the delivered machine breath can lead to either inadequate or excessive support from the ventilator. Too high cycling-off setting can result in premature breath termination with double triggering, whereas too low can lead to delayed cycling with patient discomfort and an inadequate inspiratory time causing expiratory asynchrony. Careful management of inappropriate leaks and review of the ventilator settings will help avoid further asynchrony problems [20].

Airway clearance: Multiple factors explain the dysfunction of mucociliary clearance during PMV: impaired cough related to immobility, sedation, neuromuscular blockade, and muscle weakness; excessive production of mucus or increased mucus viscosity; and decreased ciliary function due to inflammation. Several pulmonary hygiene therapies are available and should be provided to long-term mechanically ventilated patients [63].

3.2.2 Ventilatory Strategies for Difficult and Prolonged Weaning (Table 1)

Synchronized Intermittent Mandatory Ventilation (SIMV). This mode can have two different control variables, pressure or volume, and is usually associated with secondary supported breaths through pressure support (PS). The conventional way of initiating weaning in modes with intermittent mandatory sequence is to decrease the number of mandatory breaths. SIMV with or without PS represents the most common weaning mode [64, 65]. However, the contemporary literature shows clear disadvantages of this mode, and its use during weaning is not recommended, especially in adult literature, as it prolongs the time on MV with no clinical benefit observed and higher rates of asynchrony. It is hypothesized that the respiratory center is not able to adapt rapidly to changes in the workload of the respiratory system, and as mandatory support decreases, WOB generated during spontaneous breaths will remain the same as during mandatory breaths. Neuromuscular output will only begin to increase when the mandatory rate falls below 60% of full support [66–68].

Automated modes (closed-loop ventilation): These modes automatically adjust certain ventilator settings based on feedback signals. When using a closed-loop ventilation mode, critical care providers must set the targets rather than the actual ventilator settings. The ventilator measures some of the patient's physiological variables, compares them with the targets set, and, based on that, automatically adjusts certain settings to reduce the difference between the actual values and the targets. The targets can be set by the provider or determined by an algorithm, whereas the automatic adjustment is performed on a breath-by-breath basis or over several breaths. The main disadvantage of these advanced modes lies on lack of experience that can lead to inappropriate target setting. There is no evidence of the usefulness of these modes in the weaning process. Mandatory minimum ventilation (MMV) and adaptive support ventilation (ASV) are examples of closed-loop ventilation. Other modes with limited experience in the pediatric clinical practice other than for research purposes are SmartCare or Intellivent-ASV [26, 69–71].

Spontaneous modes: Pressure support (PS) and volume support (VS). With PS, the usual wean-off procedure consists of progressively decreasing the pressure level with close monitoring and assessment of exhaled tidal volume and/or WOB (accessory respiratory muscle use and patient's respiratory rate). Targeting physiologic tidal volumes (6–8 mL/kg) is preferable to avoid over-assistance and improve gas exchange. Additionally, critically ill patients often have a higher resting respiratory rate (RR); subsequently, the goal is to maintain a comfortable RR, rather than to normalize RR. However, finding the optimal balance between patient effort and the level and timing of ventilatory assist during PS remains uncertain.

VS is a special PS available in some ventilators that guarantee a minimal tidal volume (V_T) per assisted breath. VS enables to maintain the target V_T despite changes in compliance and/or resistance within the lung and airways. Thus, a target V_T of 6–8 mL/kg should be set (considering compensation for ventilator tubing and artificial dead space) and subsequently assess the decrease of peak pressure over time. Weaning with VS is semiautomatic; the PS level required to maintain the preset V_T is reduced automatically as respiratory mechanics and patient's drive improve.

Table 1 Different ventilatory strategies used for weaning patients from invasive mechanical ventilation

Assisted-control modes		
SIMV ± PS	**SIMV- P ± PS** **SIMV- V ± PS** **SIMV-PRVC ± PS**	Weaning consists of reducing the number of mandatory breaths. Adult literature does not recommend SIMV as it prolongs the time on MV without clinical benefit and higher rates of asynchrony
Automated modes	**ASV** **MMV** **SmartCare** **Intellivent-ASV**	The ventilator measures physiological variables, compares them with the target set, and automatically adjusts to reduce differences between actual values and targets. Main disadvantage is lack of experience that can lead to inappropriate target setting
Spontaneous modes	**PS**	**PS**: Pressure level is gradually reduced targeting physiologic tidal volumes (6–8 mL/kg)
	VS	**VS**: a target physiologic tidal volume should be set, and subsequently assess the decrease of peak pressure over time
Proportional modes	**NAVA**	**NAVA**: Inspiratory positive pressure provided in proportion to the electrical activity of the diaphragm.
	PAV	**PAV**: Automatically adjusts flow and volume according to changes in lung mechanics
	ATC	**ATC**: Continuous assistance provided to compensate the resistance of the endotracheal tube
"Sprinting" weaning	For patients with prolonged mechanical ventilation, weaning may be attempted by alternating periods of complete ventilatory support with shorter periods of spontaneous breathing (CPAP, PS) that are gradually increased to train the respiratory muscles	
CPAP	A primary mode of MV that provides positive airway pressure throughout the respiratory cycle. Among its indications are weaning from mechanical ventilation and even as part of SBTs	
T-piece	Oxygen delivered without positive pressure through the endotracheal tube. The T-piece allows evaluation of diaphragmatic dysfunction due to phrenic nerve injury after cardiovascular surgery, otherwise not observed while in PS	
NRS	**HFNC** **CPAP** **BiPAP**	Used as rescue therapies or electively to avoid reintubation of patients with post-extubation respiratory failure. Neuromuscular disease, cerebral palsy, brain injury, and patients with cardiac dysfunction are potential candidates who may benefit from pre-planned NRS.
Spontaneous breathing		

ASV adaptive support ventilation, *ATC* automated tube compensation, *BiPAP* bilevel positive airway pressure, *CPAP* continuous positive airway pressure, *HFNC* high-flow nasal cannula, *MMV* mandatory minute ventilation, *NAVA* neurally adjusted ventilatory assist, *NRS* noninvasive respiratory support, *P* pressure, *PAV* proportional assist ventilation, *PRVC* pressure-regulated volume controlled ventilation, *PS* pressure support, *SIMV* synchronized intermittent mandatory ventilation, *V* volume, *VS* volume support

If an exceedingly high target V_T is prescribed, this excessive support may prolong the weaning process. Hence, the general recommendation is the same as for PS weaning [72, 73].

Proportional modes: Asynchrony is a contributing factor to PMV and hinders the ventilator liberation process. Modes such as neurally adjusted ventilatory support (NAVA) or proportional assist ventilation (PAV) have demonstrated superiority in synchronization when compared to other support modes, although they have not proven their advantage in terms of weaning outcomes [74]. Automated tube compensation (ATC) is an option available only in some ventilators. This mode can assist weaning, as the ventilator provides continuous assistance to compensate for endotracheal tube (ETT) resistance. The pressure provided is adjusted according to the airflow generated by the patient. However, pediatric studies indicate that the ETT does not increase WOB during SBT [75]. With NAVA, the ventilator provides an inspiratory positive pressure in proportion to the electrical activity of the diaphragm as an indicator of the neural drive to breathe. Furthermore, NAVA reduces the risk of over-assistance compared to PS and monitors diaphragm activity. NAVA can be maintained after extubation as an NIV mode. However, it is still unclear whether NAVA enables to accelerate weaning [76–78].

With PAV, the pressure generated in the airway is proportional to the patient's effort (the greater the patient's effort, the greater the provided support). PAV automatically adjusts the flow and volume generated according to any changes in lung mechanics and facilitates synchrony between patient and ventilator. However, in studies with adult patients, there is no evidence of its superiority compared to PS. Unlike NAVA, there is limited experience in children [79–81].

Sprint weaning: Weaning is attempted by alternating periods of complete ventilatory support with shorter periods of spontaneous breathing [continuous positive airway pressure (CPAP), PS] that are gradually increased to train the respiratory muscles until sustained spontaneous breathing is steadily achieved [64]. Although it is a strategy reported in prolonged weaning, there is limited evidence of the effectiveness of this approach.

CPAP: This is a primary mode of MV that provides positive airway pressure throughout the respiratory cycle to maintain alveolar recruitment and improve oxygenation. Among its well-established indications are weaning from MV, even as part of SBTs.

T-piece trial: A different approach to assess a patient's readiness to be liberated from the ventilator is through progressively longer periods of SBTs via a T-piece (oxygen delivered without positive pressure). A survey of pediatric intensivists in the USA reported that less than 20% of providers used the T-piece for weaning [82]. Of note, a pediatric randomized clinical trial (N = 257) compared PS (10 cm H_20) with T-piece that only provides flow as a readiness test for extubation (2 h). The analysis reported no statistical difference in extubation failure rate at 48 h [50]. Moreover, T-piece enables assessment of the patient's muscle strength without ventilatory support and can identify diaphragmatic dysfunction due to phrenic nerve injury after cardiovascular surgery that otherwise would not have been noted while on PS.

Noninvasive respiratory support (NRS): High-flow nasal cannula (HFNC), CPAP, and bilevel positive airway pressure (BiPAP) are commonly used as rescue therapies to avoid reintubation of patients with post-extubation respiratory failure. But there is also a rationale to apply electively NRS for removing ETT or tracheostomy in those patients with incomplete weaning from prolonged IMV [83–85]. The use of NRS provides an alternative to IMV with the advantage of decreasing ventilator-associated pneumonia, ETT-related upper airway injury, and sedative requirements associated with side effects such as iatrogenic withdrawal syndrome or delirium. Neuromuscular patients are well-identified candidates who may benefit from BiPAP in combination with ancillary procedures (i.e., cough assist) to be liberated from IMV [86, 87]. Preplanned NRS is likely useful in other high-risk pediatric subpopulations including children with cerebral palsy, brain injury, and cardiac dysfunction. A network meta-analysis in adult population reported a lower reintubation rate with NRS compared with conventional oxygen therapy, although neither NIV nor HFNC proved superior to each other [OR 1.04 (95% CI 0.78–1.38)] [88]. In high-risk extubated adult population, HFNC was not inferior to NIV in preventing reintubation and post-extubation acute respiratory failure [89]. Conversely, a pediatric RCT reported that HFNC compared with CPAP following extubation failed to meet the non-inferiority criterion for time to liberation from respiratory support [90].

3.2.3 Respiratory Physiotherapy and Early Mobilization

Physiotherapy positively influences the weaning process in patients requiring PMV. Children with PMV in the PICU setting often develop generalized muscle weakness, which also affects respiratory muscles, especially those involved in the inspiratory phase. The resulting muscle atrophy is associated with decreased muscle mass and strength efficiency, and the predominant muscle composition has been reported to switch from type IIa fibers, with greater aerobic capacity, to type IIb fibers [91]. Evidence for the benefits of rehabilitation for critically ill patients has evolved in recent years. Adult guidelines recommend including physiotherapy in the intensive care setting to speed up the weaning process, but only indirect evidence supports the use of physiotherapy in adult patients undergoing PMV [92]. Programs focused on early mobilization and physical therapy of the critically ill patient should not only be part of ICU liberation bundles, but also be included as part of the wean-off in children with long-term MV [93].

There is some evidence that respiratory muscle weakness is a consequence of PMV. Proteolysis of the diaphragm is detectable as early as 18 h of controlled MV [62]. Even patients ventilated with spontaneous modes may be affected by atrophic changes, especially if there is an over-assistance in PS. Low inspiratory muscle strength (PiMax 20–30 cmH_2O) at the time of liberation of the ETT is associated with extubation failure in children [14, 34]. Furthermore, ultrasound studies of diaphragm thickness (a surrogate measure of inspiratory muscle strength) revealed that by the fourth day of MV, a reduction in diaphragm thickness was detected in 41% of adult patients [94].

Early mobilization prompts, through increased ventilation, endurance training of the respiratory muscles, although diaphragm dysfunction is up to twofold more frequent than limb weakness [95]. Respiratory muscle strengthening should be performed in a titrated approach according to the patient's level of weakness, followed by sufficient rest periods. Inspiratory muscle training can facilitate ventilator liberation while improving the quality of respiratory function. More specifically, strength training (high-intensity, low repetition loading) has been shown to be feasible for adult ventilator-dependent patients [96] who may even continue to benefit from training in the post-extubation period. A prerequisite for the patient is to be awake and actively participating in training, with the limitations intrinsic to the child's age and degree of neuropsychological development. Some patients will most likely be unable to participate due to sedation, withdrawal syndrome, delirium, or clinical instability. Other potential contraindications also include neuromuscular disease, hemodynamic instability, hemoptysis, or severe kyphoscoliosis [97].

Effective cough, airway humidification, and secretion clearance are equally vital to extubation success. Cough peak expiratory flow rate as the measure of cough strength can be predictive for extubation failure. To facilitate a successful liberation, cough augmentation techniques or devices, such as lung volume recruitment or assisted cough, must be used with different intensity and settings depending on an individualized approach and according to the underlying condition [44, 68].

However, despite the favorable reported data, there is still reluctance and lack of knowledge of the benefits of early mobilization and physiotherapy techniques and a moderate-high level of disagreement on the acceptable extent of activity in these critical patients. On the basis that practice among different institutions is very heterogeneous, several factors influence the lack of implementation of these measures such as 24x7 availability of physiotherapists and respiratory therapists, appropriate nurse/patient ratio, and daily rehabilitation goal collaboratively established by the interprofessional team.

3.2.4 Nutrition

Nutritional status of patients with PMV is commonly influenced by the severity of the underlying process leading to ICU admission, but in addition, malnutrition is associated with poor outcomes including prolonged duration of MV. It is seemingly important to record the anthropometric measurements of patients at PICU admission as standard of care to identify patients at high risk of malnourishment due to the robust association of undernutrition with PICU length of stay, duration of MV, and mortality [98].

Artificial nutritional support can help improve the outcomes of these patients, but per expert consensus, energy requirements, timely initiation, and attainment of energy targets should be individualized [99]. During the first days of PICU admission, there is a marked catabolic response (negative protein balance) that may result in loss of lean muscle body mass contributing to the development of muscular weakness, a key factor in hindering the weaning process. Hence, a minimum protein intake of 1.5 g/kg/d must be ensured to avoid cumulative protein deficits in critically ill children, and probably higher for infants and young children [100, 101].

Enteral nutrition is the preferred route for nutrient delivery. Implementation of specific enteral nutrition protocols tailored to a particular institution will help address barriers such as prolonged interruptions due to procedures, identification of feeding intolerance, or indications of feeding tubes (gastric versus post-pyloric). When enteral nutrition is not feasible or contraindicated, parenteral nutrition is an alternative nutritional support. In the long-term setting (home discharge, weaning or step-down unit, ward), the need for percutaneous endoscopic gastrostomy to deliver enteral nutrition in patients with PMV will be discussed with families.

3.2.5 Tracheostomy and Decannulation

Tracheostomy use is relatively common among critically ill patients requiring PMV, especially in the adult population. In adult ICUs, reported tracheostomy rates vary among 5–24% of ventilated patients and median time to tracheostomy from the start of MV ranges from 9 to 12 days [102, 103]. In children with PMV, there is also a large variation among different PICUs, but among those children who received a tracheostomy, the majority did after more than 2 weeks of MV onset, and only a minority of these patients were decannulated before PICU discharge [104].

Indications and timing of a tracheostomy in patients with PMV remain controversial. Long-term MV via a tracheostomy favors the weaning process by allowing a reduction or even withdrawal of sedatives, better comfort, earlier resumption of autonomy, and fewer life-threatening events such as accidental extubation or even allows transfer to units other than the PICU. However, performing a tracheostomy could expose a surgical intervention with risk of complications [105, 106].

Once the child tolerates ventilation through a cuffless tracheostomy (or with the cuff deflated), a one-way valve can be placed in the ventilator circuit allowing full pharyngeal exhalation while still ventilating mechanically (speaking valve) [107]. Interestingly, other authors reported their experience in transitioning children from invasive ventilation via tracheostomy to noninvasive ventilation [108].

Tracheostomy decannulation is usually considered once the child is no longer ventilator dependent. Prior to decannulation, although not mandatory, the child is usually required to tolerate increasing periods of tracheostomy capping. Additionally, if the child is deemed ready, a bronchoscopic evaluation of the entire airway and an assessment of pCO_2 (overnight end-tidal CO_2, blood gases, transcutaneous CO_2) are suggested before decannulation [109]. Then, the tracheostomy can be removed and covered with an occlusive dressing with close monitoring to identify potential complications. Of note, some institutions avoid tracheostomy decannulation during the winter season [105].

4 Noninvasive Respiratory Support (NRS) in the Weaning Process

NRS can be an alternative to ongoing IMV in patients who are deemed eligible to start the process of weaning but have failed an SBT. The patient will continue to receive support as their respiratory muscular strength recovers without being exposed to the potentially harmful effects of sedatives, which reduces the incidence of ventilator-associated pneumonia and accelerates the wean-off.

4.1 Noninvasive Positive-Pressure Ventilation (BiPAP, CPAP)

The inclusion of NIV in weaning requires pre-established criteria for initiation and failure. Three indications for NIV during weaning have been described: a) post-extubation prophylaxis in patients at high risk of reintubation (planned NIV), b) support in extubated patients with respiratory failure within the first 48 h after extubation (rescue NIV), and c) as a stand-alone weaning mode. The first two strategies aim to avoid reintubation, and the third attempts to facilitate weaning in patients with long-term MV. The CPG for pediatric ventilator liberation suggests using planned NIV in patients with high risk of extubation failure, such as children with PMV [31].

The experience in children is limited to case series with small sample size. One observational study reported that NIV was more effective in avoiding reintubation when used early in patients at high risk of extubation failure than as rescue in patients with respiratory failure. Reduction of RR and FiO_2 after 6 h was associated with NIV success [83]. Moreover, the role of NIV during the decannulation process has been reported in a selected group of pediatric patients with respiratory failure following decannulation [108, 109]. Likewise, the combination of NIV and mechanical insufflation-exsufflation devices can be used in children with NMD or acquired weakness related to critical illness to avoid permanent tracheostomy and invasive MV [44].

When NIV is used as a mode of PMV, the weaning process is also typically prolonged and highly dependent on the underlying disease. Children who likely can be weaned from CPAP or NIV are those whose disorders improve spontaneously with age, such as bronchopulmonary dysplasia, Pierre Robin syndrome, and airway malacia. In a study of 213 patients with prolonged NIV due to different causes, 58 patients (27%) could be liberated from NIV: 57% due to significant improvement with age and 43% after specific surgical intervention (adenotonsillectomy, aryepiglottic fold resection, mandibular distraction osteogenesis, etc.). Most of these children were weaned after a period of 6 months to 3 years [110].

4.2 High-Flow Nasal Cannula

HFNC is an NRS mode commonly used. This oxygen delivery system warms and humidifies at flow rates that exceed the patient's inspiratory flow. HFNC has been associated with washout of nasopharyngeal dead space, reduced resistance related to air passage through the airway, lung mucociliary clearance, and some degree of distending pressure for alveolar recruitment, compared to dry, cold gas used in conventional oxygen therapy. When compared to other methods of NRS (i.e., CPAP), HFNC is often preferred because it is better tolerated by patients [111].

In adult population, HFNC has been widely used as respiratory support after ventilator liberation to prevent extubation failure, especially in high-risk patients. But the use of HFNC has also been reported within the weaning process, as part of an SBT or as a step prior to tracheostomy decannulation [112, 113].

In neonates, weaning from invasive ventilation is one of the main indications for HFNC. Nasal CPAP is known to be superior to non-positive pressure support and is the current standard of care for NRS of very preterm infants. At present, HFNC has become an alternative to provide NRS to very preterm infants [114, 115].

In the pediatric population, HFNC has also been used to prevent or support post-extubation respiratory failure. Compared with conventional oxygen therapy, HFNC was not useful in decreasing $PaCO_2$ in an RCT of 89 infants <18 months in the first 48 h post-extubation after cardiac surgery, although HFNC was considered safe and a better option than conventional oxygen therapy to improve oxygenation [116]. However, in an RCT of acutely ill children (N = 600), HFNC was not found to be noninferior to CPAP in children extubated after IMV [90].

5 Specialized Weaning Units

The weaning process in patients with PMV can be faced in a setting other than the ICU [68]. Specialized weaning units are less costly than ICUs but offer adequate levels of multidisciplinary care. Some of them also work as part of "step-down" or transitional care units and can also serve as a bridge between hospital and long-term care facilities or home care programs. These respiratory intermediate care units not only relieve pressure on busy ICUs, but also provide multidisciplinary teams focused on the difficult-to-wean patients (pulmonary nurse practitioners, pediatric pulmonary physicians, respiratory therapists, nutritionists, speech and occupational therapists, etc.). Unlike PICUs, these units are more focused on rehabilitation and more aggressive physical therapy, with scheduled and supervised daily activities. Swallowing, which contributes to weaning, is trained, and nasogastric tube is withdrawn. Nutritional recovery is carried out. The family is more integrated into care, longer visits are allowed, and rest and sleep are respected, all of which contribute to psycho-emotional well-being and recovery. Interestingly, most experience has been reported from the adult literature, with variable weaning success and mortality rates [117, 118] although some similar experiences in pediatrics also exist [10, 105, 119]. Telemonitoring modalities have also been proposed to manage difficult wean-off [120, 121] in adult population.

6 Weaning and PMV in Specific Pediatric Subpopulations (Fig. 2)

The requirement for PMV in populations with complex chronic diseases is discussed in other chapters. In this section, we will only refer briefly to some particularities in the weaning process.

6.1 Neurocritical Conditions

Weaning in this subgroup of PMV patients is determined by clinical concerns about their impaired mental status and the risk of aspiration and acute respiratory failure, although their lung and airways are relatively unaffected. Even if an SBT is being passed, extubation success may depend on other factors, such as glottic or pharyngeal tone, and the ability to cough and clear secretions. A weak or absent cough has been found to be the most significant predictor of extubation failure in the pediatric neurocritical population, whereas neurologic status assessed by Glasgow coma scale, sedation scores, or other conventional extubation readiness parameters did not accurately predict extubation failure [122]. Secretion load (quality and quantity) and strength of cough reflex during a spontaneous or induced cough maneuver must be objectively assessed and recorded during the ERT. This approach enables a standardized management of airway clearance and the use of cough assist devices in the immediate post-extubation period.

In patients with intact cough and gag reflexes but ongoing encephalopathy that favors the development of atelectasis, NIV even during the nighttime period alone may decrease the risk of post-extubation respiratory failure [123]. Tracheostomy might be considered if two or more unsuccessful extubation attempts occur, or after a failed extubation attempt due to weak/absent cough reflex. Interestingly, tracheostomy <7 days post-injury after pediatric traumatic brain injury was associated with a decrease in ventilator days, ICU and hospital days, and airway complications compared with late tracheostomy >7 days post-injury [124].

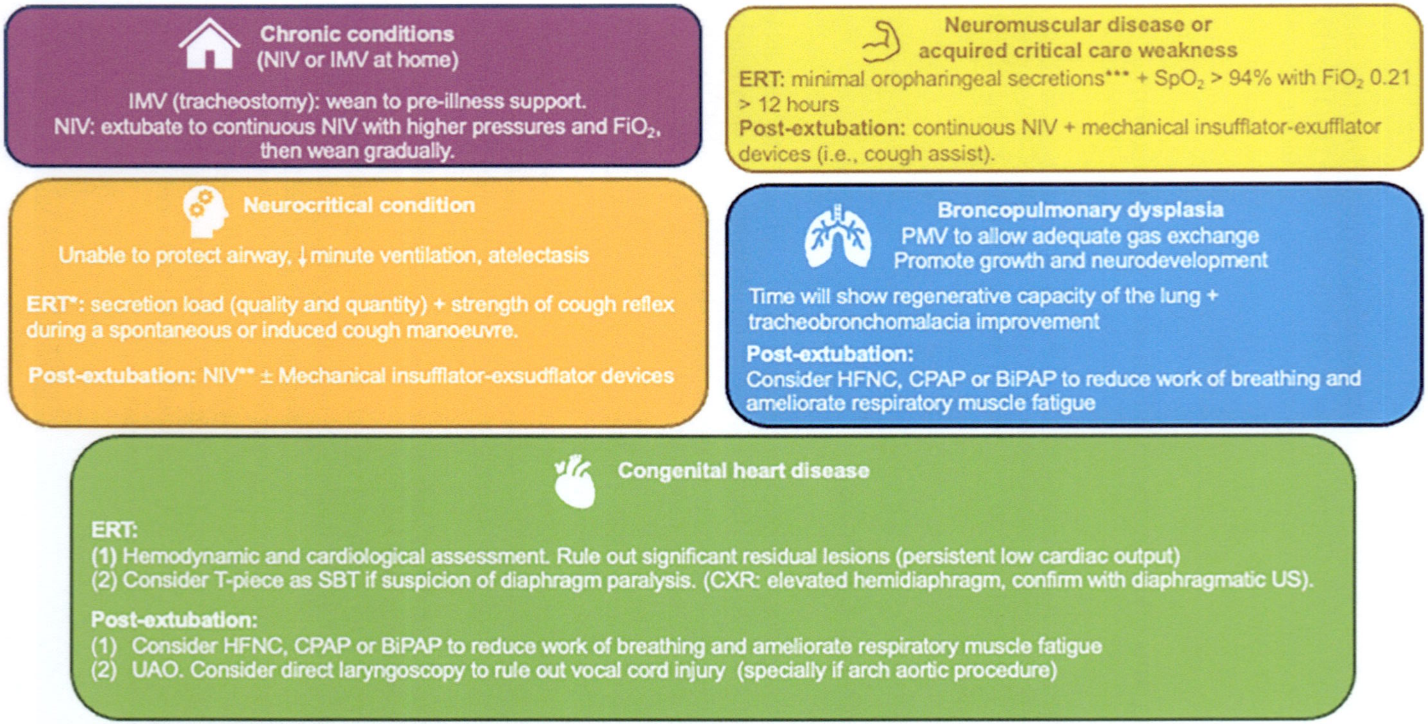

*Consider tracheostomy if ≧ 2 extubation attempts fail or despite optimal treatment for > 2 weeks. **It may be intermittent, i.e., night-time alone.
***Children > 12 years with a CPF<160 L/min more likely to fail extubation.

Fig. 2 Weaning and PMV in special pediatric subpopulations. The same general principles of weaning and extubation readiness testing are also applicable, but some criteria can be modified to avoid extubation failure in these different subsets of patients. *BiPAP* Bilevel positive airway pressure, *CPAP* continuous positive airway pressure, *CPF* cough peak flow, *CXR* chest radiograph, *ERT* extubation readiness testing, FiO_2 inspired fraction of oxygen, *HFNC* high-flow nasal cannula, *IMV* invasive mechanical ventilation, *NIV* noninvasive ventilation, *PMV* prolonged mechanical ventilation, *SBT* spontaneous breathing trial, SpO_2 oxygen saturation measured by pulse oximetry, *UAO* upper airway obstruction, *US* ultrasound

6.2 Neuromuscular Disease (NMD)

Children with NMD due to their innate muscle weakness are candidates for PMV and difficult or prolonged weaning. The same general principles of weaning and extubation readiness assessment are also applicable to them, but it is also acknowledged that some criteria should be modified to avoid extubation failure in this subgroup.

The British guidelines for the management of children with NMD (2012) specify the four criteria required to consider a patient ready for extubation: (1) presence of only minimal oropharyngeal secretions, (2) use of effective airway clearance methods such as mechanical insufflation-exsufflation devices (i.e., cough assist), (3) an oxygen saturation >94% without supplemental oxygen for >12 h, and (4) use of continuous NIV immediately after extubation [86].

Cough effectiveness can be assessed by the measurement of cough peak flow (CPF). Adults and children older than 12 years, with a CPF <160 liters/min, are not able to clear oropharyngeal secretions effectively, and extubation is likely to fail without intensive use of augmented coughing techniques and immediate use of NIV [44]. A protocol that includes NIV immediately after extubation has been used successfully in 157 adults and children with NMD who were unable to overcome conventional SBTs [44].

6.3 Congenital Heart Disease (CHD)

Early extubation of patients who undergo surgery for CHD in the operating room or within hours of PICU admission has become standard of care at many institutions (fast track). In addition to the usual benefits of early liberation of IMV, early extubation has physiological advantages for some of these patients, especially those with cavopulmonary connections (Fontan and Glenn procedures). However, a long course of IMV can be needed for other CHD complex patients after surgery. Current data suggest that extubation failure in cardiac critical care patients ranges from 10% to 27% [125, 126].

Factors other than usual that can explain extubation failure and the resulting lengthening of IMV are (1) presence of significant residual lesions that required more extensive hemodynamic and cardiological assessment during the ERT; (2) recurrent laryngeal nerve injury, especially after surgeries involving the aortic arch; and (3) diaphragmatic paralysis that should be suspected if the chest radiograph shows an elevated hemidiaphragm and warrants evaluation with diaphragmatic ultrasound. During the SBT, using the T-piece allows an assessment of the patient's actual muscle strength without ventilatory support that would not have been revealed while on PS [126, 127].

NRS is commonly used after IMV liberation, in either HFNC, CPAP, or BiPAP modes to reduce WOB and ameliorate respiratory muscle fatigue [116, 128, 129].

6.4 *Bronchopulmonary Dysplasia (BPD)*

Severe BPD (type 2) defines a subset of patients who remain dependent on IMV or NIV. The goal of long-term MV in this group of patients is to maintain the respiratory support necessary to allow the patient to grow and develop [130]. Some infants will improve and tolerate a gradual weaning from ventilatory support, others might remain dependent on NRS (BiPAP, CPAP, or HFNC), and a small group will develop chronic respiratory failure and will be candidates for tracheostomy.

The presence of tracheobronchomalacia may increase the likelihood that the infant will benefit from tracheostomy and be discharged home on chronic ventilation [105, 131, 132]. The postnatal alveolarization process and the maturation that increases cartilaginous tone and improves tracheobronchomalacia contribute to wean ventilatory support [131]. The mean age of MV liberation was 2.4 years in children with ventilator-dependent BPD, whereas tracheostomy decannulation occurred at a mean age of 3.5 years [135].

7 Weaning of Patients on Home Ventilation

Successful liberation from invasive respiratory support at home, including tracheostomy, is feasible in medically complex children at relatively young ages. In a cohort of 46 patients, the median age of liberation from home mechanical ventilation (HMV) with tracheostomy was around 2 years old, and decannulation was less than 4 years old [134]. Based on retrospective analysis of a large series of patients in a single center (N = 102) with severe BPD, it has been suggested that if a child is not off ventilator by 5 years and decannulated by age 6 years, it is unlikely to become so [135].

The whole process comprises several steps: ventilator settings progressively weaned, initiation of collar tracheostomy trials, independence of the HMV, and, finally, decannulation [135]. Clinical decisions are made based on the patient's respiratory status, although monitoring of $ETCO_2$ and peripheral venous/capillary pCO_2 may support clinical criteria [109]. The use of a speaking valve and tracheostomy capping is important but not imperative. Although evidence is lacking, bronchoscopy and polysomnography by a pulmonologist and/or otolaryngologist are options to ensure that there are no anatomic reasons precluding decannulation. Furthermore, obstructive lesions such as adenotonsillar hypertrophy, granulomas, or original airway injury should be ruled out and, if present, addressed by surgical techniques. American Thoracic Society guidelines describe "one-step" decannulation following airway evaluation [136] and observation for 24–48 h [109, 137].

Importantly, there is growing support for the use of noninvasive ventilation (NIV) to facilitate transition to decannulation. Different protocols are based on downsizing the internal diameter of the cannula, capping of the tracheostomy cannula, and progressive increase of NIV periods [138]. Some institutions switch selected patients (central congenital hypoventilation syndrome, for example) to NIV support even though they require ongoing nocturnal support [139].

Finally, families of difficult-to-wean patients must be supported through training programs for caregivers, regular hospital visits, phone follow-up, and even modalities of telemonitoring.

8 Conclusion

PMV patients might fall into the difficult-to-wean category. Overall, the liberation process in children with PMV should follow a standardized protocol and the same steps as any otherwise routine wean-off. Therefore, we recommend that weaning in patients with PMV should follow the CPG for pediatric ventilator liberation [31], despite keeping in mind the relevant nuances and the specific subpopulation to which the patient belongs.

Additionally, NRS (BiPAP, CPAP, HFNC) plays a key role in weaning, as a component of de-escalation respiratory support or as a unique component of the PMV process. Therefore, we must know how to apply the rules of weaning under these circumstances.

References

1. Sauthier M, Rose L, Jouvet P. Pediatric prolonged mechanical ventilation: considerations for definitional criteria. Respir Care. 2017;62(1):49–53.
2. Colleti J Jr, Azevedo RT, de Oliveira Caino FR, de Araujo OR. Prolonged mechanical ventilation in children: review of the definition. Pediatr Crit Care Med. 2021;22(11):e588–93.
3. Traiber C, Piva JP, Fritsher CC, Garcia PC, Lago PM, Trotta EA, Ricachinevsky CP, Bueno FU, Baecker V, Lisboa BD. Profile and consequences of children requiring prolonged mechanical ventilation in three Brazilian pediatric intensive care units. Pediatr Crit Care Med. 2009;10(3):375–80.
4. Ping Kirk AH, Sng QW, Zhang LQ, Ming Wong JJ, Puthucheary J, Lee JH. Characteristics and outcomes of long-stay patients in the pediatric intensive care unit. J Pediatr Intensive Care. 2018;7(1):1–6.
5. Marcin JP, Slonim AD, Pollack MM, Ruttimann UE. Long-stay patients in the pediatric intensive care unit. Crit Care Med. 2001;29(3):652–7.
6. Monteverde E, Fernández A, Poterala R, Vidal N, Siaba Serrate A, Castelani P, Albano L, Podestá F, Farias JA. Characterization of pediatric patients receiving prolonged mechanical ventilation. Pediatr Crit Care Med. 2011;12(6):e287–91.
7. Kneyber MC, Zhang H, Slutsky AS. Ventilator-induced lung injury. Similarity and differences between children and adults. Am J Respir Crit Care Med. 2014;190(3):258–65.
8. Mourani PM, Sontag MK. Ventilator-associated pneumonia in critically ill children: a new paradigm. Pediatr Clin N Am. 2017;64(5):1039–56.
9. Dumas HM, Hughes ML, O'Brien JE. Children dependent on respiratory support: a 10-year review from one pediatric postacute care hospital. Pediatr Pulmonol. 2020;55(8):2050–4.

10. Rogerson CM, Beardsley AL, Nitu ME, Cristea AI. Health care resource utilization for children requiring prolonged mechanical ventilation via tracheostomy. Respir Care. 2020;65(8):1147–53.
11. Venkataraman ST, Khan N, Brown A. Validation of predictors of extubation success and failure in mechanically ventilated infants and children. Crit Care Med. 2000;28(8):2991–6.
12. Kurachek SC, Newth CJ, Quasney MW, Rice T, Sachdeva RC, Patel NR, Takano J, Easterling L, Scanlon M, Musa N, Brilli RJ, Wells D, Park GS, Penfil S, Bysani KG, Nares MA, Lowrie L, Billow M, Chiochetti E, Lindgren B. Extubation failure in pediatric intensive care: a multiple-center study of risk factors and outcomes. Crit Care Med. 2003;31(11):2657–64.
13. Baisch SD, Wheeler WB, Kurachek SC, Cornfield DN. Extubation failure in pediatric intensive care incidence and outcomes. Pediatr Crit Care Med. 2005;6(3):312–8.
14. Farias JA, Alía I, Retta A, Olazarri F, Fernández A, Esteban A, Palacios K, Di Nunzio L, Fernández G, Bordón A, Berrondo C, Sheehan G. An evaluation of extubation failure predictors in mechanically ventilated infants and children. Intensive Care Med. 2002;28(6):752–7.
15. Choi AY, Kim M, Park E, Son MH, Ryu JA, Cho J. Outcomes of mechanical ventilation according to WIND classification in pediatric patients. Ann Intensive Care. 2019;9(1):72.
16. Kapnadak SG, Herndon SE, Burns SM, Shim YM, Enfield K, Brown C, Truwit JD, Vinayak AG. Clinical outcomes associated with high, intermediate, and low rates of failed extubation in an intensive care unit. J Crit Care. 2015;30(3):449–54.
17. Payen V, Jouvet P, Lacroix J, Ducruet T, Gauvin F. Risk factors associated with increased length of mechanical ventilation in children. Pediatr Crit Care Med. 2012;13(2):152–7.
18. Watson RS, Asaro LA, Hutchins L, Bysani GK, Killien EY, Angus DC, Wypij D, Curley MAQ. Risk factors for functional decline and impaired quality of life after pediatric respiratory failure. Am J Respir Crit Care Med. 2019;200(7):900–9.
19. Carlton EF, Donnelly JP, Prescott HC, Asaro LA, Barbaro RP, Watson RS, Curley MAQ, RESTORE Study Investigators. School and work absences after critical care hospitalization for pediatric acute respiratory failure: a secondary analysis of a cluster randomized trial. JAMA Netw Open. 2021;4(12):e2140732.
20. White AC. Long-term mechanical ventilation: management strategies. Respir Care. 2012;57(6):889–97. discussion 898–9.
21. Boles JM, Bion J, Connors A, Herridge M, Marsh B, Melot C, Pearl R, Silverman H, Stanchina M, Vieillard-Baron A, Welte T. Weaning from mechanical ventilation. Eur Respir J. 2007;29(5):1033–56.
22. Béduneau G, Pham T, Schortgen F, Piquilloud L, Zogheib E, Jonas M, Grelon F, Runge I, Nicolas T, Grangé S, Barberet G, Guitard PG, Frat JP, Constan A, Chretien JM, Mancebo J, Mercat A, Richard JM, Brochard L, WIND (Weaning according to a New Definition) Study Group and the REVA (Réseau Européen de Recherche en Ventilation Artificielle) Network ‡. Epidemiology of weaning outcome according to a new definition. The WIND study. Am J Respir Crit Care Med. 2017;195(6):772–83.
23. Girard TD, Alhazzani W, Kress JP, Ouellette DR, Schmidt GA, Truwit JD, Burns SM, Epstein SK, Esteban A, Fan E, Ferrer M, Fraser GL, Gong MN, Hough CL, Mehta S, Nanchal R, Patel S, Pawlik AJ, Schweickert WD, Sessler CN, Strøm T, Wilson KC, Morris PE, ATS/CHEST Ad Hoc Committee on Liberation from Mechanical Ventilation in Adults. An Official American Thoracic Society/American College of Chest Physicians Clinical Practice Guideline: liberation from mechanical ventilation in critically Ill adults. Rehabilitation protocols, ventilator liberation protocols, and cuff leak tests. Am J Respir Crit Care Med. 2017;195(1):120–33.
24. Vitacca M, Ambrosino N, Clini E, Porta R, Rampulla C, Lanini B, Nava S. Physiological response to pressure support ventilation delivered before and after extubation in patients not capable of totally spontaneous autonomous breathing. Am J Respir Crit Care Med. 2001;164(4):638–41.
25. Blackwood B, Murray M, Chisakuta A, Cardwell CR, O'Halloran P. Protocolized versus non-protocolized weaning for reducing the duration of invasive mechanical ventilation in critically ill paediatric patients. Cochrane Database Syst Rev. 2013;2013(7):CD009082.

26. Jouvet PA, Payen V, Gauvin F, Emeriaud G, Lacroix J. Weaning children from mechanical ventilation with a computer-driven protocol: a pilot trial. Intensive Care Med. 2013;39(5):919–25.
27. Abu-Sultaneh S, Hole AJ, Tori AJ, Benneyworth BD, Lutfi R, Mastropietro CW. An interprofessional quality improvement initiative to standardize pediatric extubation readiness assessment. Pediatr Crit Care Med. 2017;18(10):e463–71.
28. Krawiec C, Carl D, Stetter C, Kong L, Ceneviva GD, Thomas NJ. Challenges with implementation of a respiratory therapist-driven protocol of spontaneous breathing trials in the pediatric ICU. Respir Care. 2017;62(10):1233–40.
29. Loberger JM, Jones RM, Prabhakaran P. A respiratory therapist-driven pathway improves timeliness of extubation readiness assessment in a single PICU. Pediatr Crit Care Med. 2020;21(8):e513–21.
30. Blackwood B, Tume LN, Morris KP, Clarke M, McDowell C, Hemming K, Peters MJ, McIlmurray L, Jordan J, Agus A, Murray M, Parslow R, Walsh TS, Macrae D, Easter C, Feltbower RG, McAuley DF, SANDWICH Collaborators. Effect of a sedation and ventilator liberation protocol vs usual care on duration of invasive mechanical ventilation in pediatric intensive care units: a randomized clinical trial. JAMA. 2021;326(5):401–10.
31. Abu-Sultaneh S, Iyer NP, Fernández A, Gaies M, González-Dambrauskas S, Hotz JC, Kneyber MCJ, López-Fernández YM, Rotta AT, Werho DK, Baranwal AK, Blackwood B, Craven HJ, Curley MAQ, Essouri S, Fioretto JR, Hartmann SM, Jouvet P, Korang SK, Rafferty GF, Ramnarayan P, Rose L, Tume LN, Whipple EC, Wong JJM, Emeriaud G, Mastropietro CW, Napolitano N, Newth CJL, Khemani RG. Executive summary: International clinical practice guidelines for pediatric ventilator liberation, A PALISI network document. Am J Respir Crit Care Med. 2023;207(1):17–28. https://doi.org/10.1164/rccm.202204-0795OC.
32. Faustino EV, Gedeit R, Schwarz AJ, Asaro LA, Wypij D, Curley MA, Randomized Evaluation of Sedation Titration for Respiratory Failure (RESTORE) Study Investigators. Accuracy of an extubation readiness test in predicting successful extubation in children with acute respiratory failure from lower respiratory tract disease. Crit Care Med. 2017;45(1):94–102.
33. Parr JR, Buswell CA, Banerjee K, Fairhurst C, Williams J, O'Hare A, Pennington L, British Academy of Childhood Disability Drooling Study Development Group. Management of drooling in children: a survey of UK paediatricians' clinical practice. Child Care Health Dev. 2012;38(2):287–91.
34. Khemani RG, Sekayan T, Hotz J, Flink RC, Rafferty GF, Iyer N, Newth CJL. Risk factors for pediatric extubation failure: the importance of respiratory muscle strength. Crit Care Med. 2017;45(8):e798–805.
35. Toida C, Muguruma T, Miyamoto M. Detection and validation of predictors of successful extubation in critically ill children. PLoS One. 2017;12(12):e0189787.
36. Dionisio MT, Rebelo A, Pinto C, Carvalho L, Neves JF. Ultrasound assessment of ventilator-induced diaphragmatic dysfunction in paediatrics. Acta Medica Port. 2019;32(7–8):520–8.
37. Valverde Montoro D, García Soler P, Hernández Yuste A, Camacho Alonso JM. Ultrasound assessment of ventilator-induced diaphragmatic dysfunction in mechanically ventilated pediatric patients. Paediatr Respir Rev. 2021;40:58–64.
38. MacBean V, Jolley CJ, Sutton TG, Deep A, Greenough A, Moxham J, Rafferty GF. Parasternal intercostal electromyography: a novel tool to assess respiratory load in children. Pediatr Res. 2016;80(3):407–14.
39. van Leuteren RW, de Waal CG, de Jongh FH, Bem RA, van Kaam AH, Hutten G. Diaphragm activity pre and post extubation in ventilated critically ill infants and children measured with transcutaneous electromyography. Pediatr Crit Care Med. 2021;22(11):950–9.
40. Green J, Ross PA, Newth CJL, Khemani RG. Subglottic post-extubation upper airway obstruction is associated with long-term airway morbidity in children. Pediatr Crit Care Med. 2021;22(10):e502–12.
41. Khemani RG, Randolph A, Markovitz B. Corticosteroids for the prevention and treatment of post-extubation stridor in neonates, children and adults. Cochrane Database Syst Rev. 2009;2009(3):CD001000.

42. Iyer NP, López-Fernández YM, González-Dambrauskas S, Baranwal AK, Hotz JC, Zhu M, Zhang Y, Craven HJ, Whipple EC, Abu-Sultaneh S, Khemani RG. A network meta-analysis of dexamethasone for preventing post-extubation upper airway obstruction in children. Ann Am Thorac Soc. 2023;20(1):118–30. https://doi.org/10.1513/AnnalsATS.202203-212OC.
43. Ouellette DR, Patel S, Girard TD, Morris PE, Schmidt GA, Truwit JD, Alhazzani W, Burns SM, Epstein SK, Esteban A, Fan E, Ferrer M, Fraser GL, Gong MN, Hough CL, Mehta S, Nanchal R, Pawlik AJ, Schweickert WD, Sessler CN, Strøm T, Kress JP. Liberation from mechanical ventilation in critically ill adults: an official American College of Chest Physicians/American Thoracic Society clinical practice guideline: inspiratory pressure augmentation during spontaneous breathing trials, protocols minimizing sedation, and noninvasive ventilation immediately after extubation. Chest. 2017;151(1):166–80.
44. Bach JR, Gonçalves MR, Hamdani I, Winck JC. Extubation of patients with neuromuscular weakness: a new management paradigm. Chest. 2010;137(5):1033–9.
45. Randolph AG, Wypij D, Venkataraman ST, Hanson JH, Gedeit RG, Meert KL, Luckett PM, Forbes P, Lilley M, Thompson J, Cheifetz IM, Hibberd P, Wetzel R, Cox PN, Arnold JH, Pediatric Acute Lung Injury and Sepsis Investigators (PALISI) Network. Effect of mechanical ventilator weaning protocols on respiratory outcomes in infants and children: a randomized controlled trial. JAMA. 2002;288(20):2561–8.
46. Curley MA, Wypij D, Watson RS, Grant MJ, Asaro LA, Cheifetz IM, Dodson BL, Franck LS, Gedeit RG, Angus DC, Matthay MA, RESTORE Study Investigators and the Pediatric Acute Lung Injury and Sepsis Investigators Network. Protocolized sedation vs usual care in pediatric patients mechanically ventilated for acute respiratory failure: a randomized clinical trial. JAMA. 2015;313(4):379–89.
47. Manczur T, Greenough A, Nicholson GP, Rafferty GF. Resistance of pediatric and neonatal endotracheal tubes: influence of flow rate, size, and shape. Crit Care Med. 2000;28(5):1595–8.
48. Khemani RG, Hotz J, Morzov R, Flink RC, Kamerkar A, LaFortune M, Rafferty GF, Ross PA, Newth CJ. Pediatric extubation readiness tests should not use pressure support. Intensive Care Med. 2016;42(8):1214–22.
49. Ferguson LP, Walsh BK, Munhall D, Arnold JH. A spontaneous breathing trial with pressure support overestimates readiness for extubation in children. Pediatr Crit Care Med. 2011;12(6):e330–5.
50. Farias JA, Retta A, Alía I, Olazarri F, Esteban A, Golubicki A, Allende D, Maliarchuk O, Peltzer C, Ratto ME, Zalazar R, Garea M, Moreno EG. A comparison of two methods to perform a breathing trial before extubation in pediatric intensive care patients. Intensive Care Med. 2001;27(10):1649–54.
51. Mahmoud NMS. Predicting successful extubation rate using modified spontaneous breathing trial in PICUs. J Compr Ped. 2021;12(4):e116602.
52. Thiagarajan RR, Bratton SL, Martin LD, Brogan TV, Taylor D. Predictors of successful extubation in children. Am J Respir Crit Care Med. 1999;160(5 Pt 1):1562–6.
53. Baumeister BL, el Khatib M, Smith PG, Blumer JL. Evaluation of predictors of weaning from mechanical ventilation in pediatric patients. Pediatr Pulmonol. 1997;24(5):344–52.
54. Hulzebos E, Takken T, Reijneveld EA, Mulder MM, Bongers BC. Reference values for respiratory muscle strengh in children and adolescents. Respiration. 2018;95(4):235–43.
55. Manczur TI, Greenough A, Pryor D, Rafferty GF. Assessment of respiratory drive and muscle function in the pediatric intensive care unit and prediction of extubation failure. Pediatr Crit Care Med. 2000;1(2):124–6.
56. Abdel Rahman DA, Saber S, El-Maghraby A. Diaphragm and lung ultrasound indices in prediction of outcome of weaning from mechanical ventilation in pediatric intensive care unit. Indian J Pediatr. 2020;87(6):413–20.
57. Lee EP, Hsia SH, Hsiao HF, Chen MC, Lin JJ, Chan OW, Lin CY, Yang MC, Liao SL, Lai SH. Evaluation of diaphragmatic function in mechanically ventilated children: an ultrasound study. PLoS One. 2017;12(8):e0183560.

58. Hubble CL, Gentile MA, Tripp DS, Craig DM, Meliones JN, Cheifetz IM. Deadspace to tidal volume ratio predicts successful extubation in infants and children. Crit Care Med. 2000;28(6):2034–40.
59. Riou Y, Chaari W, Leteurtre S, Leclerc F. Predictive value of the physiological deadspace/tidal volume ratio in the weaning process of mechanical ventilation in children. J Pediatr. 2012;88(3):217–21.
60. Khemani RG. Dead space to tidal volume ratio (VD/VT) to explain extubation failure in children: the limitations of current evidence. J Pediatr. 2012;88(3):191–4.
61. Grosu HB, Lee YI, Lee J, Eden E, Eikermann M, Rose KM. Diaphragm muscle thinning in patients who are mechanically ventilated. Chest. 2021;142(6):1455–60.
62. Hooijman PE, Beishuizen A, Witt CC, de Waard MC, Girbes AR, Spoelstra-de Man AM, Niessen HW, Manders E, van Hees HW, van den Brom CE, Silderhuis V, Lawlor MW, Labeit S, Stienen GJ, Hartemink KJ, Paul MA, Heunks LM, Ottenheijm CA. Diaphragm muscle fiber weakness and ubiquitin-proteasome activation in critically ill patients. Am J Respir Crit Care Med. 2015;191(10):1126–38.
63. Krause MF, Hoehn T. Chest physiotherapy in mechanically ventilated children: a review. Crit Care Med. 2000;28(5):1648–51.
64. Newth CJ, Venkataraman S, Willson DF, Meert KL, Harrison R, Dean JM, Pollack M, Zimmerman J, Anand KJ, Carcillo JA, Nicholson CE, Eunice Shriver Kennedy National Institute of Child Health and Human Development Collaborative Pediatric Critical Care Research Network. Weaning and extubation readiness in pediatric patients. Pediatr Crit Care Med. 2009;10(1):1–11.
65. Farias JA, Fernández A, Monteverde E, Flores JC, Baltodano A, Menchaca A, Poterala R, Pánico F, Johnson M, von Dessauer B, Donoso A, Zavala I, Zavala C, Troster E, Peña Y, Flamenco C, Almeida H, Nilda V, Esteban A, Latin-American Group for Mechanical Ventilation in Children. Mechanical ventilation in pediatric intensive care units during the season for acute lower respiratory infection: a multicenter study. Pediatr Crit Care Med. 2012;13(2):158–64.
66. Chen L, Gilstrap D, Cox CE. Mechanical ventilator discontinuation process. Clin Chest Med. 2016;37(4):693–9.
67. Kacmarek RM, Branson RD. Should intermittent mandatory ventilation be abolished? Respir Care. 2016;61(6):854–66.
68. Ambrosino N, Vitacca M. The patient needing prolonged mechanical ventilation: a narrative review. Multidiscip Respir Med. 2018;13:6.
69. Kirakli C, Naz I, Ediboglu O, Tatar D, Budak A, Tellioglu E. A randomized controlled trial comparing the ventilation duration between adaptive support ventilation and pressure assist/control ventilation in medical patients in the ICU. Chest. 2015;147(6):1503–9.
70. Wysocki M, Jouvet P, Jaber S. Closed loop mechanical ventilation. J Clin Monit Comput. 2014;28(1):49–56.
71. Arnal JM, Garnero A, Novotni D, Corno G, Donati SY, Demory D, Quintana G, Ducros L, Laubscher T, Durand-Gasselin J. Closed loop ventilation mode in Intensive Care Unit: a randomized controlled clinical trial comparing the numbers of manual ventilator setting changes. Minerva Anestesiol. 2018;84(1):58–67.
72. Pierson DJ. Patient-ventilator interaction. Respir Care. 2011;56(2):214–28.
73. López-Fernandez Y, Gónzalez-Gómez JM, Morales-Martínez A, Pilar-Orive FJ, Camilo C, Winter M, Christopherson M. Pressure support and volume support ventilation. In: Medina Villanueva A, Pilar Orive J, Garcia Cuscó M, Blokpoel R, Pons M, Rimensberger P, editors. Handbook of neonatal and mechanical ventilation. 2nd ed. Las Palmas de Gran Canaria: Tesela Ediciones; 2021.
74. Kacmarek RM. Proportional assist ventilation and neurally adjusted ventilatory assist. Respir Care. 2011;56(2):140–8. discussion 149–52.
75. Burns KEA, Soliman I, Adhikari NKJ, Zwein A, Wong JTY, Gomez-Builes C, Pellegrini JA, Chen L, Rittayamai N, Sklar M, Brochard LJ, Friedrich JO. Trials directly comparing

alternative spontaneous breathing trial techniques: a systematic review and meta-analysis. Crit Care. 2017;21(1):127.
76. Vagheggini G, Mazzoleni S, Vlad Panait E, Navalesi P, Ambrosino N. Physiologic response to various levels of pressure support and NAVA in prolonged weaning. Respir Med. 2013;107(11):1748–54.
77. Harris J, Tibby SM, Endacott R, Latour JM. Neurally adjusted ventilator assist in infants with acute respiratory failure: a literature scoping review. Pediatr Crit Care Med. 2021;22(10):915–24.
78. Kallio M, Peltoniemi O, Anttila E, Pokka T, Kontiokari T. Neurally adjusted ventilatory assist (NAVA) in pediatric intensive care—a randomized controlled trial. Pediatr Pulmonol. 2015;50(1):55–62.
79. Moerer O. Effort-adapted modes of assisted breathing. Curr Opin Crit Care. 2012;18(1):61–9.
80. Sindelar R, McKinney RL, Wallström L, Keszler M. Proportional assist and neurally adjusted ventilation: clinical knowledge and future trials in newborn infants. Pediatr Pulmonol. 2021;56(7):1841–9.
81. Tirupakuzhi Vijayaraghavan BK, Hamed S, Jain A, Chimunda T, Telias I, Friedrich JO, Burns KEA. Evidence supporting clinical use of proportional assist ventilation: a systematic review and meta-analysis of clinical trials. J Intensive Care Med. 2020;35(7):627–35.
82. Mhanna MJ, Anderson IM, Iyer NP, Baumann A. The use of extubation readiness parameters: a survey of pediatric critical care physicians. Respir Care. 2014;59(3):334–9.
83. Mayordomo-Colunga J, Medina A, Rey C, Concha A, Menéndez S, Los Arcos M, Garcia I. Non invasive ventilation after extubation in paediatric patients: a preliminary study. BMC Pediatr. 2010;5(10):29.
84. Baudin F, Gagnon S, Crulli B, Proulx F, Jouvet P, Emeriaud G. Modalities and complications associated with the use of high-flow nasal cannula: experience in a pediatric ICU. Respir Care. 2016;61(10):1305–10.
85. Fioretto JR, Ribeiro CF, Carpi MF, Bonatto RC, Moraes MA, Fioretto EB, Fagundes DJ. Comparison between noninvasive mechanical ventilation and standard oxygen therapy in children up to 3 years old with respiratory failure after extubation: a pilot prospective randomized clinical study. Pediatr Crit Care Med. 2015;16(2):124–30.
86. Hull J, Aniapravan R, Chan E, Chatwin M, Forton J, Gallagher J, Gibson N, Gordon J, Hughes I, McCulloch R, Russell RR, Simonds A. British Thoracic Society guideline for respiratory management of children with neuromuscular weakness. Thorax. 2012;67(Suppl 1):i1–40.
87. Racca F, Mongini T, Wolfler A, Vianello A, Cutrera R, Del Sorbo L, Capello EC, Gregoretti C, Massa R, De Luca D, Conti G, Tegazzin V, Toscano A, Ranieri VM. Recommendations for anesthesia and perioperative management of patients with neuromuscular disorders. Minerva Anestesiol. 2013;79(4):419–33.
88. Fernando SM, Tran A, Sadeghirad B, Burns KEA, Fan E, Brodie D, Munshi L, Goligher EC, Cook DJ, Fowler RA, Herridge MS, Cardinal P, Jaber S, Møller MH, Thille AW, Ferguson ND, Slutsky AS, Brochard LJ, Seely AJE, Rochwerg B. Noninvasive respiratory support following extubation in critically ill adults: a systematic review and network meta-analysis. Intensive Care Med. 2022;48(2):137–47.
89. Hernández G, Vaquero C, Colinas L, Cuena R, González P, Canabal A, Sanchez S, Rodriguez ML, Villasclaras A, Fernández R. Effect of postextubation high-flow nasal cannula vs noninvasive ventilation on reintubation and postextubation respiratory failure in high-risk patients: a randomized clinical trial. JAMA. 2016;316(15):1565–74.
90. Ramnarayan P, Richards-Belle A, Drikite L, Saull M, Orzechowska I, Darnell R, Sadique Z, Lester J, Morris KP, Tume LN, Davis PJ, Peters MJ, Feltbower RG, Grieve R, Thomas K, Mouncey PR, Harrison DA, Rowan KM, FIRST-ABC Step-Down RCT Investigators and the Paediatric Critical Care Society Study Group. Effect of high-flow nasal cannula therapy vs continuous positive airway pressure following extubation on liberation from respiratory support in critically ill children: a randomized clinical trial. JAMA. 2022;327(16):1555–65.

91. Puthucheary ZA, Rawal J, McPhail M, Connolly B, Ratnayake G, Chan P, Hopkinson NS, Phadke R, Dew T, Sidhu PS, Velloso C, Seymour J, Agley CC, Selby A, Limb M, Edwards LM, Smith K, Rowlerson A, Rennie MJ, Moxham J, Harridge SD, Hart N, Montgomery HE. Acute skeletal muscle wasting in critical illness. JAMA. 2013;310(15):1591–600.
92. Schmidt GA, Girard TD, Kress JP, Morris PE, Ouellette DR, Alhazzani W, Burns SM, Epstein SK, Esteban A, Fan E, Ferrer M, Fraser GL, Gong MN, Hough CL, Mehta S, Nanchal R, Patel S, Pawlik AJ, Schweickert WD, Sessler CN, Strøm T, Wilson KC, Truwit JD, ATS/CHEST Ad Hoc Committee on Liberation from Mechanical Ventilation in Adults. Official Executive Summary of an American Thoracic Society/American College of Chest Physicians Clinical Practice Guideline: Liberation from Mechanical Ventilation in Critically Ill Adults. Am J Respir Crit Care Med. 2017;195(1):115–9.
93. Loberger JM, Waddell KC, Prabhakaran P, Jones RM, Lawrence MV, Bittles LA, Hill AM, O'Sheal SE, Armstrong AW, Thomas CL, Daniel LH, Tofil NM, Sasser WC, Richter RP, Rutledge CL. Pediatric ventilation liberation: bundled extubation readiness and Analgosedation pathways decrease mechanical ventilation duration and benzodiazepine exposure. Respir Care. 2022;12:respcare.09942.
94. Goligher EC, Dres M, Fan E, Rubenfeld GD, Scales DC, Herridge MS, Vorona S, Sklar MC, Rittayamai N, Lanys A, Murray A, Brace D, Urrea C, Reid WD, Tomlinson G, Slutsky AS, Kavanagh BP, Brochard LJ, Ferguson ND. Mechanical ventilation-induced diaphragm atrophy strongly impacts clinical outcomes. Am J Respir Crit Care Med. 2018;197(2):204–13.
95. Dres M, Dubé BP, Mayaux J, Delemazure J, Reuter D, Brochard L, Similowski T, Demoule A. Coexistence and impact of limb muscle and diaphragm weakness at time of liberation from mechanical ventilation in medical intensive care unit patients. Am J Respir Crit Care Med. 2017;195(1):57–66.
96. Bissett B, Gosselink R, van Haren FMP. Respiratory muscle rehabilitation in patients with prolonged mechanical ventilation: a targeted approach. Crit Care. 2020;24(1):103.
97. Hoffman M, Van Hollebeke M, Clerckx B, Muller J, Louvaris Z, Gosselink R, Hermans G, Langer D. Can inspiratory muscle training improve weaning outcomes in difficult to wean patients? A protocol for a randomised controlled trial (IMweanT study). BMJ Open. 2018;8(6):e021091.
98. de Souza MF, Leite HP, Koch Nogueira PC. Malnutrition as an independent predictor of clinical outcome in critically ill children. Nutrition. 2012;28(3):267–70.
99. Mehta NM, Skillman HE, Irving SY, Coss-Bu JA, Vermilyea S, Farrington EA, McKeever L, Hall AM, Goday PS, Braunschweig C. Guidelines for the provision and assessment of nutrition support therapy in the pediatric critically ill patient: Society of Critical Care Medicine and American Society for Parenteral and Enteral Nutrition. JPEN J Parenter Enteral Nutr. 2017;41(5):706–42.
100. Bechard LJ, Parrott JS, Mehta NM. Systematic review of the influence of energy and protein intake on protein balance in critically ill children. J Pediatr. 2012;161(2):333–9.e1.
101. Jotterand Chaparro C, Laure Depeyre J, Longchamp D, Perez MH, Taffé P, Cotting J. How much protein and energy are needed to equilibrate nitrogen and energy balances in ventilated critically ill children? Clin Nutr. 2016;35(2):460–7.
102. Freeman BD, Borecki IB, Coopersmith CM, Buchman TG. Relationship between tracheostomy timing and duration of mechanical ventilation in critically ill patients. Crit Care Med. 2005;33(11):2513–20.
103. Esteban A, Anzueto A, Alía I, Gordo F, Apezteguía C, Pálizas F, Cide D, Goldwaser R, Soto L, Bugedo G, Rodrigo C, Pimentel J, Raimondi G, Tobin MJ. How is mechanical ventilation employed in the intensive care unit? An international utilization review. Am J Respir Crit Care Med. 2000;161(5):1450–8.
104. Wakeham MK, Kuhn EM, Lee KJ, McCrory MC, Scanlon MC. Use of tracheostomy in the PICU among patients requiring prolonged mechanical ventilation. Intensive Care Med. 2014;40(6):863–70.

105. Baker CD. Long-term ventilation for children with chronic lung disease of infancy. Curr Opin Pediatr. 2019;31(3):357–66.
106. Sterni LM, Collaco JM, Baker CD, Carroll JL, Sharma GD, Brozek JL, Finder JD, Ackerman VL, Arens R, Boroughs DS, Carter J, Daigle KL, Dougherty J, Gozal D, Kevill K, Kravitz RM, Kriseman T, MacLusky I, Rivera-Spoljaric K, Tori AJ, Ferkol T, Halbower AC, ATS Pediatric Chronic Home Ventilation Workgroup. An Official American Thoracic Society clinical practice guideline: pediatric chronic home invasive ventilation. Am J Respir Crit Care Med. 2016;193(8):e16–35.
107. Sutt AL, Caruana LR, Dunster KR, Cornwell PL, Anstey CM, Fraser JF. Speaking valves in tracheostomised ICU patients weaning off mechanical ventilation—do they facilitate lung recruitment? Crit Care. 2016;1(20):91.
108. Fauroux B, Leboulanger N, Roger G, Denoyelle F, Picard A, Garabedian EN, Aubertin G, Clément A. Noninvasive positive-pressure ventilation avoids recannulation and facilitates early weaning from tracheotomy in children. Pediatr Crit Care Med. 2010;11(1):31–7.
109. Liptzin DR, Connell EA, Marable J, Marks J, Thrasher J, Baker CD. Weaning nocturnal ventilation and decannulation in a pediatric ventilator care program. Pediatr Pulmonol. 2016;51(8):825–9.
110. Mastouri M, Amaddeo A, Griffon L, Frapin A, Touil S, Ramirez A, Khirani S, Fauroux B. Weaning from long term continuous positive airway pressure or noninvasive ventilation in children. Pediatr Pulmonol. 2017;52(10):1349–54.
111. Pilar FJ, López-Fernandez YM. High-flow nasal cannula oxygen in acute respiratory post-extubation failure in pediatric patients: key practical topics and clinical implications. In: Esquinas A, editor. Noninvasive mechanical ventilation and difficult weaning in critical care. Springer; 2016.
112. Liu F, Shao Q, Jiang R, Zeng Z, Liu Y, Li Y, Liu Q, Ding C, Zhao N, Peng Z, Qian K. High-flow oxygen therapy to speed weaning from mechanical ventilation: a prospective randomized study. Am J Crit Care. 2019;28(5):370–6.
113. Hernández Martínez G, Rodriguez ML, Vaquero MC, Ortiz R, Masclans JR, Roca O, Colinas L, de Pablo R, Espinosa MD, Garcia-de-Acilu M, Climent C, Cuena-Boy R. High-flow oxygen with capping or suctioning for tracheostomy decannulation. N Engl J Med. 2020;383(11):1009–17.
114. Manley BJ, Owen LS, Doyle LW, Andersen CC, Cartwright DW, Pritchard MA, Donath SM, Davis PG. High-flow nasal cannulae in very preterm infants after extubation. N Engl J Med. 2013;369(15):1425–33. https://doi.org/10.1056/NEJMoa1300071.
115. Collins CL, Barfield C, Horne RS, Davis PG. A comparison of nasal trauma in preterm infants extubated to either heated humidified high-flow nasal cannulae or nasal continuous positive airway pressure. Eur J Pediatr. 2014;173(2):181–6.
116. Testa G, Iodice F, Ricci Z, Vitale V, De Razza F, Haiberger R, Iacoella C, Conti G, Cogo P. Comparative evaluation of high-flow nasal cannula and conventional oxygen therapy in paediatric cardiac surgical patients: a randomized controlled trial. Interact Cardiovasc Thorac Surg. 2014;19(3):456–61.
117. Lone NI, Walsh TS. Prolonged mechanical ventilation in critically ill patients: epidemiology, outcomes and modelling the potential cost consequences of establishing a regional weaning unit. Crit Care. 2011;15(2):R102.
118. Vagheggini G, Vlad EP, Mazzoleni S, Bortolotti U, Guarracino F, Ambrosino N. Outcomes for difficult-to-wean subjects after cardiac surgery. Respir Care. 2015;60(1):56–62.
119. Edwards JD, Rivanis C, Kun SS, Caughey AB, Keens TG. Costs of hospitalized ventilator-dependent children: differences between a ventilator ward and intensive care unit. Pediatr Pulmonol. 2011;46(4):356–61.
120. Ambrosino N, Vitacca M, Dreher M, Isetta V, Montserrat JM, Tonia T, Turchetti G, Winck JC, Burgos F, Kampelmacher M, Vagheggini G, ERS Tele-Monitoring of Ventilator-Dependent Patients Task Force. Tele-monitoring of ventilator-dependent patients: a European Respiratory Society statement. Eur Respir J. 2016;48(3):648–63.

121. Vitacca M, Guerra A, Assoni G, Pizzocaro P, Marchina L, Scalvini S, Balbi B. Weaning from mechanical ventilation followed at home with the aid of a telemedicine program. Telemed J E Health. 2007;13(4):445–9.
122. Cohn EC, Robertson TS, Scott SA, Finley AM, Huang R, Miles DK. Extubation failure and tracheostomy placement in children with acute neurocritical illness. Neurocrit Care. 2018;28(1):83–92.
123. Karanjia N, Nordquist D, Stevens R, Nyquist P. A clinical description of extubation failure in patients with primary brain injury. Neurocrit Care. 2011;15(1):4–12.
124. Holscher CM, Stewart CL, Peltz ED, Burlew CC, Moulton SL, Haenel JB, Bensard DD. Early tracheostomy improves outcomes in severely injured children and adolescents. J Pediatr Surg. 2014;49(4):590–2.
125. Gaies M, Tabbutt S, Schwartz SM, Bird GL, Alten JA, Shekerdemian LS, Klugman D, Thiagarajan RR, Gaynor JW, Jacobs JP, Nicolson SC, Donohue JE, Yu S, Pasquali SK, Cooper DS. Clinical epidemiology of extubation failure in the pediatric cardiac ICU: a report from the pediatric cardiac critical care consortium. Pediatr Crit Care Med. 2015;16(9):837–45.
126. Mastropietro CW, Cashen K, Grimaldi LM, Narayana Gowda KM, Piggott KD, Wilhelm M, Gradidge E, Moser EAS, Benneyworth BD, Costello JM. Extubation failure after neonatal cardiac surgery: a multicenter analysis. J Pediatr. 2017;182:190–196.e4.
127. Polito A, Patorno E, Costello JM, Salvin JW, Emani SM, Rajagopal S, Laussen PC, Thiagarajan RR. Perioperative factors associated with prolonged mechanical ventilation after complex congenital heart surgery. Pediatr Crit Care Med. 2011;12(3):e122–6.
128. Laudato N, Gupta P, Walters HL 3rd, Delius RE, Mastropietro CW. Risk factors for extubation failure following neonatal cardiac surgery. Pediatr Crit Care Med. 2015;16(9):859–67.
129. López-Fernández Y, Pilar-Orive FJ. Application of noninvasive ventilation in preventing extubation failure in children with heart disease: key topics and clinical implications. In: Esquinas A, editor. Noninvasive mechanical ventilation and difficult weaning in critical care. Springer; 2016.
130. Abman SH, Collaco JM, Shepherd EG, Keszler M, Cuevas-Guaman M, Welty SE, Truog WE, McGrath-Morrow SA, Moore PE, Rhein LM, Kirpalani H, Zhang H, Gratny LL, Lynch SK, Curtiss J, Stonestreet BS, McKinney RL, Dysart KC, Gien J, Baker CD, Donohue PK, Austin E, Fike C, Nelin LD, Bronchopulmonary Dysplasia Collaborative. Interdisciplinary care of children with severe bronchopulmonary dysplasia. J Pediatr. 2017;181:12–28.e1.
131. Hysinger EB, Friedman NL, Padula MA, Shinohara RT, Zhang H, Panitch HB, Kawut SM, Children's Hospitals Neonatal Consortium. Tracheobronchomalacia is associated with increased morbidity in bronchopulmonary dysplasia. Ann Am Thorac Soc. 2017 Sep 1;14(9):1428–35.
132. Fierro J, Piccione J, Lorch S. Clinical factors influencing time to decannulation in children with tracheostomy and ventilator dependence secondary to bronchopulmonary dysplasia. J Pediatr. 2021;228:31–5.
133. Hysinger EB, Panitch HB. Paediatric tracheomalacia. Paediatr Respir Rev. 2016;17:9–15.
134. Henningfeld JK, Maletta K, Ren B, Richards KL, Wegner C, D'Andrea LA. Liberation from home mechanical ventilation and decannulation in children. Pediatr Pulmonol. 2016;51(8):838–49.
135. Cristea AI, Carroll AE, Davis SD, Swigonski NL, Ackerman VL. Outcomes of children with severe bronchopulmonary dysplasia who were ventilator dependent at home. Pediatrics. 2013;132(3):e727–34.
136. Sherman JM, Davis S, Albamonte-Petrick S, Chatburn RL, Fitton C, Green C, Johnston J, Lyrene RK, Myer C 3rd, Othersen HB, Wood R, Zach M, Zander J, Zinman R. Care of the child with a chronic tracheostomy. This official statement of the American Thoracic Society was adopted by the ATS Board of Directors, July 1999. Am J Respir Crit Care Med. 2000;161(1):297–308.
137. de Trey L, Niedermann E, Ghelfi D, Gerber A, Gysin C. Pediatric tracheotomy: a 30-year experience. J Pediatr Surg. 2013;48(7):1470–5.

138. Guia M, Ciobanu LD, Sreedharan JK, Abdelrahim ME, Gonçalves G, Cabrita B, Alqahtani JS, Duan J, El-Khatib M, Diaz-Abad M, Wittenstein J, Karim HMR, Bhakta P, Ruggeri P, Garuti G, Burns KEA, Soo Hoo GW, Scala R, Esquinas A, International Association of Non Invasive Ventilation. The role of non-invasive ventilation in weaning and decannulating critically ill patients with tracheostomy: a narrative review of the literature. Pulmonology. 2021;27(1):43–51.
139. Trang H, Samuels M, Ceccherini I, Frerick M, Garcia-Teresa MA, Peters J, Schoeber J, Migdal M, Markstrom A, Ottonello G, Piumelli R, Estevao MH, Senecic-Cala I, Gnidovec-Strazisar B, Pfleger A, Porto-Abal R, Katz-Salamon M. Guidelines for diagnosis and management of congenital central hypoventilation syndrome. Orphanet J Rare Dis. 2020;15(1):252.

Prolonged and Long-Term Mechanical Ventilation in Children with Cardiac Diseases

Tadahito Kato and Atsushi Kawaguchi

1 Introduction

In recent years, improvements in surgical techniques for pediatric cardiac disease and medical management of heart failure have significantly improved the prognosis for children with heart disease [1]. On the other hand, an increasing number of patients require prolonged or long-term ventilatory support due to the diversification of treatment and residual surgical complications [2, 3]. The development of mechanical ventilators has also contributed to this situation by improving the types of respiratory support and the mobility of various devices [4]. Therefore, healthcare professionals responsible for the care of children with cardiac disease need to be familiar with a range of management options, from invasive ventilation in the intensive care unit to noninvasive ventilation (NIV) and home oxygen therapy.

Understanding cardiopulmonary interactions and circulatory and respiratory physiology is essential for respiratory management in pediatric cardiac disease. Respiratory support in cardiac disease has several cardiovascular benefits, including improved oxygenation due to pulmonary edema and pleural effusion, reduced oxygen consumption due to reduced respiratory effort and load, reduced left ventricular (LV) afterload, and improved pulmonary hypertension due to improved oxygenation and ventilation [5, 6]. However, in certain cases, such as congenital heart disease with a left-to-right shunt, supplemental oxygen may have a negative effect on hemodynamics by worsening pulmonary congestion. In addition, positive-pressure ventilation, such as the Fontan circulation, may worsen by inhibiting systemic venous return and pulmonary blood flow [7, 8]. It should also be recognized that unnecessary home mechanical ventilation (MV) should be avoided, as long-term

T. Kato (✉) . A. Kawaguchi
Division of Pediatric Critical Care, Department of Pediatrics,
St Marianna University, Kawasaki, Japan
e-mail: tadahito.kato@marianna-u.ac.jp; atsushi.kawaguchi@marianna-u.ac.jp

A. Kawaguchi et al. (eds.), *Prolonged and Long-Term Mechanical Ventilation in Children*, https://doi.org/10.1007/978-981-97-8903-0_9

mechanical ventilation and home mechanical ventilation can limit the patient's physical activity and thus development, in addition to being an economic problem. This chapter summarizes issues and concepts related to prolonged mechanical ventilation (PMV) in the pathophysiology of pediatric cardiac failure and acquired heart disease as a typical chronic heart disease and postoperative congenital heart disease as an acute condition.

2 Theory of Positive Ventilatory Support in Pediatric Cardiac Diseases

2.1 Respiratory Support in Left-Heart Failure

The main principles of mechanical ventilatory support in patients with left-heart failure are to improve oxygenation, reduce the work of breathing, and reduce left ventricular afterload. In a patient with left-heart failure, left ventricular end-diastolic pressure increases as left ventricular function deteriorates. This results in increased left atrial pressure, pulmonary venous pressure, and pulmonary capillary pressure. This causes fluid leakage from the capillaries into the lung interstitium, causing pulmonary edema and worsening oxygenation due to increased ventilation-perfusion (VQ) mismatch. Furthermore, the increased work of breathing due to reduced pulmonary and thoracic compliance from fluid retention increases oxygen consumption, leading to further worsening of heart failure.

Positive-pressure ventilation, including NIV, can improve oxygenation by dilating alveoli collapsed by fluid. Positive-pressure ventilation in left-heart failure also has a beneficial effect on circulatory dynamics by increasing the intrathoracic pressure. LV afterload is influenced by intrathoracic pressure. Especially during spontaneous breathing in pulmonary edema, exertional breathing produces a large negative pressure in the thoracic cavity. For example, if a negative pressure of 10 mmHg is applied, a force of 110 (100 + 10) mmHg is required in the LV to produce a systolic pressure of 100 mmHg. If a positive pressure of 10 mmHg is applied to the intrathoracic pressure by positive-pressure ventilation, the LV only needs to generate a transmural pressure of 90 (100–10) mmHg to produce the same blood pressure, resulting in a reduction in afterload [9].

Thus, in the setting of left ventricular failure, positive-pressure ventilation has advantages not only in terms of respiratory dynamics but also in terms of circulatory dynamics and can be a treatment for both respiratory and circulatory failure. In addition, reducing the respiratory workload will further reduce the cardiac workload if oxygen consumption can be reduced. However, there are insufficient data to conclude whether long-term positive-pressure ventilation is beneficial in the treatment of children with left-heart failure and to what extent it improves their prognosis, for example by avoiding heart transplantation or reducing its progression.

2.2 Congenital Heart Disease with Increased Pulmonary Blood Flow

In a biventricular circulation without shunt lesions, the benefits of MV support should be significant, and it makes sense in the management of heart failure. However, as many congenital heart disease (CHD) patients have some form of intracardiac shunt, the balance between systemic and pulmonary circulation must always be a consideration in the respiratory management of patients with CHD.

In CHD, a left-to-right shunt with increased pulmonary blood flow is a major cause of pulmonary congestion. It is important to understand that unlike left-heart failure caused by left ventricular dysfunction or valvular insufficiency, heart failure with increased pulmonary blood flow due to shunting is caused by inefficient circulation compared to normal biventricular circulation. For example, in a ventricular septal defect, blood flow from the left ventricle not only supplies systemic circulation via the aorta but also flows through the defect to the pulmonary artery, resulting in increased volume overload of the left ventricle.

Here is a simple example. First, assume that the cardiac output required for the left ventricle in a shunt-free biventricular circulation to supply the systemic circulation is 1. If the blood flow to the aorta and the blood flow to the pulmonary artery via the VSD are 1:1 (Qp/Qs = 2), then the total blood flow from the left ventricle (cardiac output) is 2. Thus, the left ventricle is subjected to twice the normal volume load due to this inefficient circulation. In this condition, if decompensated, left atrial and pulmonary venous pressures would be elevated even with normal left ventricular function. This would result in pulmonary edema.

The size of the defect is the most critical factor in determining the amount of shunt flowing from the left ventricle to the pulmonary artery. The balance between pulmonary and systemic vascular resistance is also important. Decreased pulmonary vascular resistance leads to worsening heart failure by increasing the left-to-right shunt across the defect. Oxygen saturation, CO_2, and lung volume are important factors in determining pulmonary vascular resistance (PVR). In heart failure with pulmonary edema and increased pulmonary blood flow, oxygen administration is contraindicated because it decreases PVR. Positive-pressure ventilation is often as useful as in normal left-heart failure, but the effect on PVR must be considered. The effects of positive-pressure ventilation on PVR are discussed below.

2.3 Right Ventricular Failure, Right Heart Bypass

Respiration significantly affects both PVR and systemic venous return. In addition, PVR and systemic venous return are critical factors that affect systemic circulation, especially in patients with right ventricular (RV) failure, such as after repair of tetralogy of Fallot (ToF) and after right-heart bypass surgery, such as the Glenn or Fontan operations. In addition, PVR directly affects venous return in right-heart bypass patients and also has a major impact on the systemic circulation as RV afterload in right-heart failure patients.

Oxygen saturation, CO_2, and lung volume are important factors in defining PVR; here, we discuss the relation between lung volume and PVR (Fig. 1). PVR is lowest when lung volume is close to functional residual capacity (FRC), which is the volume at the end of passive expiration of normal tidal breathing. As the lung volume decreases below FRC, the caliber of the extra-alveolar vessels decreases due to the lack of radial traction from the surrounding pulmonary interstitium, leading to an increase in PVR. In addition, hypoxia due to collapsed alveoli also causes pulmonary vasoconstriction, further increasing PVR. These are alleviated by alveolar expansion. Conversely, overexpansion causes alveolar vessels to be compressed by the alveoli, again increasing PVR. The sum of these two factors determines PVR; the relation follows the curve shown in the graph. In other words, PVR increases whether the lung volume is too large or too small [10].

During spontaneous breathing, inspiration creates a negative intrathoracic pressure (ITP) that reduces right atrial (RA) and RV transmural pressures and promotes venous return. The effect is more pronounced in patients with RV failure and right-heart bypass, such as the Fontan circulation. In contrast, during positive-pressure ventilation, ITP becomes positive, which inhibits venous return and may lead to organ congestion and decreased cardiac output due to inadequate LV preload. Thus, spontaneous breathing often has more advantages for circulation dependent on venous return. Therefore, the importance of avoiding positive-pressure ventilation, including early postoperative extubation, is emphasized in patients after repair of ToF and in those with Fontan circulation [8] [11]. However, if there is significant

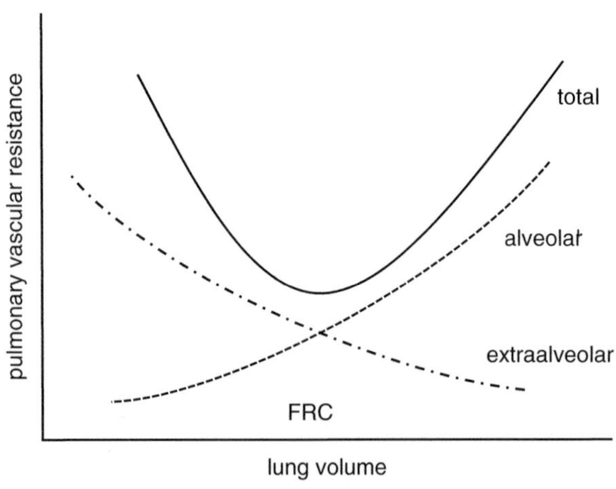

Fig. 1 The relation between pulmonary vascular resistance (PVR) and lung volume. As lung volume increases, the resistance of the alveolar vessels rises due to the distension of the alveoli. Meanwhile, the radial traction provided by the expanding lung distends the extra-alveolar vessels, leading to a decrease in the resistance of the extra-alveolar vessels. Total PVR becomes a U-shaped curve because of the combined effect of lung expansion on alveolar and extra-alveolar vessels, which is minimized at around the functional residual capacity (FRC)

alveolar collapse due to atelectasis or pleural effusion, this may cause an increase in PVR. In such cases, appropriate positive-pressure ventilation to expand the alveoli may decrease PVR as described before. Therefore, respiratory management should be designed to facilitate pulmonary circulation in each case. Although there is a lack of high-quality clinical evidence and consensus regarding the setting of positive end-expiratory pressure (PEEP) in cardiac patients undergoing MV, it is recommended that adequate PEEP (3–5 cmH_2O) be applied to maintain sufficient lung volume [12].

2.4 *Patients on Ventricular Assist Devices*

In recent years, the management of patients on extracorporeal life support has shifted from long-term MV to extubation and rehabilitation [13, 14]. Recent device advances have also allowed for long-term management of ventricular assist device (VAD) patients [15]. Although the majority of bridge-to-transplant patients are treated with a left ventricular assist device (LVAD) alone, it is important to note that RV failure may still be present after LVAD implantation. If RV failure is underestimated, the RV may not be able to accept the venous return produced by the increased cardiac output supported by the LVAD [16]. RV failure may cause respiratory compromise due to the development of pleural effusion and/or upper airway edema, which may prevent patients from weaning from respiratory support. It is important to balance the left and right heart, and sometimes a biventricular assist device should be used [17]. Although there are limited data on prolonged MV in patients after VAD implantation, LVAD implantation without a right VAD has been reported to be a risk factor for prolonged MV [18].

2.5 *Long-Term Prognosis and Harms of PMV in Heart Failure*

In addition to providing respiratory support, positive-pressure ventilation may also be beneficial for the circulation. The efficacy of MV in heart failure has been demonstrated, particularly in NPPV for acute heart failure [19]. However, there is currently a paucity of high-quality evidence on the prognosis and efficacy of prolonged MV in cardiac disease, both in children and adults. In a study investigating the effects of NIV in adults with heart failure, long-term NIV was shown to reduce systemic vascular resistance, increase cardiac output, and promote left ventricular reverse remodeling in patients with heart failure [20, 21]. It has also been suggested that the improvement in respiratory and circulatory function may provide a benefit by reducing sympathetic nerve activity [13]. A single-center study reported that long-term adaptive servo-ventilation (ASV) reduced arrhythmias, cardiac-related events, and cardiac arrest in chronic heart failure [22, 23].

The Canadian Continuous Positive Airway Pressure for Central Sleep Apnea and Heart Failure Trial (CANPAP) was a randomized controlled trial that evaluated the effects of CPAP in 258 heart failure patients with central sleep apnea. It reported an improvement in nocturnal oxygen saturation (SaO_2), a reduction in sympathetic nervous activity, and an increase in left ventricular ejection fraction (LVEF) and 6-min walk distance, but no improvement in heart transplant-free survival [24].

The SERVE-HF trial also evaluated the efficacy of long-term MV in heart failure with reduced ejection fraction complicated by sleep-disordered breathing in a randomized, controlled trial. The study compared all-cause mortality and lifesaving cardiovascular interventions such as heart transplantation, VAD implantation, resuscitation after sudden cardiac arrest, and hospitalization for worsening heart failure in the NIV group with those in the non-NIV group. The NIV group had a higher mortality rate than the control group [25]. Overall, there has been no high-quality evidence supporting favorable outcomes with NIV in adults with heart failure.

MV itself has the adverse effect of causing lung injury, such as barotrauma. In addition, long-term ventilation in cardiac disease may also reduce cardiac output due to lower LV preload caused by inhibition of venous return by continuous application of unnecessarily high expiratory positive airway pressure. It has also been suggested that respiratory alkalosis caused by hyperventilation may lead to hypokalemia, which may induce cardiac arrhythmias. Positive airway pressure is particularly likely to decrease cardiac output in heart failure patients with low pulmonary capillary wedge pressures and no pulmonary congestion [26].

This has led to advocacy for the importance of patient selection and optimization of device settings to improve long-term outcomes in heart failure patients. First, patients without pulmonary congestion (PCWP <12 mmHg) are unlikely to benefit from NIV. In addition, special care should be taken when introducing NIV and adjusting settings in patients with reduced EF (LVEF <45%).

In addition, the optimal setting is likely to vary from patient to patient. According to a report in adult patients with HF, PEEP should be adjusted to achieve maximum cardiac output while reducing pulmonary congestion. The method is to titrate PEEP and determine the optimal setting by measuring PCWP and cardiac output [27]. Stroke volume estimated by transthoracic echocardiography (calculated as left ventricular outflow tract area x LV outflow velocity-time integral) can also be used for noninvasive monitoring and readjustment of PEEP, which may improve long-term prognosis [28].

Children are more likely than adults to undergo pathophysiologic changes due to growth and development. In the case of single ventricle physiology, the stage of palliation may also cause significant changes in circulatory dynamics. In addition, in patients with significant RV failure or passive flow-dependent pulmonary circulation such as Glenn and Fontan, PEEP has a greater impact on the pulmonary and systemic circulation, requiring more careful ventilator settings.

2.6 PMV in Children After Cardiac Surgery

Since the 1990s, early tracheal extubation after pediatric cardiac surgery in the operating room or intensive care unit has become common. The safety of early extubation has also been established in neonates, early infants, and after surgery with cardiopulmonary bypass (CPB) for complex cardiac defects. Early tracheal extubation has the benefit of shortening ICU and hospital stays and reducing costs [29–31]. The benefits are particularly significant after bidirectional Glenn and Fontan operations, where withdrawal of positive-pressure ventilation is expected to reduce pulmonary artery pressure and improve hemodynamics [8].

However, due to significant hemodynamic changes from pre- to postoperative, inhibition of chest wall mechanics from open chest surgery, and lung damage from inflammation associated with CPB, children after cardiac surgery may require PMV [32, 33]. High morbidities such as ventilator-associated pneumonia and cost burden issues occur in children receiving PMV [34].

Neonates and early infants tend to have longer postoperative ventilation times after cardiac surgery than older patients. In contrast, patients with single ventricle physiology after bidirectional Glenn (BDG) or Fontan surgery have shorter ventilation times because extubation is more commonly performed in the operating room. Although the criteria for PMV vary with age and disease, it is important to recognize the risk factors for patients with PMV preoperatively, intraoperatively, and early postoperatively.

2.7 PMV After Biventricular Repair

Many studies have defined PMV as a ventilation period of 48 h to 7 days or longer, and using this definition, approximately 10% of patients will require PMV after cardiac surgery, and PMV itself has been reported to be associated with mortality [35–37].

In a study of 722 postoperative cardiac patients with CAD, preoperative predictors of PMV included young age and congestive heart failure [35]. In another validation of 411 postoperative patients with CAD, 103 (25%) had moderate MV (>61 h) and 38 had PMV (>7 days). In this study, when examining factors that occurred within 24 h of surgery, duration of CPB, intraoperative transfusion, post-CPB PaO_2/FiO_2 ratio, and fluid intake on the first day were associated with the duration of mechanical ventilation. Blood urea nitrogen level, delayed sternal closure, and tracheobronchomalacia were independent predictors of PMV for more than 7 days [36].

Furthermore, in 362 postoperative patients after complex cardiac surgery (risk adjustment in congenital heart surgery-1 > or = 3), the median duration of MV was 1.5 days, and 41 (11%) required PMV for more than 7 days. The following criteria were considered independent risk factors for prolonged mechanical ventilation in this study: younger age (<30 days), greater severity of illness on postoperative admission, healthcare-associated infection, major noncardiac structural anomalies, noninfectious pulmonary complications such as pleural effusion and pneumothorax, and need for reintervention [37].

2.8 Postoperative Cardiac PMVed Neonates and Early Infants

PMV has been defined as a postoperative ventilation period of 72–96 h or longer in the majority of relevant studies in neonates and young infants. In a multicenter retrospective study of 275 neonates, PMV (>96 h) was found in 89 patients (32%). The Vasoactive-Ventilation-Renal (VVR) score (ventilation index (VI) + vasoactive-inotrope score (VIS) + delta Cre (change in Cre from baseline×10)) was reported to be independently associated with PMV and can be used as a reliable predictor. VI and VIS are calculated as follows: VIS = dopamine dose [μg/kg/min] + dobutamine dose [μg/kg/min] + 100 × epinephrine dose [μg/kg/min] + 10 × milrinone dose [μg/kg/min] + 10,000 × vasopressin dose [U/kg/min] + 100 × norepinephrine dose [μg/kg/min], and VI = ([ventilator respiratory rate] × [peak inspiratory pressure − positive end-expiratory pressure] × Paco2)/1000. The VVR score is calculated at 0, 6, and 12 hours after admission. If the peak value is greater than or equal to 35 within 12 postoperative hours, patients should be considered at increased risk for VVR [38].

In a study of 172 postoperative cardiac patients aged 3 months or younger, 61 required PMV (>72 h). In this study, RACHS-1 (Risk Adjustment for Surgery for Congenital Heart Disease), nosocomial pneumonia, low cardiac output syndrome, postoperative fluid retention, and extubation failure were reported as risk factors for PMV [3].

2.9 PMV After Fontan Operation

In post-Fontan children, PMV is often defined as MV more than 12–24 h postoperatively, with reported risk rates ranging from 17% to 38%. Predictors of PMV in preoperative characteristics include younger age at surgery, heterotaxy syndrome, fenestration, smaller branch pulmonary artery size, and advanced atrioventricular valve regurgitation. Fenestration and branch pulmonary artery size indicate a poor pulmonary vascular bed and a suboptimal Fontan circuit.

Predictors of intraoperative data included intraoperative maximal vasoactive-inotropic score (VIS), prolonged CPB, aortic cross-clamp time, and minimum temperature during CPB. Higher VIS indicates impaired ventricular function, and longer aortic cross-clamp time indicates the need for atrioventricular valve repair. These are among the most important factors in Fontan hemodynamics. Postoperative characteristics including postoperative prothrombin time, alkaline phosphatase, total bilirubin level, postoperative fluid resuscitation, higher inotropic score, and treatment for pulmonary hypertension have been reported as predictors of PMV [39–41].

3 Specific Complications After Pediatric Cardiac Surgery

3.1 *Recurrent Nerve Palsy and Vocal Fold Immobility*

Aortic arch surgery carries a risk of recurrent laryngeal nerve injury, and postoperative vocal cord dysfunction (VCD) can be problematic. VCD can lead to feeding difficulties and aspiration. VCD occurs in approximately 5% of neonates and infants under 90 days of age and is unilateral in 75% of cases. It is usually complicated by aortic arch surgery (77%), but can also occur in non-aortic arch surgery. It is reported to be associated with feeding tube use, PMV, and surgical airways [42].

3.2 *Diaphragmatic Paralysis*

Phrenic nerve injury (PNI) is a critical complication in patients after cardiac surgery, reported to occur in 0.3–12.8% of cases [43]. It is rarely caused by direct dissection of the phrenic nerve and is most often due to transient neuropraxia caused by traction, cold water, or heat from electrocautery [44]. It can complicate various surgical procedures such as correction of ToF, arterial switch, closure of ventricular septal defect, Blalock-Taussig shunt, bidirectional Glenn, and Fontan operation [43, 45, 46]. In older children, diaphragmatic paralysis (DP) may be compensated by intercostal muscles. However, neonates and young infants are more likely to be affected by DP, leading to respiratory distress and respiratory failure, which can cause PMV [47]. Especially in postoperative Glenn and Fontan patients, DP can also inhibit passive venous blood flow on the lesion side and has significant circulatory effects such as pleural effusion in the early postoperative period and chronic ascites in the remote period [48].

3.3 *Diagnosis*

DP may be suspected if ventilator weaning is difficult or if the affected diaphragm is elevated on chest radiography. Fluoroscopy and ultrasound are useful for definitive diagnosis. Fluoroscopy has the advantage of simultaneously visualizing bilateral diaphragmatic motion over the respiratory cycle and has historically been considered the gold standard. However, it has disadvantages such as the need for transport to the cath lab and radiation exposure.

Bedside ultrasound has been reported to be more accurate than fluoroscopy, with sensitivity and specificity greater than 90% [44, 49]. The subcostal sagittal and posterior axillary longitudinal views are superior for evaluating the left and right diaphragms separately, while the subxiphoid coronal plane can evaluate both diaphragms simultaneously. If both diaphragms can be visualized, additional fluoroscopy is unnecessary in most patients. A retrospective observational study reported that ultrasound was less accurate than fluoroscopy in differentiating paradoxical diaphragm motion from paralysis due to lower sensitivity [50]. However, there is a report that M-mode in subcostal view combined with B-mode allows for a more objective evaluation and is more accurate in paradoxical motion [44].

3.4 Management

Diaphragmatic plication should be considered in cases of repeated reintubation, failure to wean from the ventilator, recurrent lung infections, and persistent respiratory distress [45]. In patients diagnosed with diaphragm paralysis, 19–67% have been reported to undergo plication surgery [43, 47, 51, 52]. The time from cardiac surgery to plication varies widely, with a median of 8–21 days, depending on the institution, and there are currently no widely accepted criteria [43, 45, 53].

In other words, it is unclear when to perform plication because DP does not always significantly affect respiratory status or may resolve spontaneously. One observational study reported the benefit of early plication (approximately 10 days after cardiac surgery) to prevent PMV [49, 53]. However, many patients may be able to avoid plication with a conservative approach [51] [52].

3.5 Prognosis and Recovery Rate

Evidence for recovery of diaphragmatic motion in the remote postoperative period is scarce, with only a few reports. In a follow-up study of 72 patients with DP, 40 plicated and 32 non-plicated, the rate of recovery of diaphragmatic motion was similar, 60% in the plicated group and 55% in the non-plicated group [46]. In a study of 46 children who underwent plication, fluoroscopic follow-up at an average of 16 months after surgery showed that the motion of the plicated diaphragm had recovered up to 77% of the contralateral side's excursion [53].

3.6 Bilateral Diaphragmatic Paralysis

Bilateral diaphragmatic paralysis (BDP) requires a different management strategy than unilateral DP. It has a worse prognosis and more limited clinical evidence compared to unilateral cases. In one report of seven bilateral cases, the median age was 2 months (0.6–12 months). In this report, five patients had paradoxical motion after recovery of one side of the diaphragm and underwent plication. The remaining two patients did not have paradoxical motion after unilateral recovery and were successfully weaned from the ventilator. The median duration of ventilation was 48 days (20–90 days), and no patient required a tracheostomy [54].

There is a case report of using NPPV in BDP to successfully avoid prolonged endotracheal intubation [55]. Nevertheless, in some cases, especially in BDP, tracheostomy may be necessary if diaphragmatic movement does not recover over a long period of time. However, tracheostomy itself has been reported to be associated with mortality, and it is unclear at what point tracheostomy should be performed [56].

4 Summary

In pediatric cardiac patients, the duration of MV should be evaluated in the context of different pathophysiology depending on the condition and underlying disease, that is, from the use of ventilators for circulatory support in patients with heart failure to the support of lung disease that occurs during the course of cardiac care. The definition of PMV after congenital heart surgery is also unique and requires caution in interpreting scientific evidence. Further clinical evidence is needed to help guide safe PMV and avoid unnecessary PMV in this cohort of children with cardiac disease.

References

1. Baumgartner H, et al. 2020 ESC guidelines for the management of adult congenital heart disease. Eur Heart J. 2021;42(6):563–645.
2. Temur B, et al. Outcomes of home mechanical ventilation with tracheostomy after congenital heart surgery. Cardiol Young. 2021;31(9):1484–8.
3. Shi S, et al. Perioperative risk factors for prolonged mechanical ventilation following cardiac surgery in neonates and young infants. Chest. 2008;134(4):768–74.
4. Fauroux B, et al. ERS statement on paediatric long-term noninvasive respiratory support. Eur Respir J. 2022;59(6):2101404.
5. Fessler, H.E., et al., Mechanism of reduced LV afterload by systolic and diastolic positive pleural pressure. J Appl Physiol (1985), 1988. 65(3): p. 1244–1250.

6. Imran TF, et al. Effect of continuous positive airway pressure treatment on pulmonary artery pressure in patients with isolated obstructive sleep apnea: a meta-analysis. Heart Fail Rev. 2016;21(5):591–8.
7. Williams DB, et al. Hemodynamic response to positive end-expiratory pressure following right atrium-pulmonary artery bypass (Fontan procedure). J Thorac Cardiovasc Surg. 1984;87(6):856–61.
8. Lofland GK. The enhancement of hemodynamic performance in Fontan circulation using pain free spontaneous ventilation. Eur J Cardiothorac Surg. 2001;20(1):114–8. discussion 118–9.
9. Buda AJ, et al. Effect of intrathoracic pressure on left ventricular performance. N Engl J Med. 1979;301(9):453–9.
10. Shekerdemian L, Bohn D. Cardiovascular effects of mechanical ventilation. Arch Dis Child. 1999;80(5):475–80.
11. Bronicki RA, et al. Hemodynamics and cerebral oxygenation following repair of tetralogy of Fallot: the effects of converting from positive pressure ventilation to spontaneous breathing. Congenit Heart Dis. 2010;5(5):416–21.
12. Kneyber MCJ, et al. Recommendations for mechanical ventilation of critically ill children from the Paediatric Mechanical Ventilation Consensus Conference (PEMVECC). Intensive Care Med. 2017;43(12):1764–80.
13. Cucchi M, et al. Awake extracorporeal life support and physiotherapy in adult patients: a systematic review of the literature. Perfusion. 2023;38(5):939–58. https://doi.org/10.1177/02676591221096078.
14. Anton-Martin P, et al. Extubation during pediatric extracorporeal membrane oxygenation: a single-center experience. Pediatr Crit Care Med. 2014;15(9):861–9.
15. Kanaya T, et al. Impact of long-term support with Berlin heart EXCOR® in pediatric patients with severe heart failure. Pediatr Cardiol. 2019;40(6):1126–33.
16. Farrar DJ, et al. Right heart interaction with the mechanically assisted left heart. World J Surg. 1985;9(1):89–102.
17. Saeed D. Right ventricular failure and biventricular support strategies. Cardiol Clin. 2018;36(4):599–607.
18. Prodhan P, et al. Risk factors for prolonged mechanical ventilation for children on ventricular assist device support. Ann Thorac Surg. 2015;99(5):1713–8.
19. Masip J, et al. Noninvasive ventilation in acute cardiogenic pulmonary edema: systematic review and meta-analysis. JAMA. 2005;294(24):3124–30.
20. Haruki N, et al. Comparison of acute and chronic impact of adaptive servo-ventilation on left chamber geometry and function in patients with chronic heart failure. Eur J Heart Fail. 2011;13(10):1140–6.
21. Takama N, Kurabayashi M. Effectiveness of adaptive servo-ventilation for treating heart failure regardless of the severity of sleep-disordered breathing. Circ J. 2011;75(5):1164–9.
22. Yoshihisa A, et al. Impact of adaptive servo-ventilation on cardiovascular function and prognosis in heart failure patients with preserved left ventricular ejection fraction and sleep-disordered breathing. Eur J Heart Fail. 2013;15(5):543–50.
23. Iwaya S, et al. Suppressive effects of adaptive servo-ventilation on ventricular premature complexes with attenuation of sympathetic nervous activity in heart failure patients with sleep-disordered breathing. Heart Vessel. 2014;29(4):470–7.
24. Arzt M, et al. Suppression of central sleep apnea by continuous positive airway pressure and transplant-free survival in heart failure: a post hoc analysis of the Canadian continuous positive airway pressure for patients with Central Sleep Apnea and Heart Failure Trial (CANPAP). Circulation. 2007;115(25):3173–80.
25. Cowie MR, et al. Adaptive servo-ventilation for central sleep apnea in systolic heart failure. N Engl J Med. 2015;373(12):1095–105.
26. Bradley TD, et al. Cardiac output response to continuous positive airway pressure in congestive heart failure. Am Rev Respir Dis. 1992;145(2 Pt 1):377–82.

27. Imamura T, Nitta D, Kinugawa K. Optimization of pressure settings during adaptive servo-ventilation support using real-time heart rate variability assessment: initial case report. BMC Cardiovasc Disord. 2017;17(1):11.
28. Sekiguchi H, et al. A novel optimized adaptive servo-ventilation setting for a patient with severe heart failure based on the echocardiogram: a case report. Eur Heart J Case Rep. 2022;6(3):ytac074.
29. Heinle JS, Diaz LK, Fox LS. Early extubation after cardiac operations in neonates and young infants. J Thorac Cardiovasc Surg. 1997;114(3):413–8.
30. Kloth RL, Baum VC. Very early extubation in children after cardiac surgery. Crit Care Med. 2002;30(4):787–91.
31. Neirotti RA, et al. Early extubation in congenital heart surgery. Heart Lung Circ. 2002;11(3):157–61.
32. Harrison AM, et al. Failed extubation after cardiac surgery in young children: prevalence, pathogenesis, and risk factors. Pediatr Crit Care Med. 2002;3(2):148–52.
33. Clark SC. Lung injury after cardiopulmonary bypass. Perfusion. 2006;21(4):225–8.
34. Fischer JE, Allen P, Fanconi S. Delay of extubation in neonates and children after cardiac surgery: impact of ventilator-associated pneumonia. Intensive Care Med. 2000;26(7):942–9.
35. Ben-Abraham R, et al. Predictors for mortality after prolonged mechanical ventilation after cardiac surgery in children. J Crit Care. 2002;17(4):235–9.
36. Székely A, et al. Intraoperative and postoperative risk factors for prolonged mechanical ventilation after pediatric cardiac surgery. Paediatr Anaesth. 2006;16(11):1166–75.
37. Polito A, et al. Perioperative factors associated with prolonged mechanical ventilation after complex congenital heart surgery. Pediatr Crit Care Med. 2011;12(3):e122–6.
38. Cashen K, et al. Multicenter validation of the vasoactive-ventilation-renal score as a predictor of prolonged mechanical ventilation after neonatal cardiac surgery. Pediatr Crit Care Med. 2018;19(11):1015–23.
39. Luo Q, et al. Risk factors for prolonged mechanical ventilation after total cavopulmonary connection surgery: 8 years of experience at Fuwai hospital. J Cardiothorac Vasc Anesth. 2020;34(4):940–8.
40. Salvin JW, et al. Factors associated with prolonged recovery after the Fontan operation. Circulation. 2008;118(14 Suppl):S171–6.
41. Song Y, et al. Predictive factors contributing to prolonged recovery in patients after Fontan operation. BMC Pediatr. 2022;22(1):501.
42. Gorantla SC, et al. Current epidemiology of vocal cord dysfunction after congenital heart surgery in young infants. Pediatr Crit Care Med. 2019;20(9):817–25.
43. Joho-Arreola AL, et al. Incidence and treatment of diaphragmatic paralysis after cardiac surgery in children. Eur J Cardiothorac Surg. 2005;27(1):53–7.
44. Gil-Juanmiquel L, et al. Bedside ultrasound for the diagnosis of abnormal diaphragmatic motion in children after heart surgery. Pediatr Crit Care Med. 2017;18(2):159–64.
45. Akay TH, et al. Diaphragmatic paralysis after cardiac surgery in children: incidence, prognosis and surgical management. Pediatr Surg Int. 2006;22(4):341–6.
46. Smith BM, et al. Course, predictors of diaphragm recovery after phrenic nerve injury during pediatric cardiac surgery. Ann Thorac Surg. 2013;96(3):938–42.
47. Floh AA, et al. The advantage of early plication in children diagnosed with diaphragm paresis. J Thorac Cardiovasc Surg. 2017;154(5):1715–1721.e4.
48. Ovroutski S, et al. Paralysis of the phrenic nerve as a risk factor for suboptimal Fontan hemodynamics. Eur J Cardiothorac Surg. 2005;27(4):561–5.
49. Parmar D, et al. Early diagnosis of diaphragm palsy after pediatric cardiac surgery and outcome after diaphragm plication—a single-center experience. Ann Pediatr Cardiol. 2021;14(2):178–86.
50. Miller SG, Brook MM, Tacy TA. Reliability of two-dimensional echocardiography in the assessment of clinically significant abnormal hemidiaphragm motion in pediatric cardiothoracic patients: comparison with fluoroscopy. Pediatr Crit Care Med. 2006;7(5):441–4.

51. Georgiev S, et al. Phrenic nerve injury after paediatric heart surgery: is aggressive plication of the diaphragm beneficial? Eur J Cardiothorac Surg. 2013;44(5):808–12.
52. Denamur S, et al. Outcome analysis of a conservative approach to diaphragmatic paralysis following congenital cardiac surgery in neonates and infants: a bicentric retrospective study. Interact Cardiovasc Thorac Surg. 2021;33(4):597–604.
53. Baker CJ, et al. Hemidiaphragm plication after repair of congenital heart defects in children: quantitative return of diaphragm function over time. J Thorac Cardiovasc Surg. 2008;135(1):56–61.
54. Bhaskar P, et al. Bilateral diaphragmatic palsy after congenital heart surgery: management options. Cardiol Young. 2016;26(5):927–30.
55. Kovacikova L, Dobos D, Zahorec M. Non-invasive positive pressure ventilation for bilateral diaphragm paralysis after pediatric cardiac surgery. Interact Cardiovasc Thorac Surg. 2009;8(1):171–2.
56. Cotts T, et al. Tracheostomy after pediatric cardiac surgery: frequency, indications, and outcomes. J Thorac Cardiovasc Surg. 2011;141(2):413–8.

Prolonged Mechanical Ventilation in Children Born with Prematurity

Analía Fernández and Yolanda M. López-Fernández

1 Introduction

When chronic lung disease of prematurity was described for the first time by Northway et al. [1], over 50 years ago, lung injury was the result of postnatal mechanical ventilation and oxygen therapy in infants born before 36 weeks of gestation. Advances in neonatal intensive care have led to the survival of extremely preterm infants [2] with lungs structurally and biochemically immature that suffer from a severe developmental arrest of alveolar and microvascular growth [3]. The subsequent impaired lung growth and postnatal injury of the lung and airways caused lifesaving invasive and noninvasive ventilatory support and oxygen therapy, resulting in a new form of bronchopulmonary dysplasia (BPD). In the most severely affected neonates, it will lead to chronic respiratory failure, prolonged mechanical ventilation, and tracheostomy, providing the support necessary to grow and develop [3, 4].

The incidence of BPD increases as the gestational age (GA) decreases and varies between NICUs, ranging between 15% and 65%, and has been reported up to 77% in infants born ≤32 weeks of GA [2, 5]. Even with significant improvements in perinatal care including surfactant treatment, administration of antenatal corticosteroids, and ventilatory strategies, the incidence of BPD did not decrease, likely due to the survival of the most immature infants. Therefore, the number of patients with BPD requiring tracheostomy and prolonged mechanical ventilation (PMV) has been increasing significantly over the decades, from 0.7 to 2 per 100,000 to 6.3 per 100,000 children

A. Fernández (✉)
Pediatric Intensive Care Unit, Hospital General de Agudos "C. Durand", Ciudad Autónoma de Buenos Aires, Argentina

Y. M. López-Fernández
Pediatric Intensive Care Unit, Department of Pediatrics, Cruces University Hospital, Biocruces-Bizkaia Health Research Institute, Bizkaia, Spain
e-mail: yolandamarg.lopezfernandez@osakidetza.eus

A. Kawaguchi et al. (eds.), *Prolonged and Long-Term Mechanical Ventilation in Children*, https://doi.org/10.1007/978-981-97-8903-0_10

[6–8]. Several studies describe a marked reduction in predischarge mortality of infants with tracheostomy-dependent BPD from 50% to 15–14% [4–9]. In the preterm population, especially those with very low birth weight, risk factors associated with extubation failure are lower gestational age, lower 5-min Apgar score, use of total parenteral nutrition (TPN) with delayed full enteral feeding, PMV (>7 days), and use of inotropes, among others. Although the mechanisms by which the use of inotropes affects extubation success are unknown, hemodynamic instability may affect pulmonary and cerebral maturity. Thus, extubation failure in preterm infants affects subsequent respiratory morbidity (BPD), but a higher rate of intraventricular hemorrhage (IVH) has also been reported [10–12]. Children with BPD and PMV might be transferred from the NICU to a PICU or a post-acute care facility to adequate or initiative ventilatory support with home portable ventilators. Most children with BPD can be liberated from MV, but some of them will require home respiratory support [13].

To define PMV for this group of patients, we use chronological age or corrected age [14]. In neonates, age can be counted from birth (chronological) or using the corrected age, reducing the number of weeks born before 40 weeks of gestation to the chronological age. Sauthier et al. [14] propose that the corrected age should be used in the definition of pediatric PMV to standardize the maturation stage of neonates, in cohorts that include premature and term neonates, the usual case in PICUs. Pediatric PMV will not include within 21 consecutive days before 37 weeks of gestational age. This means that the definition of pediatric PMV could not be applied before 40 weeks of gestational age [14].

Children with BPD might also require PICU and PMV after being discharged from NICU. Hospitalization rates for infants with BPD are higher than those of the general population and preterms without BPD. They also have substantial risk for ICU readmissions and often require prolonged mechanical ventilation and extensive healthcare resources and incur high treatment costs. One of the most frequent reasons for readmission is respiratory illness, including reactive airway disease, pneumonia, and respiratory syncytial virus infection, and ranges between 43 and 63% of hospital admissions during the first 2 years of life [15, 16]. Fraser et al. in a retrospective review of 13 years in one PICU in England reported that 10% of the patients requiring MV for more than 28 days were patients with an acute respiratory infection and BPD [17]. Chronic lung diseases had been associated with failed extubation [18]. A prolonged mechanical ventilation course may be caused by a failed extubation. Despite the lung injury caused by BPD, this condition is not often described among the risk factors for higher extubation failure [19–22], and its association with extubation failure was only reported in one study [23].

2 BPD Definitions

A persistent challenge in the study and treatment of BPD is the lack of an effective definition. BPD was first described by Northway et al. in 1967 based on radiographic and pathological evidence of pulmonary disease (opacification, atelectasis, cysts, radiolucency) observed in late preterm neonates (mean gestational age of 34 weeks) following prolonged exposure to supplemental oxygen and mechanical ventilation [1]. The

National Heart, Lung, and Blood Institute (NHLBI) in 1978 sponsored a workshop that defined BPD as 28 days of oxygen exposure with characteristic radiographic changes. Shennan et al., after following 600 infants with birth weights <1500 g for 2 years, proposed a change in the time of evaluation of oxygen requirement at 36 weeks postmenstrual age (PMA), since it better predicted adverse pulmonary outcomes [24]. Surfactant treatment changed the outcomes of premature infants and the histology of their lungs. Even when the number of alveoli and capillaries was reduced, airway injury and inflammation were less prominent, and fewer areas of hyperinflation, parenchymal fibrosis, and focal collapse were observed. Improvement in neonatal treatment of premature infants caused a shift in BPD prevalence to very-low-birth-weight infants with pronounced alveolar and vascular "growth arrest" and led to the distinction of a new form of BPD [6]. Therefore, in 2000, the National Institute of Child Health and Human Development (NICHD), NHLBI, and Office of Rare Diseases (ORD) proposed the new definition of BPD [25]. This definition assesses for BPD at 36 weeks PMA in infants <32 weeks gestation who required supplemental oxygen for at least 28 days. An abnormal radiograph was no longer required. This definition also stratified BPD severity, based on the amount of supplemental oxygen and mode of respiratory support at 36 weeks of GA, in mild, moderate, or severe cases. The definition includes "room air challenge test" that consists of the withdrawal of supplemental oxygen for 1 h. If their oxygen saturation drops below 90%, they can be defined as having BPD by this definition. They include a physiologic assessment rather than the oxygen requirement since the last one is subjective and provider dependent. New devices of noninvasive support were developed after the definition, as well as infants dead before 36 weeks of GA caused by severe forms of BPD have no room in this definition, which motivates the latest revision of the definition in 2016 focused on respiratory outcomes during early life. Therefore, a new definition was proposed in 2018 at a conference conducted by the NIH Eunice Kennedy Shriver National Institute of Child Health and Human Development (NICHD) [26]. The NICHD definition includes infants born ≤32 weeks of GA who require ventilator support (invasive or noninvasive) for more than three consecutive days, to maintain arterial oxygen saturation above 90% at 36 weeks PMA and the confirmation of lung disease with an abnormal radiograph. Invasive positive-pressure dependence at 36 weeks, regardless of the degree of hypoxemia, has recently been shown to be the strongest predictor of death and serious respiratory morbidity during the first 2 years of life. The disease severity is classified into three groups, with grade III being the most severe form of BPD. Grade III (A) includes infants who died because of parenchymal lung disease and respiratory failure. Like previous definitions, this definition struggles with early identification of BPD, which might help in the decision of applying targeted therapies to the most at-risk infants [26].

3 BDP Pathophysiology

Pulmonary development has five stages: embryonic (4–6 weeks GA), pseudoglandular (5–17 weeks GA), canalicular (16–25 weeks GA), saccular (24–32 weeks GA), and alveolar stages (from 33 GA weeks to infancy) [27]. During the embryonic stage, the larynx, trachea, and main bronchi develop; during the pseudoglandular stage, the generation of the bronchial tree up to the terminal bronchioles occurs, with the formation of an arterial system; while during the canalicular and saccular stages, the differentiation between the conductive pathways and alveoli begins. The production of pulmonary surfactant starts at 24 weeks GA. In the alveolar phase, the division of the saccules into alveoli occurs. The alveolar division process continues throughout childhood. BPD is a consequence of the early interruption of the lung development process and postnatal lung injuries. Those different forms of lung injury are caused by different mechanisms with specific molecular pathways. These mechanisms may affect, in a relatively specific way, airways, alveoli, vessels, interstitium, and lymphatic systems, giving rise to different clinical phenotypes of BPD [28]. The pulmonary development process can be interrupted in the canalicular or saccular phase, and consequently the structural alteration of the lung is more severe during the lower gestational age.

But current definitions involve infants born at or before 32 weeks of gestation. Two main pathways lead to birth before 32 weeks of gestation: infection/inflammation (chorioamnionitis, pre-labor rupture of membranes) and dysfunctional placentation associated with hypertensive disorders of pregnancy and intrauterine growth restriction. Inflammation cytokines and mediators influence the regulation of alveolar development, angiogenesis, and airway remodeling and induce sustained abnormalities of distal lung growth and pulmonary hypertension. Placental dysfunction is caused by a complex interplay of pro- and antiangiogenic factors, oxidative stress, and other pathways providing impairment in alveolar and lung vascular growth, even in the absence of postnatal factors [29]. Low oxygen tension during embryonic and fetal development is essential for proper vascular development and lung morphogenesis. The excessive postnatal increase in oxygen tension downregulates the expression of the hypoxia-inducible factor (HIF)-regulated genes (HRGs) that causes a disturbance of the overall developmental program [30].

After birth, oxidative stress (OS) alters the molecular pathways involved in lung development, leading to impaired alveolarization, pulmonary microvascular remodeling, smooth muscle hyperplasia, and moderate fibrosis. OS causes excessive apoptosis of type II pneumocytes and induces an imbalance of mesenchymal-epithelial signaling that leads to the transdifferentiation of pulmonary alveolar lipofibroblasts into myofibroblasts. Lipofibroblasts protect the alveolus from oxidative damage, while myofibroblasts are unable to maintain lung epithelial cell growth and differentiation, resulting in alveolarization [31].

3.1 Pathogenesis of Parenchymal Disorders

There are several injuries with specific manifestations that affect the lung parenchyma, referred to as phenotypes [28].

The *parenchymal phenotype* of BPD is characterized by larger and fewer alveoli and reduced alveolar surface area, resulting in emphysema with areas of hyperinflation and fibrous interstitial abnormalities, and leading to impaired gas exchange due to the arrest of development of the alveolus [32]. Pulmonary mechanics shows increased compliance with obstructive airflow limitation. Alveolar septation and alveolar multiplication that take place from 36 weeks of GA until 3 years of life improve parenchymal injury allowing the weaning of respiratory support [33]. This phenotype could be found in computed tomography, alone or in combination with others, in up to 78% of patients with severe BPD [34].

Interstitial phenotype shows an increase in fibrotic tissue and widening of the interstitial spaces, with lower compliance of the lung and without an obstructive pattern. Interstitial injury may be worsened by the capillary leak from inflammation due to infection, respiratory distress syndrome (RDS), or ventilator-induced lung injury (VILI) [28].

Congestive phenotype is a consequence of immature and inadequate pulmonary lymphatic drainage. Infants are prone to pulmonary edema that might affect surfactant activity and result in atelectasis and decrease compliance of the lung [28].

3.2 Pathogenesis of Acquired Airway Disorders in Premature Infants

The anatomical maturation of the fetal airways precedes alveolar development, but the airways are immature at birth and highly susceptible to damage before the maturational process is complete [35].

The endotracheal tube (ETT) can cause ischemic necrosis in the contact area of the laryngeal surface. The movement of the ETT against the mucosa also contributes to upper airway injury [35]. It can result in granuloma formation, subglottic stenosis, and cricoarytenoid fixation, and in more severe and rare cases, complications like tracheal rupture and retropharyngeal abscess occur [36].

Positive-pressure ventilation (PPV) imposes physical forces on the immature airways and may cause marked airway deformation of the relatively compliant airways. These cause changes in the airway chondrocytes and in extracellular matrix expression, which might delay the growth and differentiation of the conducting airways. This results in increased tracheal diameter, and thinning of airway cartilage and smooth muscle, which exacerbate the congenital weakness of the premature airway wall, resulting in increased collapsibility and decreased resistance to deformation. After prolonged PPV, tracheomegaly and tracheobronchomalacia (TBM) could develop in premature infants. In infants who required prolonged intubation, failed extubation is often the first sign of developing acquired airway problems when an infant with minimum ventilator support develops significant respiratory distress soon after extubation with or without stridor, or episodes of apnea/bradycardia/desaturation (A/B/D). Episodic cyanotic spells might be caused by airway collapse due to severe tracheo- and/or bronchomalacia [35].

Airway obstruction due to small airway constriction is present in most infants with established BPD. Studies have suggested that prematurity may be associated with neutrophilic airway inflammation and oxidative stress later in life rather than with eosinophilic inflammation as seen in children with asthma [37]. Only a subset of infants will respond to bronchodilator therapy with B-agonists, and a trial of bronchodilator therapy is indicated to assess response. In patients with responsiveness to B agonists, steroids upregulate B-adrenergic receptors, and for this reason, inhaled steroids remain indicated in those patients [35].

3.3 Pulmonary Arterial Hypertension

Pulmonary hypertension is associated with higher morbidity and mortality in BPD infants, especially in the first 6 months after the initial diagnosis. Several factors including antenatal exposure to oxidative stress or fetal growth restriction, and postnatal stress, such as hyperoxia, aggressive ventilation, or sepsis, may alter vascular development and vascular remodeling with smooth muscle cell proliferation and contribute to a significant reduction in the cross-sectional area of the pulmonary vascular bed, with an increase in pulmonary vascular resistance that leads to pulmonary arterial hypertension [39]. The vascular phenotype of BPD appears to be strongly associated with the endotype of placental vascular dysfunction. Retrospective studies show that late pulmonary hypertension may occur in up to 17–43% of infants with BPD and that the mortality rate of the condition may be as high as 14–38% [28].

Computed tomography angiogram enables precise and objective delineation of the tracheobronchial pathology, in addition to the evaluation of the adjacent cardiovascular system and lung parenchyma. Newer CT techniques such as dynamic and volumetric imaging have increased the sensitivity and accuracy in the diagnosis of airway stenosis and malacia [38].

Wu et al. [40], in a retrospective study of a cohort of preterm infants with severe BPD, describe that approximately 12% of the included infants had pure parenchymal lung disease, 8% had pulmonary hypertension, and 7% had large airway disease as a major cause for their oxygen dependency. The most common phenotypic presentation (32%) was the co-occurrence of all three components [40].

Postnatal steroids (PSs) prevent progression to BPD and facilitate weaning of ventilator-dependent infants, but PS use is also associated with an increased incidence of neurodevelopmental impairment, even assuming that BPD itself increases the risk of neurodevelopmental impairment. In a recent study, PS in infants at high risk of BPD was associated with increased rates of gross motor abnormalities at two years of corrected age, regardless of the type of steroid [41].

On the other side, it seems sensible to consider genetic testing (with its inherent limitations) and lung biopsy in addition to imaging in infants with atypical BPD. As a diffuse lung disease, the clinical characteristics of BPD may be similar to a wide range of disorders under the category of childhood interstitial lung disease (ChILD). Some lung biopsies from infants with atypical forms of BPD have been diagnosed of pulmonary interstitial glycogenosis that responds favorably to high doses of systemic steroids [42].

4 BPD Ventilatory Strategies

Ventilatory strategies in the early postnatal period or in a patient admitted to the PICU with a respiratory reagudization are primarily aimed at avoiding lung injury and prioritize weaning support whenever possible. To avoid VILI, fast weaning to noninvasive ventilation is targeted during the acute phase in neonates. However, in patients with severe BPD, weaning may not be accomplished, and prolonged invasive support may be required [39]. The goals of care and the strategies are strikingly different between protective and chronic ventilation. Chronic ventilation aims to support the severely affected neonate's breathing and enable the infant to grow and develop. Appropriate ventilator strategies for established chronic lung disease account for the observed pathophysiology. In these patients, the complex interplay of large and small airways as well as the heterogeneity of lung parenchymal disease needs to be considered [43–45].

In the parenchymal phenotype, the lung is a heterogeneous tissue with regional differences in compliance and resistance. Emphysematous regions are relatively slow-emptying compartments of the lung with longer respiratory time constants that require substantially higher tidal volumes and longer inspiratory and expiratory times for optimal ventilation of these compartments. Additionally, the diameter of the proximal airways decreases, and the resistance increases during expiration. Airway closure may occur due to tracheomalacia or bronchomalacia. Flow–volume curves often exhibit expiratory flow limitation because of the expiratory collapse of poorly supported small airways. The use of high PEEP values will keep the airway open and can be titrated by observing the flow–volume graphics, increasing the level of PEEP until the expiratory flow limitation is resolved. The use of higher PEEP values in the presence of air trapping facilitates the complete emptying of the airways during expiration, especially in the slow compartment section. To avoid the risk of air trapping, higher PEEP values should be administered with low ventilator rates and adequate expiratory time. When inappropriate PEEP values are selected, the lungs become hyperinflated, causing increased pulmonary vascular resistance, increased work of breathing, increased oxygen demand, and hypercapnia. In the presence of intrinsic PEEP, the infant is not able to trigger the ventilator, resulting in air hunger and agitation. Careful monitoring and evaluation of pressure-volume, volume-flow, and time-flow graphs during the ventilation of these infants are critical [44–48].

Ventilatory strategy in the chronic phase of a parenchymal phenotype requires a larger tidal volume (10–12 mL/kg), given slowly (inspiratory time ≥ 0.6 s) to more evenly distribute breaths throughout the heterogeneous lung and reduce air hunger. Slower respiratory rates mitigate air trapping ($\leq$20 breaths per minute), and higher values of PEEP allow optimal management of airway disease. Even in those without large airway malacia, higher PEEP may be necessary to match the intrinsic PEEP. In interstitial and congestive phenotypes, the ventilatory strategy includes lower tidal volumes (6–8 mL/kg) and higher Ti and higher PEEP values to prevent atelectasis. FiO_2 should target higher SpO_2 to prevent pulmonary hypertension and desaturation spells (92–96%) [45, 46].

Some centers utilize neurally adjusted ventilatory assist (NAVA) ventilation to improve synchrony. There are some important considerations regarding NAVA ventilation. The patient must have an intact central drive and requires an esophageal catheter. The potential role of NAVA ventilation, either invasive or noninvasive, in preterm infants during both the acute and chronic stages of developing BPD appears to offer interesting results according to Shetty et al. [49]. Although the NAVA mode does not change BPD rates, infants receiving NAVA or NIV-NAVA have favorable outcomes in terms of extubation failure rates, duration of invasive ventilation, total duration of mechanical ventilation, and total length of stay.

BPD and Liberation of Invasive Respiratory Support

Pulmonary growth will allow a progressive reduction of ventilatory settings. Careful attention must be paid to the impact that this reduction has on the infant's respiratory stability, work of breathing, growth, and developmental progress. Weaning off ventilator support reduces the morbimortality associated with mechanical ventilation, but weaning the respiratory support too quickly may result in a significant increase in work of breathing and affects growth, and the healing process, and may even exacerbate lung disease and pulmonary hypertension.

Extubation to noninvasive ventilation may be attempted, and if the patient tolerates extubation and remains stable, noninvasive support could be weaned. Continuous positive airway pressure (CPAP) is often used to wean infants from mechanical ventilation. Although some studies showed that NCPAP facilitates extubation as compared with oxygen, others found no difference [50–55]. However, a recent meta-analysis favors the use of prophylactic NCPAP post-extubation from mechanical ventilation [56]. In a randomized controlled trial comparing the efficacy of synchronized nasal intermittent positive-pressure ventilation (SNIPPV) versus NCPAP as modes of extubation in the weaning of premature infants ≤34 weeks from prolonged mechanical ventilation, Khalafet et al. reported that 94% of infants who were randomized to receive SNIPPV were extubated successfully as compared with 60% of those on NCPAP (P.01) [56].

During weaning, if noninvasive support is only required for a portion of each day, it may be considered for the treatment of BPD. But some patients will not tolerate extubation or noninvasive support as a means of weaning. In these cases, prolonged ventilation through a tracheostomy should be considered. Long-term continuous noninvasive ventilation interferes with developmental progress and tends to be less secure than an invasive tracheostomy (Fig. 1).

There is an increase in tracheostomy rates in extremely low-birth-weight infants. But timing and indication of tracheostomy remain controversial. It is indicated in infants with severe upper airway disease [8, 56]. In infants with severe BPD who need long-term ventilatory support, earlier tracheostomy (before 120 days of life) may be associated with better outcomes [57, 58]. Once the patient is stabilized with chronic ventilation strategies, the need for a tracheostomy is warranted. It seems reasonable to evaluate the patient, give more time for stabilization, and intend weaning of respiratory support. But when consecutive attempts to wean support fail, tracheostomy should be considered. Once the tracheostomy has been placed, a

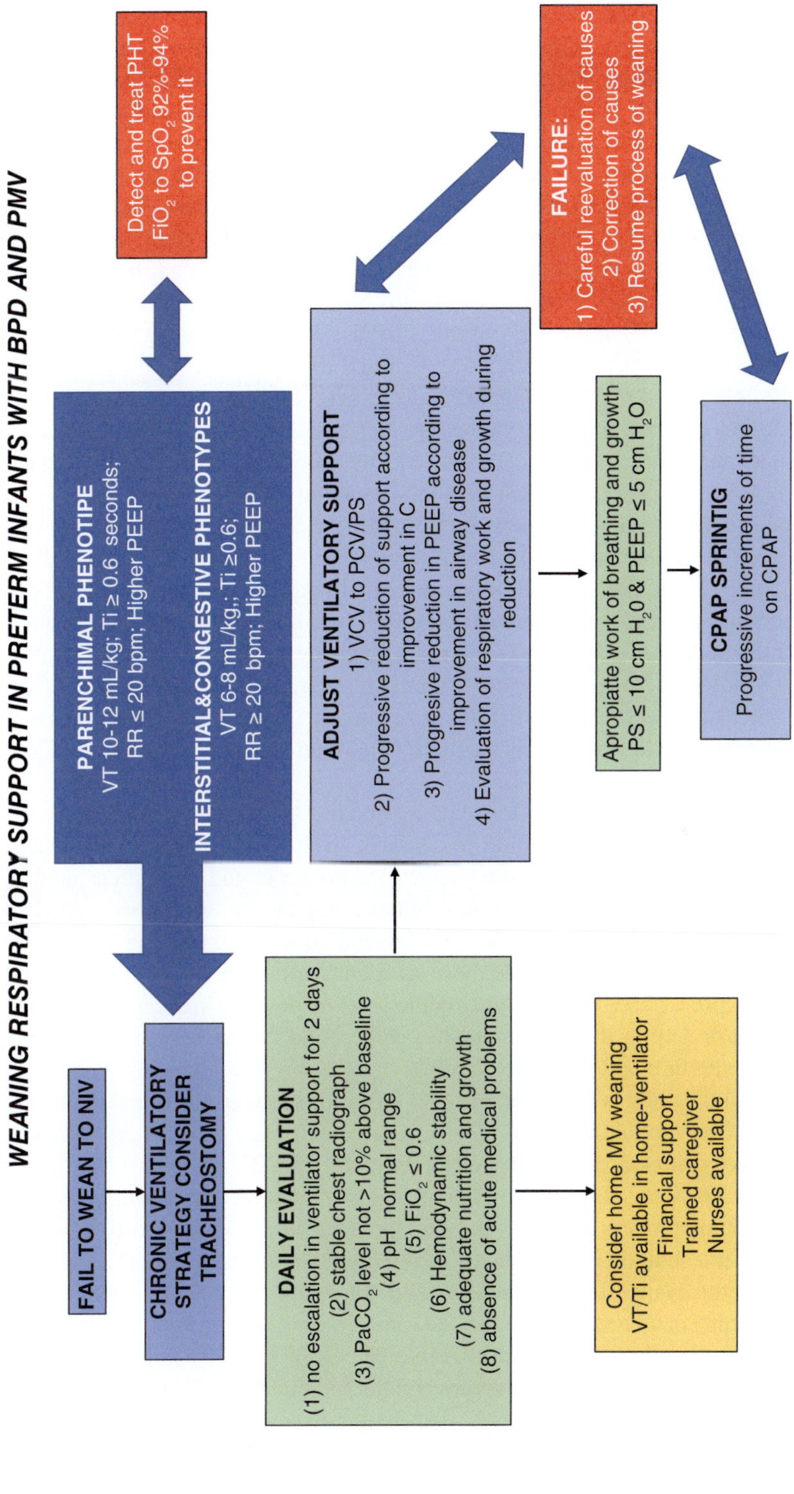

Fig. 1 Algorithm for weaning respiratory support in preterm infants with BPD and PMV. *BPD*, bronchopulmonary dysplasia, *bpm* breaths per minute, *C* compliance, *CPAP* continuous positive airway pressure, FiO_2 inspired fraction of oxygen, *MV* mechanical ventilation, *NIV* noninvasive ventilation, *PCV* pressure control ventilation, *PEEP* positive end-expiratory pressure, *PHT* pulmonary hypertension, *PMV* prolonged mechanical ventilation, *PS* pressure support, *RR* respiratory rate, SpO_2 peripheral oxygen saturation, *VCV* volume control ventilation, *VT* tidal volume, *Ti* inspiratory time

period of very close observation is necessary to ensure that the stoma matures and heals properly. When the patient stabilizes, sedation may be weaned, and weaning of mechanical ventilation process could be considered [57–59].

In 2006, O'Brien et al. reported a consensus detailing a structured approach to weaning children from mechanical ventilation in a post-acute care setting. This consensus was performed by physicians and nurse practitioners from the Specialized Pediatric Applied Research Collaborative (SPARC), a group of post-acute pediatric specialty hospitals in the eastern USA. It was noted early that, since there are no prospective studies, the guidelines should be necessarily based on a limited number of prior retrospective studies and on consensus opinion. They proposed a Weaning Severity Index and a Weaning Algorithm for the assessment and implementation of the weaning process. When children are admitted to a PICU or a post-acute care facility to continue ventilatory support and evaluate weaning, a complete assessment of airway patency, pulmonary function, nutritional status, and goals; tolerance of handling and rehabilitation therapies; and neurological status should be performed to guide the proper moment to initiate weaning [60].

The criteria for weaning readiness proposed by the SPARC consensus are (1) no escalation in ventilator support within 2 days prior to weaning; (2) stable chest radiograph; (3) blood $PaCO_2$ level not more than 10% above baseline; (4) blood pH within normal range; (5) supplemental FiO_2 of 0.6 or lower; (6) stable blood pressure over the previous 5–7 days; (7) heart rate no greater than 95% maximal normal for age; (8) tolerance of adequate nutrition; (9) absence of active infection, acute pain, or other medical problems that might negatively impact the weaning process; and (10) reported understanding by the family/guardian and all healthcare providers of the desirability of weaning [60].

There are different approaches to weaning used most commonly in the PICU: (1) performing a spontaneous breathing trial (SBT) [61]; (2) decreasing mechanical support to a low level of pressure-support (PS) ventilation; and (3) decreasing to a minimal set rate of synchronized intermittent mandatory ventilation (SIMV) [61–64]. SIMV is reported to be the least favored strategy among the three [65]. Weaning strategies for children in the post-acute care setting should proceed slowly. The weaning process begins by adjusting the level of positive inspiratory pressure (PIP/PS) and/or setting the ventilator rate. If the child tolerates weaning, further reduction in pressure and/or the set ventilator rate of breathing can be done every 2–3 days until the child is ready for a trial of CPAP or spontaneous breathing trials. Then time off the ventilator (sprinting) is gradually increased, as tolerated. Weaning from ventilatory support during sleep is the last step (Fig. 2).

During that process, if the patient does not continue to meet the weaning readiness, the weaning process may have to be temporarily stopped and investigation for causes of failure should be performed. Failure often is multifactorial, so a detailed and protocolized evaluation of respiratory and non-respiratory factors must be performed. Weaning can be resumed when the causes are corrected, and the patient has reached a new baseline. Although reversible causes of weaning failure are often identified, some chronic and more severe conditions might influence the prognosis [66]. In patients with BPD criteria that required invasive MV at term and

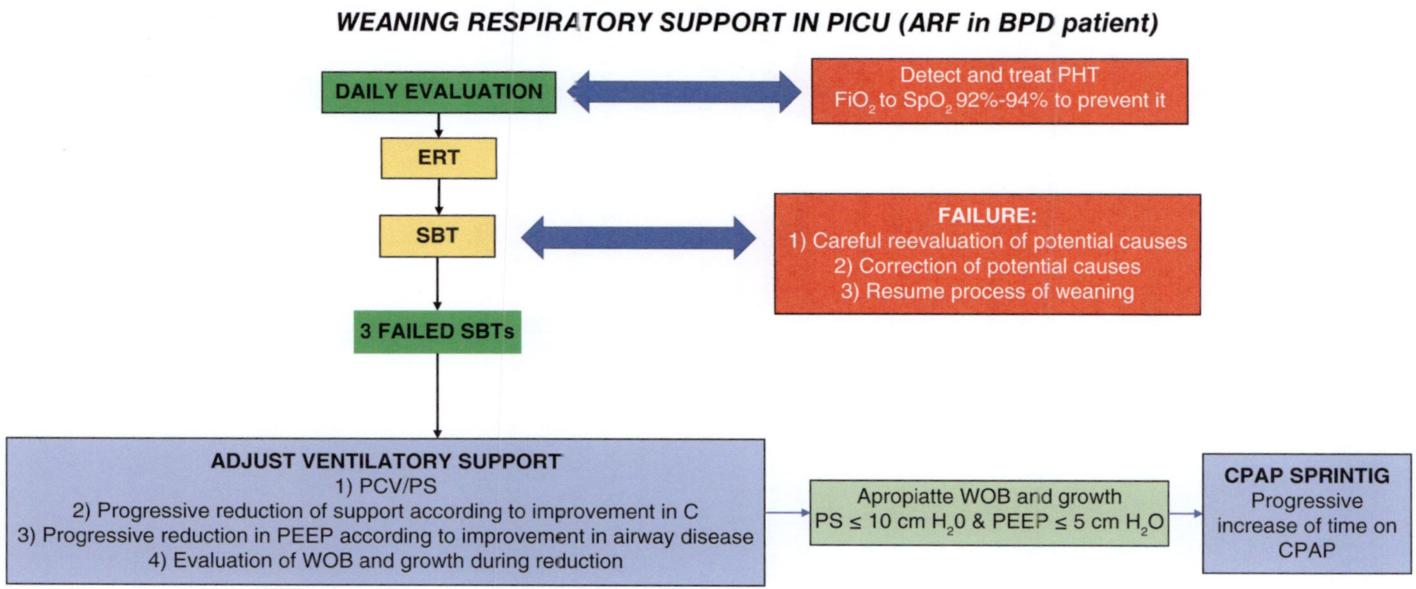

Fig. 2 Algorithm for weaning respiratory support in PICU (ARF in BPD patient). *ARF* acute respiratory failure, *BPD* bronchopulmonary dysplasia, *C* compliance, *CPAP* continuous positive airway pressure, *ERT* extubation readiness test, FiO_2 inspired fraction of oxygen, *PCV* pressure control ventilation, *PEEP* positive end-expiratory pressure, *PHT* pulmonary hypertension, *PICU* pediatric intensive care unit, *PS* pressure support, *SBT* spontaneous breathing test, SpO_2 peripheral oxygen saturation, *WOB* work of breathing

supplemental oxygen and/or with disproportionate respiratory symptoms, and in patients with incomplete criteria and/or atypical features, further investigation is warranted. It includes an echocardiogram (diagnosis of pulmonary hypertension [PHT] and cardiac defect), pulmonary tomography, and consideration of dual pathology (surfactant genetics, sweat test, ciliary brushing, immune panel). If no additional cause is found, and there is no improvement with supportive therapy, a lung biopsy might be considered [67].

Depending on availability, some patients could be transferred from PICU to a post-acute care facility. Despite the suspected cost and clinical advantages of weaning children with ventilator dependency in a post-acute inpatient setting, only a few studies have reported weaning outcomes [68, 69].

In a retrospective analysis of six post-acute care centers, O'Brien et al. reported that 41% of patients requiring PMV were admitted due to BPD. Children who were successfully weaned were mostly premature infants with BPD. Of them, 66% were weaned from MV at discharge [70]. Kharasch et al. reported that 30% of children in inpatient pulmonary rehabilitation weaned from continuous ventilator dependency to less than 12 hours per day of support. They also found that weaning was more likely achieved in premature infants with bronchopulmonary dysplasia (BPD) than with children with other conditions [71].

Not all severe BPD patients could be completely weaned off mechanical ventilation; some may be advanced to portable equipment or progressed to less critical levels of ventilation, while others could be weaned to a less invasive mode of support [72, 73]. A reduction of hours of ventilator use per day should allow a child to attend school, participate in family life, and minimize the need for constant adult supervision. Of note, in selected cases, there are sufficient family, financial, and healthcare resources to discharge a child who is ventilator dependent home before being fully weaned. Once an infant with BPD has transitioned successfully to a home ventilator, focus can be shifted toward patient discharge. This process requires a change in the focus of care, preparing the child and family for discharge to home through educating family caregivers, ordering durable medical equipment, and recruiting home nursing [74, 75] (Fig. 3).

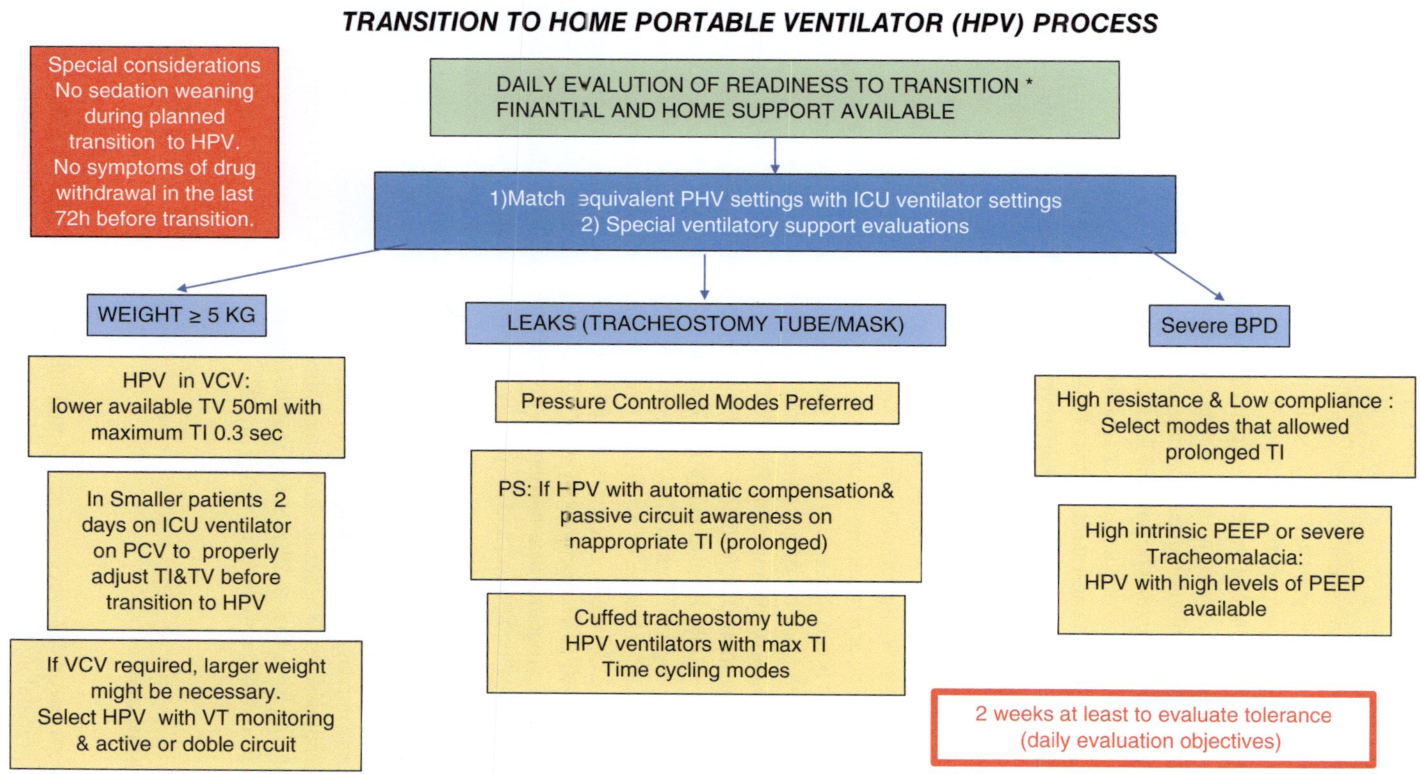

Fig. 3 Algorithm for transition to home portable ventilation process. *HPV* home portable ventilation, *ICU* intensive care unit, *VCV* volume control ventilation, *PCV* pressure control ventilation, *TV* tidal volume, *TI* inspiratory time, *PEEP* pressure end-expiratory pressure, * daily evaluation criteria Fig. 1

5 BPD and Ventilatory Support at Home

Once a child is stable and ventilated with chronic ventilation strategies on an ICU ventilator via tracheostomy, providers may begin discussing the timing and approach to transitioning to a home or portable ventilator. There are no established criteria for when to attempt this transition, and there is a significant variation in the procedure between institutions. Willis et al. recently reported that a standardized protocol for transitioning to a portable home ventilator reduced the time to a successful transition [76]. Transition to home ventilators might not be possible for smaller patients, since several home ventilators have the limitation that for smaller set tidal volumes, maximum inspiratory time (minimum flow) could be too short for the chronic ventilatory strategy. Alternatives for these patients include waiting for the child to grow and be given a larger tidal volume, using a pressure control ventilation to deliver the tidal volume in longer inspiratory time (in children with stable conditions), using newer home ventilator models which have been designed without inspiratory time limits, and weaning to CPAP via tracheostomy.

If the transition to a home ventilator fails, the patient may require additional time on the PICU ventilator. Waiting could be frustrating for both providers and families, but the child must be stable and breathing comfortably to grow and develop. Programs to discharge children to home who are chronically ventilated via tracheostomy need to follow the most recent evidence-based guidelines from the American Thoracic Society (ATS), the United Kingdom, or the Australian Pediatric Respiratory Group [77–79]. Changes to ventilator settings immediately before discharge have been associated with hospital readmission and should be avoided [80]. Guidelines strongly recommended that an "awake, trained caregiver" should always accompany a ventilated child. Pulse oximetry monitoring may add a degree of safety, but devices (including home ventilators) may fail to alarm [81, 82]. Family caregivers should be educated to competently perform all routine care as well as to appropriately respond to emergencies [83, 84]. Even formal home ventilation programs face barriers in discharging patients including obtaining appropriate medical equipment, and the paucity nursing resources for home health care. Programs may benefit from standardizing the discharge process and adding dedicated expert coordinators to their teams [85, 86]. Resources should be devoted to identifying and treating the significant traumatic stress in families. Families with technology-dependent children at home report fatigue, reduced quality of life, and depression. Sufficient quality home nursing resources may help to mitigate these issues and may also reduce hospital readmissions [87, 88]. In-home mortality does occur in this population with reports ranging from 15% to 20%. Safety may be improved by use of in-home telemedicine and, potentially, remote monitoring [11, 85].

6 Conclusion

Infants born before 32 weeks of gestational age may develop BPD influenced by different prenatal and postnatal factors. Therefore, BPD may display different phenotypes, affecting in various ways the airway and the lung parenchyma. Severe forms of BPD may require prolonged mechanical ventilation. In this scenario, a ventilatory strategy needs to be adjusted to the predominant phenotype. Weaning could be attempted in stable children, and close attention should be paid to develop and grow during this process. NIV could be a valuable tool to allow weaning from MV. Indications for tracheostomy include lesions of the upper airway and repeated weaning failure. Home mechanical ventilation could be offered to those patients who failed weaning, but it requires appropriate home ventilation programs and resources.

References

1. Northway WH, Rosan RC, Porter DY. Pulmonary disease following respiratory therapy of hyaline-membrane disease. Bronchopulmonary dysplasia. N Engl J Med. 1967;276(7):357–68.
2. Stoll BJ, Hansen NI, Bell EF, et al. Trends in care practices, morbidity, and mortality of extremely preterm neonates, 1993–2012. JAMA. 2015;314(10):1039–51.
3. Jobe AJ. The new BPD: an arrest of lung development. Pediatr Res. 1999;46(6):641–3.
4. Gien J, Kinsella J, Thrasher J, Grenolds A, Abman SH, Baker CD. Retrospective analysis of an Interdisciplinary Ventilator Care Program intervention on survival of infants with ventilator-dependent bronchopulmonary dysplasia. Am J Perinatol. 2017;34(2):155–63.
5. Jobe AH, Bancalari E. Bronchopulmonary dysplasia. Am J Respir Crit Care Med. 2001;163:1723–9.
6. Amirnovin R, Aghamohammadi S, Riley C, Woo MS, Del Castillo S. Analysis of a pediatric home mechanical ventilator population. Respir Care. 2018;63(5):558–64.
7. Simonds AK. Home ventilation. Eur Respir J. 2003;22(Supplement 47):38s–46s.
8. Overman AE, Liu M, Kurachek SC, et al. Tracheostomy for infants requiring prolonged mechanical ventilation: 10 years' experience. Pediatrics. 2013;131(5):e1491–6.
9. Lee JH, Smith PB, Quek MB, Laughon MM, Clark RH, Hornik CP. Risk factors and in-hospital outcomes following tracheostomy in infants. J Pediatr. 2016;173:39–44.
10. Park SJ, Bae MH, Jeong MH, et al. Risk factors and clinical outcomes of extubation failure in very early preterm infants: a single-center cohort study. BMC Pediatr. 2023;23(1):36.
11. Chawla S, Natarajan G, Shankaran S, Eunice Kennedy Shriver National Institute of Child Health and Human Development Neonatal Research Network, et al. Markers of successful extubation in extremely preterm infants, and morbidity after failed extubation. J Pediatr. 2017;189:113–119.e2.
12. Manley BJ, Doyle LW, Owen LS, et al. Extubating extremely preterm infants: predictors of success and outcomes following failure. J Pediatr. 2016;173:45–9.
13. Rogerson CM, Beardsley AL, Nitu ME, Cristea AI. Health care resource utilization for children requiring prolonged mechanical ventilation via tracheostomy. Respir Care. 2020;65(8):1147–53.
14. Sauthier MJ, Rose L, Jouvet P. Pediatric prolonged mechanical ventilation: considerations for definitional criteria. Respir Care. 2017;62(1):49–53.
15. Chye JK, Gray PH. Rehospitalization and growth of infants with bronchopulmonary dysplasia: a matched control study. J Paediatr Child Health. 1995;31(2):105–11.
16. Furman L, Baley J, Borawski-Clark E, Aucott S, Hack M. Hospitalization as a measure of morbidity among very low birth weight infants with chronic lung disease. J Pediatr. 1996;128(4):447–52.
17. Fraser J, Henrichsen T, Mok Q, Tasker RC. Prolonged mechanical ventilation as a consequence of acute illness. Arch Dis Child. 1998;78:253–6.
18. Kurachek SC, Newth CJ, Quasney MW, et al. Extubation failure in pediatric intensive care: a multiple-center study of risk factors and outcomes. Crit Care Med. 2003;31:2657–64.

19. Edmunds S, Weiss I, Harrison R. Extubation failure in a large pediatric ICU population. Chest. 2001;119:897–900.
20. Faustino EV, Gedeit R, Schwarz AJ, Asaro LA, et al. Accuracy of an extubation readiness test in predicting successful Extubation in children with acute respiratory failure from lower respiratory tract disease. Crit Care Med. 2017;45(1):94–102.
21. Johnston C, de Carvalho WB, Piva J, et al. Risk factors for extubation failure in infants with severe acute bronchiolitis. Respir Care. 2010;55(3):328–33.
22. Simonassi J, Bonora Sanso JP. Prevalence of extubation and associated risk factors at a tertiary care pediatric intensive care unit. Arch Argent Pediatr. 2019;117(2):87–93.
23. Kilba F, Salie S, Morrow B. Risk factors and outcomes of extubation failure in a South African tertiary paediatric intensive care unit. South Afr J Crit Care. 2022;38(1):26–32.
24. Shennan AT, Dunn MS, Ohlsson A, Lennox K, Hoskins EM. Abnormal pulmonary outcomes in premature infants: prediction from oxygen requirement in the neonatal period. Pediatrics. 1988;82:527–32.
25. Bancalari E, Claure N, Sosenko IRS. Bronchopulmonary dysplasia: changes in pathogenesis, epidemiology and definition. Semin Neonatol. 2003;8:63–71.
26. Higgins RD, Jobe AH, Koso-Thomas M, et al. Bronchopulmonary dysplasia: executive summary of a workshop. J Pediatr. 2018;197:300–8.
27. Joshi S, Kotecha S. Lung growth and development. Early Hum Dev. 2007;83:789–94.
28. Pierro M, Van Mechelen K, van Westerin-Kroom E, et al. Endotypes of prematurity and phenotypes of Bronchopulmonary dysplasia: Toward personalized neonatology. J Pers Med. 2022;12:687.
29. Jensen EA, Schmidt B. Epidemiology of bronchopulmonary dysplasia. Birth Defects Res A Clin Mol Teratol. 2014;100(3):145–57.
30. Hilgendorff A, O'Reilly MA. Bronchopulmonary dysplasia early changes leading to long-term consequences. Front Med (Lausanne). 2015;2:2.
31. Cannavò L, Perrone S, Viola V, Marseglia L, Di Rosa G, Gitto E. Oxidative stress and respiratory diseases in preterm newborns. Int J Mol Sci. 2021;22:12504.
32. Coalson JJ. Pathology of bronchopulmonary dysplasia. Semin Perinatol. 2006;30:179–84.
33. Thunqvist P, Tufvesson E, Bjermer L, Winberg A, Fellman V, Domellöf M, Melén E, Norman M, Hallberg J. Lung function after extremely preterm birth-a population-based cohort study (EXPRESS). Pediatric Pulmonol. 2018;53:64–72. [CrossRef]
34. Ochiai M, Hikino S, Yabuuchi H, Nakayama H, Sato K, Ohga S, Hara T. A new scoring system for computed tomography of the chest for assessing the clinical status of bronchopulmonary dysplasia. J Pediatr. 2008;152:90–5.
35. Zhang H, Zhang J, Zhao S. Airway damage of prematurity: the impact of prolonged intubation, ventilation, and chronic lung disease. Semin Fetal Neonatal Med. 2016;21(4):246–53. https://doi.org/10.1016/j.siny.2016.04.001. Epub 2016 Apr 26.
36. Wei JL, Bond J. Management, and prevention of endotracheal intubation injury in neonates. Curr Opin Otolaryngol Head Neck Surg. 2011;19:474e7.
37. Teig N, Allali M, Rieger C, Hamelmann E. Inflammatory markers in induced sputum of school children born before 32 completed weeks of gestation. J Pediatr. 2012;161:1085e90.
38. Tan JZ, Crossett M, Ditchfield M. Dynamic volumetric computed tomographic assessment of the young paediatric airway: initial experience of rapid, noninvasive, four-dimensional technique. J Med Imaging Radiat Oncol. 2013;57:141e8.
39. Abman SH. The dysmorphic pulmonary circulation in bronchopulmonary dysplasia: a growing story. Am J Respir Crit Care Med. 2008;178(2):114–5.
40. Wu KY, Jensen EA, White AM, Wang Y, Biko DM, Nilan K, Fraga MV, Mercer-Rosa L, Zhang H, Kirpalani H. Characterization of disease phenotype in very preterm infants with severe Bronchopulmonary dysplasia. Am J Respir Crit Care Med. 2020;201:1398–406.
41. Zayat N, Truffert P, Drumez E, EPICE Research Group, et al. Systemic steroids in preventing bronchopulmonary dysplasia (BPD): neurodevelopmental outcome according to the risk of BPD in the EPICE cohort. Int J Environ Res Public Health. 2022;19(9):5600.

42. Callaway DA, Wang Y, Lingappan K, et al. Lung biopsy in infants with severe bronchopulmonary dysplasia. Pediatr Pulmonol. 2023;58(7):2068–75.
43. Gien J, Abman SH, Baker CD. Interdisciplinary care for ventilator-dependent infants with chronic lung disease. J Pediatr. 2014;165(6):1274–5.
44. Sindelar R, Shepherd EG, Ågren J, et al. Established severe BPD: is there a way out? Change of ventilatory paradigms. Pediatr Res. 2021;90(6):1139–46.
45. Baker CD. Mechanical ventilation during chronic lung disease. Clin Perinatol. 2021;48(4):881–93.
46. Chen IL, Chen HL. New developments in neonatal respiratory management. Pediatr Neonatol. 2022;63(4):341–7.
47. Hysinger EB, Panitch HB. Paediatric tracheomalacia. Paediatr Respir Rev. 2016;17:9–15.
48. Napolitano N, Jalal K, McDonough JM, et al. Identifying and treating intrinsic PEEP in infants with severe bronchopulmonary dysplasia. Pediatr Pulmonol. 2019;54(7):1045–51.
49. Shetty S, Evans K, Cornuad P, et al. Neurally adjusted Ventilatory assist in very prematurely born infants with evolving/established Bronchopulmonary dysplasia. AJP Rep. 2021;11(4):e127–31.
50. Chan V, Greenough A. Randomized trial of methods of extubation in acute and chronic respiratory distress. Arch Dis Child. 1993;68:570–2.
51. So B-H, Tamura M, Mishina J, Watanabe T, Kamoshita S. Application of nasal continuous positive airway pressure to early extubation in very low birth weight infants. Arch Dis Child. 1995;72:F191–3.
52. Tapia JL, Bancalari A, Gonzalez A, Mercado ME. Does continuous positive airway pressure during weaning from intermittent mandatory ventilation in very low birth weight infants have risks or benefits? A controlled trial. Pediatr Pulmonol. 1995;19:269–74.
53. Davis P, Jankov R, Doyle L, Henschke P. Randomised, controlled trial of nasal continuous positive airway pressure in the extubation of infants weighing 600 to 1250 g. Arch Dis Child Fetal Neonatal Ed. 1998;79:F54–7.
54. Robertson NJ, Hamilton PA. Randomised trial of elective continuous positive airway pressure (CPAP) compared with rescue CPAP after extubation. Arch Dis Child Fetal Neonatal Ed. 1998;79:F58–60.
55. Davis P, Henderson-Smart D. Post-extubation prophylactic nasal continuous positive airway pressure in preterm infants: systematic review and meta-analysis. J Paediatr Child Health. 1999;35:367–71.
56. Nabeel Khalaf M, Brodsky N, Hurley J, Bhandari V. A prospective randomized, controlled trial comparing synchronized nasal intermittent positive pressure ventilation versus nasal continuous positive airway pressure as modes of extubation. Pediatrics. 2001;108(1):13–7.
57. Serra A, Cocuzza S, Longo MR, Grillo C, Bonfiglio M, Pavone P. Tracheostomy in childhood: new causes for an old strategy. Eur Rev Med Pharmacol Sci. 2012;16(12):1719–22.
58. Mandy G, Malkar M, Welty SE, et al. Tracheostomy placement in infants with bronchopulmonary dysplasia: safety and outcomes. Pediatr Pulmonol. 2013;48:245e9.
59. DeMauro SB, D'Agostino JA, Bann C, et al. Developmental outcomes of very preterm infants with tracheostomies. J Pediatr. 2014;164:1303e10.e2.
60. O'Brien J, BirnkranT D, Dumas HM, et al. Weaning children from mechanical ventilation in a post-acute care setting. Pediatr Rehabil. 2006;9(4):365–72.
61. Farias JA, Alia I, Esteban A, Golubicki AN, Olazarri FA. Weaning from mechanical ventilation in pediatric intensive care patients. Intensive Care Med. 1998;24:1070–5.
62. Keogh S, Courtney M, Coyer F. Weaning from ventilation in paediatric intensive care: an intervention study. Intensive Crit Care Nurs. 2003;19:186–97.
63. Hughes MR, Smith CD, Tecklenburg FW, Habib DM, Hulsey TC, Ebeling M. Effects of a weaning protocol on ventilated pediatric intensive care unit (PICU) patients. Top Health Inf Manage. 2001;22:35–43.
64. Randolph AG, Wypij D, Venkataraman ST, Hanson JH, Gedeit RG, Meert KL, Luckett PM, Forbes P, Lilley M, Thompson J, Pediatric Acute Lung Injury and SepsisInvestigators (PALISI)

Network, et al. Effect of ventilator weaning protocols on respiratory outcomes in infants and children: a randomized controlled trial. JAMA. 2002;288:2561–8.
65. Hess D. Ventilator modes used in weaning. Chest. 2001;120:474S–6S.
66. White AC. Long-term mechanical ventilation: management strategies. Respir Care. 2012;57(6):889–97.
67. Wright MFA, Wallis C. Investigation and management of the long-term ventilated premature infant. Early Hum Dev. 2018;126:10–7.
68. Ambrosio I, Woo M, Jansen M, Keens T. Safety of hospitalized ventilator-dependent children outside of the intensive care unit. Pediatrics. 1998;102:1221–2.
69. Buschbacher R. Outcomes and problems in pediatric pulmonary rehabilitation. Am J Phys Med Rehabil. 1995;74:287–93.
70. O'Brien JE, Dumas HM, Haley SM, Ladenheim B, Mast J, Burke SA, Birnkrant DJ, Whitford K, Palazzo R, Neufeld JA, Kharasch VS. Ventilator weaning outcomes in chronic respiratory failure in children. Int J Rehabil Res. 2007;30(2):171–4.
71. Kharasch V, Haley S, Dumas H, Ludlow L, O'Brien J. Oxygen and ventilator weaning during inpatient pediatric pulmonary rehabilitation. Pediatr Pulmonol. 2003;35:280–7.
72. DeWitt PK, Jansen MT, Ward SL, Keens TG. Obstacles to discharge of ventilator-assisted children from the hospital to home. Chest. 1993;103:1560–5.
73. Noyes J. Barriers that delay children and young people who are dependent on mechanical ventilators from being discharged from hospital. J Clin Nurs. 2002;11:2–11.
74. Edwards JD, Rivanis C, Kun SS, Caughey AB, Keens TG. Costs of hospitalized ventilator-dependent children: differences between a ventilator ward and intensive care unit. Pediatr Pulmonol. 2010;46(4):356–61.
75. Baker CD, Martin S, Thrasher J, et al. A standardized discharge process decreases length of stay for ventilator-dependent children. Pediatrics. 2016;137(4):e20150637.
76. Willis LD, Lowe G, Pearce P, et al. Transition from an ICU ventilator to a portable home ventilator in children. Respir Care. 2020;65:1791–9.
77. Sterni LM, Collaco JM, Baker CD, et al. An official American Thoracic Society clinical practice guideline: pediatric chronic home invasive ventilation. Am J Respir Crit Care Med. 2016;193(8):e16–35.
78. Jardine E, Wallis C. Core guidelines for the discharge home of the child on long-term assisted ventilation in the United Kingdom. UK Working Party on Paediatric Long Term Ventilation. Thorax. 1998;53:762–7.
79. Nixon GM, Edwards EA, Cooper DM, et al. APRG Home Ventilation Guideline APRG-TSANZ_2007.doc. 2008:1–38.
80. Kun SS, Edwards JD, Ward SL, Keens TG. Hospital readmissions for newly discharged pediatric home mechanical ventilation patients. Pediatr Pulmonol. 2012;47(4):409–14.
81. Sherman JM, Davis S, Albamonte-Petrick S, et al. Care of the child with a chronic tracheostomy. This official statement of the American Thoracic Society was adopted by the ATS Board of Directors, July 1999. Am J Respir Crit Care Med. 2000;161:297–308.
82. Kun SS, Nakamura CT, Ripka JF, Davidson Ward SL, Keens TG. Home ventilator low-pressure alarms fail to detect accidental decannulation with pediatric tracheostomy tubes. Chest. 2001;119(2):562–4.
83. Amin R, Parshuram C, Kelso J, et al. Caregiver knowledge and skills to safely care for pediatric tracheostomy ventilation at home. Pediatr Pulmonol. 2017;52(12):1610–5.
84. Agarwal A, Marks N, Wessel V, et al. Improving knowledge, technical skills, and confidence among pediatric health care providers in the management of chronic tracheostomy using a simulation model. Pediatr Pulmonol. 2016;51(7):696–704.
85. Edwards EA, O'Toole M, Wallis C. Sending children home on tracheostomy dependent ventilation: pitfalls and outcomes. Arch Dis Child. 2004;89(3):251–5.
86. Amin R, Sayal A, Syed F, et al. How long does it take to initiate a child on long-term invasive ventilation? Results from a Canadian pediatric home ventilation program. Can Respir J. 2015;22(2):103–8.

87. Sobotka SA, Dholakia A, Berry JG, et al. Home nursing for children with home mechanical ventilation in the United States: key informant perspectives. Pediatr Pulmonol. 2020;55(12):3465–76.
88. Tearl DK, Cox TJ, Hertzog JH. Hospital discharge of respiratory technology-dependent children: role of a dedicated respiratory care discharge coordinator. Respir Care. 2006;51(7):744–9.

Prolonged Mechanical Ventilation in Children with Neuromuscular Disease

Mirella Piera Gaboli

1 Introduction

Neuromuscular diseases (NMDs) are a heterogeneous group of diseases affecting the anterior horn cell of the spinal cord, neuromuscular junction, peripheral nerves, and muscles. NMDs cause physical respiratory insufficiency mainly due to weakness of respiratory muscle (including the diaphragm, intercostal and accessory muscles of respiration), often complicated with progressive lung compromise [28]. For the purpose of respiratory medicine, many other diseases that are not traditionally considered NMDs by neurologists, such as spinal cord injury, stroke, mitochondrial diseases, and some central nervous system conditions, may have similar or related respiratory effects. Thus, many of the issues discussed in this chapter may apply to a much larger patient group.

In children with NMDs, respiratory failure is a life-threatening complication both in acute and chronic settings, whose standard management includes intermittent positive-pressure mechanical ventilation (MV) physiotherapy and cough assistance, techniques that compensate for respiratory musculature weakness and improve secretion clearance. Pronged mechanical ventilation (PMV) may be required virtually in all patients suffering from NMDs at some point, including for symptom relief (e.g., breathlessness) in end-of-life palliative care.

M. P. Gaboli (✉)
University Hospital Virgen del Rocío, Sevilla, Spain

University of Seville, Sevilla, Spain

IBIS (Instituto de Biomedicina de Sevilla), Sevilla, Spain

Pediatric Respiratory Medicine and Pediatric Intensive Care Unit Consultant, Home ventilation program, University Hospital Virgen del Rocio, Sevilla, Spain
e-mail: mirellap.gaboli.sspa@juntadeandalucia.es

A. Kawaguchi et al. (eds.), *Prolonged and Long-Term Mechanical Ventilation in Children*, https://doi.org/10.1007/978-981-97-8903-0_11

Among children with chronic respiratory failure requiring long-term MV, those affected by neurological conditions and/or neuromuscular diseases represent up to 75% of pediatric patients receiving PMV, with consistency between countries and series [17, 18, 24, 26, 33].

Moreover, PMV in children with NMDs may be intended to increase the quality of life, facilitate discharge home, or palliate dyspnea. Several studies have already demonstrated that long-term MV in children diagnosed with an NMD and respiratory failure is associated with increased survival to adulthood [1, 10]. Transitioning from pediatric to the adult healthcare system is a challenging issue for children with NMDs on PMV and health professionals taking care of them [10, 23].

2 Respiratory Pathophysiology of Neuromuscular Disease in Children

The ability to sustain spontaneous ventilation can be viewed as a balance between the performance of the respiratory muscles on one side and the respiratory load, determined by the lung, thoracic, and airway mechanics, on the other side, with the two components being controlled by the central respiratory drive. The weakness of the respiratory muscles is the leading cause of the imbalanced ventilation observed in neuromuscular diseases. There is also a moderate increase in respiratory load due to progressive stiffening of the lung, rib cage, and scoliosis [14]. Despite the increase in central respiratory controller, which tries to drive the respiratory muscles more forcefully, alveolar hypoventilation, characterized by an increase in carbon dioxide and a decrease in oxygenation, occurs when the respiratory muscles are too weak to cope with the respiratory load (see Fig. 1).

It is often difficult to evaluate the weakness of the respiratory muscles, as well as cough effectiveness and sleep-disordered breathing, especially in noncooperative children. Nevertheless, to assess changes in respiratory muscle strength and respiratory load is regarded as crucial in NMDs.

2.1 Respiratory Muscle Strength

The assessment of lung function and respiratory muscle performance is classically based on volitional noninvasive tests, able to determine lung volumes and maximal static pressures and flows. The measurement of forced vital capacity (FVC) with forceful maneuver, or of vital capacity (VC), not requiring a forceful maneuver but still measuring the maximum amount of air an individual can expel from the lungs after maximum inhalation, is a global assessment of respiratory muscle capacity (inspiratory and expiratory). A drop in VC while supine of 19% suggests diaphragm weakness and possibly need for respiratory support during sleep. In patients with

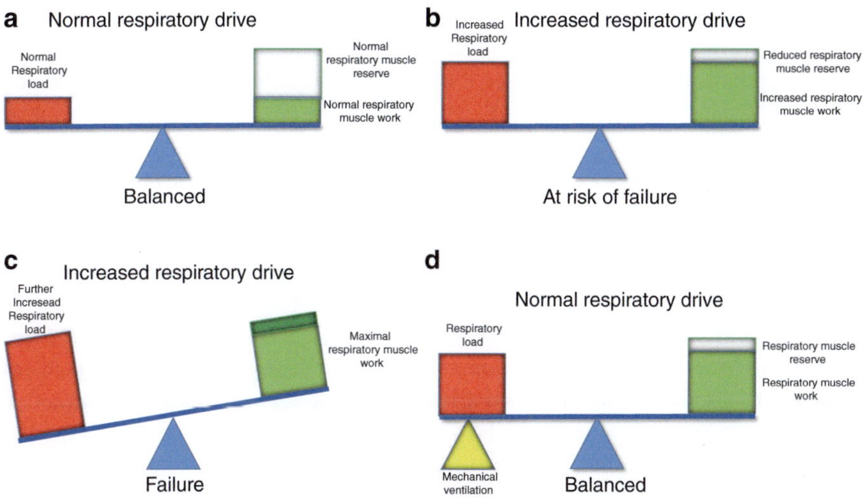

Fig. 1 Respiratory system in neuromuscular patients. (A) In normal subjects or in an early stage of neuromuscular disease during spontaneous ventilation, respiratory load (i.e., lung, rib cage, and thoracic airway mechanics) is low, and only a small proportion of respiratory muscle capacity is necessary to counter it. In this balanced situation, the respiratory drive is also normal, with more activity during wakefulness and less during sleep. (B) With the progression of the disease, muscular strength decreases and respiratory load increases, mainly due to the stiffness of the lung and rib cage, scoliosis, and changes in the muscle constitution. An increase in respiratory drive occurs to compensate for the increased respiratory load with almost maximal respiratory muscle effort and no functional capacity left. (C) An additional increase in respiratory load, such as observed in respiratory infection, or a progression of the underlying disease with weaker respiratory muscles causes respiratory failure, as respiratory muscle work cannot increase any further in spite of an increased respiratory drive. (D) Respiratory support, mainly mechanical ventilation, can restore a balanced respiratory system, mainly assisting or replacing respiratory muscle activity (CC-BY license, modified from Ref. [15])

bilateral diaphragm paralysis, VC may drop by up to 50%. Sniff nasal inspiratory pressure (SNIP) appears to be a reproducible measurement, not requiring a firm mouth seal, useful in patients with bulbar dysfunction. CV and SNIP measurements have sensitivity to rank the disease progression [12, 14]. Maximum static inspiratory and expiratory pressures (PImax and PEmax) highly correlated with VC in children with NMD and PImax of <4.0 kPa (or < 40.8 cmH_2O) were associated with sleep-disordered breathing (SDB), and PImax of <2.5 kPa (or < 25.5 cmH_2O) was associated with nocturnal hypoventilation [12, 13].

In noncooperative children, the transdiaphragmatic pressure (Pdi), measured as the difference between the gastric and the esophageal pressures, is a promising tool, although invasive, to assess diaphragm strength in NMDs [14]. In addition, given the difficulties performing spirometry, increased resistance, and reduced respiratory reactance, in patients with more restrictive lung function, oscillometry may be a promising substitute of spirometry [31].

The onset and progression of the weakness are quite variable and can be acute, as in the setting of spinal cord injury, or very gradual, as in milder forms of muscular dystrophy. It is crucial to monitor the progression towards respiratory failure by assessing respiratory muscle strength over time, every 3–6 months, in patients with NMDs [7].

2.2 Cough Function Abnormalities

Impairment of cough function is also common in NMDs and is caused by (1) inspiratory muscle weakness that leads to a reduction in the volume of intrathoracic gas available to remove secretions from airways; (2) expiratory muscle weakness that reduces peak expiratory flow and FVC; and, mainly when bulbar symptoms are present, (3) impaired glottic function that reduces the intra-airway gas compression and impairs the rapid opening of the glottis and the patency of the upper airway during coughing [12]. Cough function is crucial to maintain airway clearance and to prevent infections that often worsen respiratory insufficiency by increasing work of breathing, hypoxemia, and hypercarbia. Cough function is best assessed using a handheld peak flow meter and can be performed even in young children. A value of 160 L/min or less is associated with inadequate clearance of secretions. A measured value of 270 L/min when a patient is well and without infection has been reported to drop to values 160 L/min during illness. It should prompt initiation of cough assistance, which may precede in weeks or months the indication of noninvasive ventilation. Patients with cough failure and bulbar involvement may also be unable to manage secretions and saliva. This is instead due to difficulty managing the secretions through swallowing or expectoration than due to the volume of secretions [7].

2.3 Respiratory Abnormalities During Sleep

Sleep-disordered breathing (SDB) is prevalent in individuals with NMD and reduced lung volumes. The gold standard test to diagnose SDB in children is a polysomnography (PSG). However, other tests, including oximetry and capnography, are also used in clinical practice worldwide, given the often-limited access to PSG.

Nocturnal hypoventilation is generally seen prior to diurnal hypoventilation and respiratory failure. The definition of nocturnal hypoventilation in pediatric patients has been debated, as limited studies exist linking secondary end-organ damage to specific levels of carbonic dioxide (CO_2) in children. The most commonly utilized definition in children arises from the American Academy of Sleep Medicine (AASM), which defines it as pCO_2 of >50 mmHg for 25% or more of total sleep time during a polysomnogram, but transcutaneous measurement of pCO_2 ($PtcCO_2$)

is currently being considered as the most appropriate tool. Nocturnal hypoventilation is diagnosed in an NMD patient with slightly different sensitivity when the peak value of $PtcCO_2$ is >50 mmHg, the percentage of $PtcCO_2$ is >50 mmHg > 2% of nighttime recording, or the nocturnal $PtcCO_2$ is >10 mmHg above waking baseline level [25]. Nocturnal hypoventilation correlates poorly with oxygenation index, even when conservative value definition of nocturnal hypoxia is used, such as the mean SpO_2 level being below 90% for greater than 2% of the total recording time [6].

Respiratory events, such as obstructive or central hypopneas and apneas, are also widespread in individuals with NMDs. Obstructive events (OSA) are defined as partial (hypopnea) or complete (apnea) airway closure resulting in sleep fragmentation and/or gas exchange abnormalities. The same disruption occurs in central events but is a result of cessation (apnea) or shallow breaths (hypopnea) being taken without evidence of upper airway obstruction (CSA) [12].

Children with NMD may be at risk for all types of SDB, depending on their specific NMD diagnosis. For example, children with congenital myotonic dystrophy have a higher risk of CSA, while those with Duchenne muscular dystrophy (DMD) may have OSA and/or nocturnal hypoventilation. Nocturnal hypoventilation is a result of inadequate minute ventilation during sleep that is typically secondary to reduced muscle strength; other factors can also contribute to this, such as scoliosis and obesity. Weakness of upper airway muscles increases upper airway collapsibility causing obstruction, while reduced intercostal and diaphragm strength can lead to shallow breathing characteristic of central events. Additionally, this respiratory instability further predisposes such children to central events.

A patient with a neuromuscular diagnosis who has symptoms of sleep-disordered breathing and meets at least one of the criteria in Table 1 qualifies for a nocturnal noninvasive support device [7].

Thus, the result of a "normal" PSG should not serve as a barrier to proactive use/approval of NIV in NMD. The "abnormal" PSG may be a late result in the evolution of the disease when the individual has already advanced disease and is at risk of cumulative morbidity and mortality.

Table 1 Criteria for considering initiation of prolonged noninvasive mechanical ventilation for NMD patients breathing an inspired oxygen fraction of 0.21 (not oxygen supplemented)

1.	Diurnal, awake $PaCO_2$ more than 45 mm Hg
2.	Demonstrates sleep desaturation, defined as the mean SpO_2 level being below 90% for greater than 2% of the total recording time
3.	Demonstrated sleep hypercapnia, defined as the mean PetCO2 ($PtCO_2$) level ≥ 45 mmHg or a $PetCO_2$ ($PtCO_2$) level ≥ 50 mmHg for greater than 2% of the total recording time
4.	Maximal inspiratory pressure less than 40 cm H_2O (< 25 cmH_2O)*
5.	FVC less than 50% predicted
6.	Decrease in FVC from sitting to supine position ≥19%
7.	Recurrent acute respiratory exacerbations
8.	Daily drowsiness, irritability, moodiness, and headache due to unrefreshing sleep

*Criteria between parenthesis indicated that nocturnal ventilation is recommended

2.4 Reductions in Respiratory System Compliance

In NMDs, the reduction in respiratory system compliance varies according to the time of disease onset: onset in infancy is associated with a risk of impaired lung and chest wall growth, accounting for thoracic deformity and kyphoscoliosis. The changes in respiratory system compliance are a result of (1) the progressive loss of VC with alveolar collapse and microatelectasis; (2) the changes in both the chest wall muscles and the joints of the thoracic cage; and (3) the kyphoscoliosis, mostly in post-polio syndrome, spinal muscular atrophy, and muscular dystrophies. The reduction in respiratory system compliance contributes to an increase in the elastic work of breathing that stresses already weak muscles and may increase the risk of respiratory failure [7].

3 Respiratory Support for Children with Neuromuscular Diseases

Noninvasive mechanical ventilation at positive pressure is the most common long-term respiratory support in neuromuscular patients and will be discussed in details. Albeit far less common, the negative-pressure ventilation (NPV) is still an alternative for same children [5]. The strength of this technique is the ability to guarantee a breathing completely analogous to the natural one, by means of a negative-pressure ventilator and either a cuirass or a poncho. The ventilator first applies a negative pressure forcing the movement of the diaphragm downwards while the rib muscles tend to enlarge the thorax: this process generates lung expansion by generating a lower intrathoracic pressure than the external one; subsequently, the ventilator exerts positive pressure forcing the air inside the chamber, to compress the chest and empty the lungs. The cuirass negative-pressure ventilators were primarily beneficial in children with NMD and severe thoracic scoliosis because they may have their own cuirass built from a plaster prototype of the chest and abdomen. Cuirass ventilators are easy to put on and suitable for home use, designed to ensure a good quality of life and normal daily activities. In general, NPV may preserve physiological functions, such as speech, cough, swallowing, and feeding, and its major advantage is the prevention of endotracheal intubation and its related problems. A limitation is the lack of upper airway protection and the risk of upper airway obstruction due to instability.

It is worthy of note that, rather than treating or curing the respiratory insufficiency of NMD patients, the different mechanical ventilation techniques may offer different levels of respiratory support according to the patient's degree of respiratory failure. Mechanical devices are meant to ameliorate the quality of life, mainly by reducing respiratory load and improving airway clearance, which results in improved daytime function, reduced frequency of hospitalization for acute respiratory insufficiency, and decreased morbidity and mortality [2]. Mechanical ventilation has been shown to change the natural history of some NMDs, such as DMD [4] (see Fig. 1).

3.1 Nocturnal Ventilatory Support

As mentioned, most progressive NMDs result in nocturnal hypoventilation that precedes diurnal respiratory failure. Therefore, sleep ventilator support, mainly noninvasive ventilation, should be initiated when a patient presents with sleep symptoms and has either a positive sleep study or meets at least one of the criteria in Table 1. Nocturnal noninvasive ventilation has been shown to improve patency of the upper airways and sleep-disordered breathing, reduce daytime somnolence and irritability, reset the sensitivity of central chemoreceptors, normalize gas exchange, reduce symptoms due to chronic hypoventilation, and, therefore, improve quality of life [2].

Devices: Appropriate ventilatory support devices for nocturnal mechanical ventilation have bi-level mode with a backup respiratory rate (RR). Many modes of bi-level support are available, including pressure support (spontaneous/timed, S/Tmode), pressure control, and volume-targeted modes such as average volume-assured pressure support (AVAPS) and intelligent volume-assured pressure support. It has not been determined at this time if any of these modes is clinically superior, but recently volume-assured pressure support (VAPS) mode was associated with an improvement in adherence to nocturnal MV in children with NMD compared to S/T mode [30]. Continuous positive airway pressure (CPAP) is not appropriate for patients with NMDs, unless only OSA events can be documented with neither hypoventilation nor central events, which CPAP will not treat. In the bi-level with a backup rate (BPAP S/T) mode, expiratory pressures (EPAP) should be set at low values, starting at 4–5 cm H_2O and titrated according to the upper airway obstruction. Inspiratory pressure (IPAP) should be adjusted to produce a tidal volume of 8–10 mL/kg; occasionally, IPAP levels up to 20 cmH_2O are needed in obesity or patients with very restrictive lung disease. The backup RR is adjusted approximately five breaths less than average sleeping RR of the child, unless insufficient inspiratory triggering of the ventilator by the child is observed [15]. Using inbuilt software, giving the readouts in real time or downloaded may help clinicians optimize the ventilator setting and objectively monitor patient adherence to the treatment [15].

Interfaces: Several mask options include nasal, oronasal, or total face masks and lip-seal devices that can be used for nocturnal noninvasive MV. Nasal masks are preferred by many patients with NMDs, as they allow children to speak while wearing the mask. Although interface technologies have developed dramatically, a close follow-up of complications such as skin breakdown, significant air leaks, and patient intolerance is still necessary. Having more than one type of mask may reduce the risk of skin wounds [7].

Effectiveness: The effectiveness of nocturnal MV in patients with NMDs should result in improved sleep symptoms and normalized CO_2 levels. Titration sleep studies may be needed if settings do not result in an adequate response. In children, humidification of the circuit is recommended to improve respiratory comfort and prevent drying of bronchial secretions. The effectiveness of nocturnal NIV in prolonging survival in the NMD population has been evaluated most commonly in the context of spinal muscular atrophy and DMD, with observational studies, being that truly randomized studies with sham ventilation may not be ethical in this patient population [10]. When nocturnal MV fails to provide the required support and improve SBD, a tracheostomy and invasive MV may be considered [3].

3.2 *Diurnal Ventilation*

The respiratory muscles in patients with progressive NMDs will continue to weaken, and when diurnal dyspnea, difficulty in normal secretion clearance, fatigue, or difficulty in concentration occur, NIV may be necessary even during the day. Then, laboratory findings may include elevated CO_2 despite adequate nocturnal sleep therapy and a further drop in FCV. However, no absolute values of FVC or PImax have been identified to trigger the need for diurnal ventilation (DV), and they very much depend on the natural history of the diseases [14].

Diurnal ventilation can be accomplished with mask ventilation and a bi-level device, tracheostomy and invasive ventilation, negative-pressure mechanical ventilation, or mouthpiece ventilation (MPV), in which a ventilator, on demand of the patient that makes a sip or "kiss" effort, delivers the breath via a mouthpiece interface [5, 7]. In MPV, the ventilator is generally set to deliver either an assured volume, usually around 6–8 ml/kg, or a programmed pressure support (PS) which allows a similar tidal volume. Breathing frequency and therefore minute ventilation are decided by the patient. The low-pressure and apnea alarms will need to be turned off, and the EPAP should be set to 0 cmH_2O. Among the advantages of MPV compared with nasal and oronasal interfaces are that there is no risk of skin breakdown and that it produces less speech interference. MPV is interesting for patients requiring daytime ventilation and may be used as an alternative in patients wanting to avoid a tracheostomy. Nevertheless, when bulbar involvement is too severe, or NIV expertise is not available, tracheostomy placement will need to be considered. Among the side effects of MPV, several patients have reported gastric distension, increased salivation, and vomiting.

In addition, MPV may be used to perform breath stacking by taking multiple breaths without complete exhalation in between the breaths, which can improve cough function, increasing VC and the volume of gas for cough [7].

Intermittent abdominal pressure ventilation, a form of noninvasive negative-pressure mechanical ventilation, may be feasible in children with NMD as diurnal ventilation, but seems less effective than positive-pressure NIV. The only available evidence comes from a few reported cases in adults [27].

3.3 Cough Management

The need for some cough augmentation technique to save management of secretions usually occurs earlier than the initiation of NIV in children with NMDs. In adults, a peak cough flow (PCF) of 270 L/min is suggested as the value below which cough augmentation interventions should be considered, and when PCF is less than 160 L/min, commencing mechanical insufflator-exsufflator is recommended [8]. In children, PCF evaluation requires little cooperation, but data on PCF values within the pediatric population are scarce. Two studies have demonstrated that PCF ratios change with age in children, and data on the 5th percentile for PCF in healthy children younger than 10 years of age are less than or equal to 270 L/min.

Moreover, PCF values in children of the same age may change according to specific NMD diagnosis. Knowledge of the PCF variability allows for individualization of therapy with cough augmentative techniques based on the nature of the disease and clinical course rather than using an arbitrary age cutoff ([19]). A recent study, aimed to describe the level of agreement and correlation between measures of PEF, FVC, and PCF in South African children with NMD, identified that the cutoff PCF values of <160 L.min^{-1} and < 270 L.min^{-1} corresponded with a PEF of <160 L.min^{-1} and < 250 L.min^{-1} and an FVC of <1.2 L and < 1.8 L, respectively, good predictors of the threshold levels of PCF generally associated with ineffective cough and respiratory morbidity [21].

There are several ways in which the cough can be augmented. The first is through lung volume recruitment maneuvers, where the patient stacks one breath on top of another. Breath stacking can be accomplished by glossopharyngeal breathing, or MPV, or through a resuscitator bag, whereby an assistant can deliver repeated breaths with the patient retaining air by closing the glottis after the breath is delivered. This increases the gas volume allowing breath stacking in the lungs and results in a higher respiratory system elastic recoil pressure, thus increasing the PCF. The second method of increasing cough effectiveness is the manually assisted cough. In this maneuver, an abdominal or lateral rib cage thrust applied during the exhalation portion of the cough can increase the cough peak flow. The combination of breath stacking using lung volume recruitment and manually assisted cough can be used together with better results than either alone. A mechanical insufflation-exsufflation (MI-E) device can be used with manual cough augmentation techniques and, occasionally in very weak patients, with oral secretion suctioning [21, 22].

Although the regular use of NIV improves airway clearance, the most crucial time for using these techniques is during a respiratory tract infection, with the increase of secretions. However, as for NIV, the patients and caregivers must practice cough augmentation maneuvers regularly [7, 32].

3.4 Improving Respiratory System Compliance

The chest wall and lung in individuals with NMDs can exhibit reduced compliance over time due to disease sequelae. The regular use of NIV stabilizes the chest wall, prevents atelectasis, and slows the chest wall deformity and the decline in lung function [9]. Nevertheless, there is a good deal of interest in methods to prevent or reverse this loss of compliance [29]. The mainstay of these efforts has been a treatment to inflate the respiratory system by augmenting the inspiratory capacity above the volume the patient can achieve without assistance. The thought is that this would be like a range of motion exercise, as seen in physical therapy. The augmentation of inspiratory capacity has been accomplished through breath stacking, much like cough augmentation [32]. In one short-term study in adult subjects with NMD, a single session of ten lung volume recruitment maneuvers increased total respiratory system compliance by approximately 40%. However, this returned to baseline after less than 2 h. No data are available about children with NMDs, but because lung volume recruitment maneuvers entail low risk, most experts suggest performing them regularly [4, 7].

4 Prolonged Mechanical Ventilation in Patients with NMD Treated with Disease Modifier Drugs

Advances in treatment for NMD hold promise for children with conditions such as Duchenne muscular dystrophy (DMD) or spinal muscular atrophy (SMA), but not just for them. The ability to target the disease gene or its encoded messenger RNAs (mRNAs) with antisense oligonucleotides (ASOs) or with gene replacement has significantly increased the patient's survival and has changed their respiratory expectations [16]. Moreover, accurate genetic diagnosis, early in the disease process, will allow these treatments to be most effective, and newborn screening (NBS) is an interesting approach for this purpose. A so-called proactive approach soon after the diagnosis has been advocated as an effective way to decrease mobility and mortality related to respiratory insufficiency, at least in patents with SMA type 1. A proactive respiratory care includes a more aggressive screening for hypoventilation and impaired airway clearance with proactive treatment earlier in the course of a condition, mainly through respiratory physiotherapy with mechanical support and through PMV, ideally noninvasive but also invasive ventilation. This will result in improved quality of life as well as in longevity [20].

5 Care of NMD Children on Prolonged Mechanical Ventilation

PMV is a technically challenging treatment whose aim is to be performed domiciliary, hopefully at school and in other daily life activities of a child with NMD, if needed. NIV is almost always the first option, and it is usually initiated in the hospital during a short hospitalization or in the outpatient clinic with efficacy and compliance comparable to an in-hospital initiation. As NIV will be administered initially during sleep, overnight monitoring of sleep with the optimal setting(s), at least with an assessment of overnight gas exchange, is recommended. This sleep study can be postponed until the patient is adapted to NIV and ideally able to sleep at least 6 h with his device, and may be done in the sleep laboratory or domiciliary. Training the caregivers and the patient is essential and should include disease-specific care. Compliance with NIV is a significant issue and relies mainly on correct NIV prescription, both in time and setting, so that the child and the family may experience the positive effects of the therapy rather than the care burden. PMV in children with NMDs is almost always lifelong-lasting support that might change in the same technical aspects. However, so far, no curative treatment has allowed for MV discontinuation, except for terminal palliative care purposes [1, 10].

5.1 Monitoring and Evaluation of Noninvasive Ventilation

There are no validated guidelines for the monitoring or long-term follow-up of children with NIV, but an update on current practice is contained in the chapter "*Evaluations of Home Ventilated Children*" in this book. The timing of the follow-up visits depends on the age and the medical condition of the child. A proposed practice consists of at least a visit, if a sleep study is impossible, 1 month after the initiation, and then every 2–6 months by outpatient visits, with at least two checkups per year, including a complete sleep study with NIV. Overnight SpO_2 with $PtcCO_2$ recording during NIV may be done at home and evaluated at each visit as NMD patients may remain hypercapnic during sleep with NIV or experience a rapid disease progression. NIV should be optimized in each visit by simple measures such as changing the interface or the ventilator settings.

The simultaneous analysis of the inbuilt ventilator software and the overnight gas exchange gives valuable information on essential issues such as objective compliance, unintentional leaks, respiratory rate, patient triggering of the ventilator, airway pressures, tidal and minute volume, and residual respiratory events [15].

NIV may be associated with side effects that should be monitored carefully. Among the most common that are related to the interface are skin injury due to pressure sores, eye irritation due to unintentional air leaks, and facial deformity in young children. Most side effects of ventilation masks can be minimized by using at least two different interfaces in each child and by preventive care of the skin.

Other side effects are less common and may be caused by the positive pressure. Aerophagia, gastric distension, and gastroesophageal reflux may be observed with high inspiratory pressures or in the case of patient-ventilator asynchrony. These abdominal side effects may be managed by optimizing ventilator setting at each visit and/or correcting patient-ventilator asynchrony and/or the use of an abdominal girdle. Unintentional leaks may be associated with discomfort, poor NIV tolerance, and poor sleep quality with arousals [15].

5.2 *Noninvasive Ventilation Failure and Indication of Invasive Support*

Even if NIV is very effective, it may be difficult to apply "around the clock" on a long-term basis.

In children requiring NIV during the daytime, MPV may be impossible in young children and difficult to accept in older children. Some expert teams have a successful experience with NIV in totally ventilator-dependent children with NMD. However, others consider that the child should be able to breathe spontaneously, without NIV, for a minimal time per day in order to be able to be safely maintained at home [15].

A tracheostomy represents a possible and individualized option for children with a progressive NMD that should be prepared and discussed thoroughly with the child (when possible) and his family.

Within this context, determining a child's best interests has to consider "balancing benefit and burdens of treatment and outcomes." In some children and their families, the transition from NIV to a tracheostomy may be associated with a too high burden concerning the improvement in the quality of life of the child and his family. NIV may then be used as part of a palliative care approach without excessively prolonging a poor or unbearable quality of life. Noteworthily, a tracheostomy for invasive MV was not always associated with a decrease in quality of life as evaluated by the patients themselves [17].

Tracheostomy is often recommended for patients with severe bulbar symptoms, poor control of oral secretions resulting in recurrent aspiration pneumonia, patients in whom NIV has been unsuccessful at improving gas exchange, and patients that perceive a better quality of life without a facial interface or, simply, patient and family preference.

Among the limitation of invasive MV through a tracheostomy tube, the impact on phonation, increased risk of lower respiratory infections from bacterial colonization of the airway, impossibility to dive, and difficulties in swimming and in performing physiotherapy in water should be mentioned [3].

5.3 *Impact on Survival and Transition to Adult Care*

In the last years, it has become evident that prolonged MV is associated with increased survival in children with a range of NMDs and respiratory failure. Therefore, an increased number of patients reach adulthood and transition to adult care facilities, with various complications not previously described in and important implications for healthcare planning [10]. Patients with NMDs on PMV in age to transition to adult require complex multidisciplinary management and significant efforts to achieve the proper transition. The US Department of Health and Human Service's Maternal and Child Health Bureau (MCHB) recommends six core elements of healthcare transition that may require more than 24 months to be fulfilled. These include (1) introducing transition policy; (2) developing a registry for transition tracking and monitoring; (3) initiating healthcare transition planning; (4) preparing young adults and families with transition readiness assessments; (5) transfer to adult care; and (6) integrating young adults into adult care [11]. Nevertheless, no guidelines are available for transition from pediatric to adult pulmonary care in patients with NMDs. Therefore, research, program development, and healthcare policy implementation are necessary to enhance the quality of life of young adults with NMDs and chronic respiratory failure [23].

6 Summary

NMDs are a heterogeneous group of conditions, often congenital, with a still limited option of curative treatment that ultimately may affect each muscle of the body, including the respiratory muscles, leading to respiratory failure. The morbidity and mortality due to progressive respiratory decline have a great impact on the quality and quantity of life. A better understanding of the pathophysiology of respiratory failure in NMD patients has allowed for the development of new technologies applied in diagnosing and supporting breath disturbances, both at night and during the day. Ventilatory support is often noninvasive, with volume support or pressure support ventilation, and it is delivered via a mask interface at night and a mouthpiece when awake. As the number of hours for MV necessarily increases, tracheostomy for invasive ventilation "long day clock" may be an option. Cough assistance and cough increase technique should be regarded as a complement to PMV, to improve secretion management and lung volume recruitment.

Finally, PMV and cough management may help maintain lung function over time, and there is a large amount of data suggesting that many of these individuals' life span has increased with these respiratory care interventions. New challenges are appearing, including transitioning to adult care facilities, progressive decline in health, and loss of independence as they approach adulthood.

References

1. AlBalawi MM, Castro-Codesal M, Featherstone R, Sebastianski M, Vandermeer B, Alkhaledi B, Bedi PK, Abusido T, MacLean JE. Outcomes of long-term noninvasive ventilation use in children with neuromuscular disease: systematic review and meta-analysis. Ann Am Thorac Soc. 2022;19(1):109–19.
2. Alexiou S, Piccione J. Neuromuscular disorders and chronic ventilation. Semin Fetal Neonatal Med. 2017;22:256e259.
3. Amaddeo A, Khirani S, Griffon L, Teng T, Lanzeray A, Fauroux B. Non-invasive ventilation and CPAP failure in children and indications for invasive ventilation. Front Pediatr. 2020;8:544921.
4. Annane D, Orlikowski D, Chevret SAnnane D, Orlikowski D, Chevret S. Nocturnal mechanical ventilation for chronic hypoventilation in patients with neuromuscular and chest wall disorders. Cochrane Datab Syst Rev. 2014;12:CD001941.
5. Annunziata A, Coppola A, Polistina GE, Imitazione P, Simioli F, Lanza M, Cauteruccio R, Fiorentino G. Daytime alternatives for non-invasive mechanical ventilation in neuromuscular disorders. Acta Myol. 2021;40:51–60.
6. Ayhan Y, Karatoprak EY, Onay ZR, Can Oksay S, Girit S. Assessment of nocturnal hypoventilation by different methods and definitions in children with neuromuscular disease: oxycapnography and blood gas analysis. Medeni Med J. 2021;36:106–16.
7. Benditt JO. Respiratory care of patients with neuromuscular disease. Respir Care. 2019;64:679–88.
8. Chatwin M, Simonds AK. Long-term mechanical insufflation-Exsufflation cough assistance in neuromuscular disease: patterns of use and lessons for application. Respir Care. 2020;65:135–43.
9. Chatwin M, Bush A, Simonds AK. Outcome of goal-directed non-invasive ventilation and mechanical insufflation/exsufflation in spinal muscular atrophy type I. Arch Dis Child. 2011;96:426–32.
10. Chatwin M, Tan HL, Bush A, Rosenthal M, Simonds AK. Long term non-invasive ventilation in children: impact on survival and transition to adult care. PLoS One. 2015;10(5):e0125839.
11. Cheng CP, Panitch HB, Hansen-Flaschen J. Transition of patients with neuromuscular disease and chronic ventilator-dependent respiratory failure from pediatric to adult pulmonary care. Paediatr Respir Rev. 2020;33:3–8.
12. Chiang J, Kevan Mehta K, Amin R. Respiratory diagnostic tools in neuromuscular disease. Respirology. 2018;5:78–95.
13. Fauroux B. Respiratory muscle testing in children. Res Rev. 2003;4:243–9.
14. Fauroux B, Khirani S. Neuromuscular disease and respiratory physiology in children: putting lung function into perspective. Respirology. 2014;19(6):782–91.
15. Fauroux B, Khirani S, Griffon L, Teng T, Lanzeray A, Amaddeo A. Non-invasive ventilation in children with neuromuscular diseases. Front Pediatr. 2020;8:482.
16. Fitzgerald DA, Doumit M, Abel F. Changing respiratory expectations with the new disease trajectory of nusinersen treated spinal muscular atrophy [SMA] type 1. Paediatr Respir Rev. 2018 Sep;28:11–7.
17. González Cortés R, Bustinza Arriortua A, Pons Ódena M, García Teresa MA, Cols Roig M, Gaboli M, García Martinez S, Oñate Vergara E, García Urabayen D, Castillo Serrano A, López González J, Salcedo Posadas A, Rodríguez Nuñez A, Luna Paredes MC, Hernández G. Domiciliary mechanical ventilation in children: a Spanish multicentre study. An Pediatr. 2013;78(4):227–33.
18. Hov B, Andersen T, Toussaint M, Vollsæter M, Mikalsen IB, Indrekvam S, Hovland V. Prevalence of long-term mechanical insufflation-exsufflation in children with neurological conditions: a population-based study. Dev Med Child Neurol. 2021;63:537–44.
19. Kotwal N, Shukla PJ, Perez GF. Peak cough flow in children with neuromuscular disorders. Lung. 2020;198:371–5.

20. Lavie M, Diamant N, Cahal M, Sadot E, Be'er M, Fattal-Valevski A, Sagi L, Domany KA, Amirav I. Nusinersen for spinal muscular atrophy type 1: real-world respiratory experience. Pediatr Pulmonol. 2021 Jan;56(1):291–8.
21. Morrow BM, Angelil L, Forsyth J, Huisamen A, Juries E, Corten L. The utility of using peak expiratory flow and forced vital capacity to predict poor expiratory cough flow in children with neuromuscular disorders. S Afr J Physiother. 2019;75:1296.
22. Morrow B, Argent A, Zampoli M, Human A, Corten L, Toussaint M. Cough augmentation techniques for people with chronic neuromuscular disorders (review). Cochrane Database Syst Rev. 2021;4(4):CD013170.
23. Onofri A, Tan HL, Cherchi C, Pavone M, Verrillo E, Ullmann N, Testa MBC, Cutrera R. Transition to adult care in young people with neuromuscular disease on non-invasive ventilation. Ital J Pediatr. 2019;45:90.
24. Park M, Jang H, Sol IS, Kim SY, Kim YS, Kim YH, Sohn MH, Kim KW. Pediatric home mechanical ventilation in Korea: the present situation and future strategy. J Korean Med Sci. 2019;34:e268.
25. Pautrat J, Khirani S, Boulé M, Ramirez A, Beydon N, Fauroux B. Carbon dioxide levels during polygraphy in children with sleep-disordered breathing. Sleep Breath. 2015;19:149–57.
26. Pavone M, Verrillo E, Onofri A, Caggiano S, Chiarini-Testa MB, Cutrera R. Characteristics and outcomes in children on long-term mechanical ventilation: the experience of a tertiary pediatric center in Rome. Ital J Pediatr. 2020;46:12.
27. Puricelli C, Volpato E, Sciurello S, Nicolini A, Banfi P. Intermittent abdominal pressure ventilation: feasibility and efficacy in neuromuscular disease. A case report. Monaldi Arch Chest Dis. 2021;91:1828.
28. Silva IS, Pedrosa R, Azevedo IG, Forbes AM, Fregonezi GAF, Dourado Junior MET, Lima SRH, Ferreira GMH. Respiratory muscle training in children and adults with neuromuscular disease (Review). Cochrane Datab Syst Rev. 2019;2019(9):CD011711.
29. Simonds AK, Parker RA, Branthwaite MA. The effect of intermittent positive-pressure hyperinflation in restrictive chest wall disease. Respiration. 1989;55(3):136–43.
30. Sunkonkit K, Al-Saleh S, Chiang J, Hamilton A, Medin D, Syed F, Mocanu C, Qazi A, Ambreen M, Amin R. Volume-assured pressure support mode for noninvasive ventilation: can it improve overnight adherence in children with neuromuscular disease? Sleep Breath. 2021;25:1843–50.
31. Veldhoen ES, Roos JH, Bekkema R. Oscillometry: A substitute of spirometry in children with neuromuscular diseases? Pediatr Pulmonol. 2022;57(7):1618–24.
32. Veldhoen ES, Vercoelen F, Ros L, Verweij-van den Oudenrijn LP, Wösten-van Asperen RM, Hulzebos EH, Bartels B, Gaytant MA, van der Ent K, Ludo van der Pol W. Short-term effect of air stacking and mechanical insufflation-exsufflation on lung function in patients with neuromuscular diseases. Chron Respir Dis. 2022;19:14799731221094619.
33. Zenteno D, Torres-Puebla G, Navarro X, Rivas C, Tapia J, Rodríguez-Núñez I, Cepeda J. Experience in a pediatric prolonged mechanical ventilation unit from a public hospital in Chile. Arch Argent Pediatr. 2021;119:25–31.

Prolonged Mechanical Ventilation in Children with Known Respiratory Disease

María Ángeles García-Teresa

1 Congenital Central Hypoventilation Syndrome (CCHS)

Congenital central hypoventilation syndrome (CCHS), also known as "Ondine's curse," is a very rare genetic disorder of the autonomic nervous system (ANS) characterized by the loss of autonomic control of respiration during non-REM sleep or, in the most severe cases, throughout the sleep cycle and even during waking hours (Table 1) [1–3]. Ventilatory responses to hypoxemia and hypercapnia are altered or absent. The innate mechanisms of respiratory drive are absent/attenuated in CCHS, and patients lack sense of asphyxia. They will not respond to hypoxemia and/or hypercapnia with increased work of breathing (retractions, deeper breaths, increased respiratory rate). Lack of sense of shortness of breath can threaten their life and neurodevelopment if profound hypoxemia is not detected. Also, children diagnosed of CCHS suffer from severe cyanotic breath-holding spells requiring manual ventilation for recovery [4–6].

CCHS may be associated with other ANS dysregulation disorders, including Hirschsprung disease (known as Haddad syndrome), sinus pauses and bradycardia, neural crest-derived tumors, and ocular disorders, among others. It is caused by heterozygous mutations in the PHOX2B gene. Several genotypes have been identified, which could condition respiratory severity. Ventilator dependence usually begins after birth (early-onset CCHS), although in some cases, hypoventilation remains undetected or misinterpreted, leading to delayed diagnosis (later onset CCHS). Later onset cases usually have the 20/24 or 20/25 polyalanine repeat mutation (PARM) genotype with milder hypoventilation [6].

Ventilatory support is life support and for lifetime, so weaning off should not be attempted. Adequate ventilation should be provided at any time: during sleep and wakefulness if necessary due to acute illness, which can be conditioning 24-h

M. Á. García-Teresa (✉)
Pediatric Intensive Care Unit, Niño Jesús University Children's Hospital, Madrid, Spain

A. Kawaguchi et al. (eds.), *Prolonged and Long-Term Mechanical Ventilation in Children*, https://doi.org/10.1007/978-981-97-8903-0_12

Table 1 Diseases in pediatric population suitable for home mechanical ventilation (HMV) [3]

Central nervous system (CNS) disorders
Congenital and acquired disorders affecting the control of the respiratory center
Congenital central hypoventilation syndrome, ROHHAD
Central hypoventilation secondary to a metabolic disease like carnitine and pyruvate kinase deficiencies; syndromes like Leigh, Moebius, and Prader-Willi; tumor; trauma; stroke; asphyxia; or infection
Myelomeningocele and Arnold-Chiari malformation
Spinal muscular atrophy
Spinal cord injury
Neuromuscular disorders
Congenital hypotonias
Myasthenia gravis and congenital myasthenic syndromes
Phrenic and diaphragmatic palsy
Myopathies
Muscular dystrophy
Guillain-Barré syndrome
Botulism
Diaphragmatic hernia
Skeletal disorders
Kyphoscoliosis
Thoracic wall deformities
Congenital and acquired cardiopathies
Respiratory disorders
Upper airway obstruction
Sleep-related respiratory disorders: Hypoventilation and obesity syndrome, obstructive sleep apnea (OSA).
Craniofacial syndromes (Pierre Robin, Treacher Collins)
Laryngotracheomalacia
Tracheoesophageal fistula
Subglottic stenosis
Arnold-Chiari malformation
Vocal cord paralysis
Bronchopulmonary disorders
Bronchopulmonary dysplasia
Cystic fibrosis
Pulmonary hypoplasia
Complications from infectious or chemical pneumonias
Sequelae of pediatric acute respiratory distress syndrome
Pulmonary fibrosis
Metabolic disorders
Glycogenoses
Mucopolysaccharidoses

dependence, or during intercurrent events. After sedation, even if the patient is awake, ventilatory support may be necessary. Children with CCHS require optimized MV at home to survive and/or achieve optimal neurodevelopmental outcomes. Early diagnosis and continuous monitoring of their respiratory status are key to prevent complications and sequelae secondary to hypoxemia and hypercapnia [4].

1.1 Ventilatory Support Requirements

1.1.1 Targets [4, 5]

To achieve normal oxygenation (SpO_2 95%) and a normal range for PCO2, ideally 4.6–6.0 kPa (35–45 mmHg). Continuous noninvasive measurement of transcutaneous/end-tidal PCO2 and pulse oximetry are recommended for setting ventilation. The normal ventilation objective should be applied to all patients, regardless of age, whether newborn or older. Therefore, the pulmonary protection strategy with permissive hypercapnia, common at NICU, is harmful for patients with CCHS, whether with noninvasive ventilation (NIV), endotracheal tube, or tracheostomy.

Typically, patients diagnosed of CCHS have a healthy lung, so hypoxia without respiratory infection means hypoventilation. In case of hypoxia, oxygen therapy should not be administered, but properly set ventilation or connection to assisted ventilation should be preferred. Oxygen therapy alone improves oxygenation but may further aggravate hypoventilation and result in coma.

At home, overnight monitoring pulse oximetry with alarms is recommended, and periodic recordings of end-tidal or transcutaneous PCO_2 should be obtained. Cardiorespiratory monitors should not be used because they do not detect hypoventilation or obstructed apneas. Continuous night observation by caregivers is recommended, especially during mask ventilation.

Modalities of Ventilatory Support [4, 5]

Four types are available: positive-pressure ventilation via tracheostomy, positive-pressure ventilation via mask (mask ventilation), phrenic nerve pacing, and negative-pressure ventilation. The choice of technique is based on aspects such as the age of patient, age of ventilation onset, hours/day on ventilation, disease severity, institution experience, and preferences of patient and families. Decision should be individualized for each patient at each stage of life, taking into account the benefits and risks of each technique (Table 2) [4, 7]. Different techniques can be combined in the same patient at the same time or at different ages [6].

Tracheostomy ventilation is the commonest method of ventilatory support in the first years of life. Different authors and the American Thoracic Society (ATS) recommend ventilation by trach during the early years of life due to its safety and in order to guarantee optimal neurodevelopmental outcomes, avoiding switching to

Table 2 Benefits and risks of different types of ventilation support in CCHS [4]

	Benefits	Risks
Tracheostomy	Decreases dead space and airway resistance Enables prolonged continuous mechanical ventilation Provides effective ventilation at baseline and during infections Prevents obstructive apneas The airway is secured Easy connection and disconnection Uses portable, battery-operated ventilators (favors mobility) Prevents obstructive apneas	Invasive ventilation Requires specialized care and long training Increases cost Daily tracheostomy care Risk of phonation and speech development delays Potential stigma May interfere with feeding Complications: Infection, accidental decannulation obstruction, granuloma, tracheomalacia, tracheo-cutaneous fistula after decannulation
Mask ventilation	Noninvasive ventilation Easy handing Short training, facilitating discharge home Avoids tracheostomy Uses portable, battery-operated ventilators (favors mobility) Reduces stigmatization, better self-image Allows speech development	Potential ineffective ventilation due to leakage, upper airway obstruction, or asynchrony The airway is not secured More limited interfaces in infants and younger children Difficult to be used more than 18 hours a day Potential discomfort, pressure sores, pain, and non-cooperation that increase the risk of self-disconnection Risk of facial deformation due to prolonged use Needs high degree of carer surveillance during sleep May require temporary intubation during infection or other challenges Potential for aspiration

(continued)

Table 2 (continued)

	Benefits	Risks
Phrenic nerve pacing	Enables mobility during ventilation Psychological well-being as the patient is independent and the breathing is "more physiological" breathing Avoids mask-related facial deformation Possibility of decannulation	Surgical procedure for implanting electrodes and receiver Requires highly experienced medical centers Can cause OSA requiring mask ventilation, when decannulated Pacer malfunction Surgery is needed for replacement of electrode or receiver The airway is not secured There is no alarm to alert carers to antenna-receiver uncoupling in some devices Not indicated under one 1 year old Pacing >12–16 hours a day is not recommended. May require alternative or additional form of ventilation support during illness
Negative-pressure ventilation	Noninvasive ventilation Avoids tracheostomy. Easy handling Short training, facilitating discharge If used just overnight, the patient is device-free during the day Costs less than tracheostomy. The face is free Avoids mask-related facial deformation	Ventilation is less effective Lack of portability The patient is not accessible for assessment and care (according to devices) Can cause OSA requiring mask ventilation The airway is not secured Can cause aspiration in patients with swallowing disorders Can cause back/shoulder pain and difficulty sleeping related to supine positioning Can cause skin irritation and a sense of feeling chilled May require alternative or additional form of ventilation support during illness

CCHS congenital central hypoventilation syndrome; *OSA* obstructive sleep apnea

mask before age 6–8 years [5]. However, this is subject to controversy [4, 8] as there are no studies analyzing the impact of the choice of ventilatory support modality on neurodevelopment.

Tracheostomy is performed as soon as technically possible after diagnosis in newborns and young infants. Uncuffed cannulas are recommended in infants and children to reduce the risk of tracheomalacia and to ease speech. Cuffed cannulas may be required in children during intercurrent severe lower respiratory infections. Adult patients are more likely to use them to avoid leaks during assisted ventilation. The cannula size should be adjusted as the child grows. Smaller cannulas are generally preferred as long as adequate ventilation is provided. According to European guidelines, indications for bronchoscopy in tracheostomized CCHS patients are as follow: (i) before decannulation; (ii) if symptoms, such as airway bleeding, breath-holding spells, pain, cyanosis or desaturation during cannula changes, wheezing, recurrent infections, intolerance to a speaking valve or plugged tracheostomy cannula, change in voice quality; (iii) every 3–6 months in infants and young children in the first 2 years after tracheostomy inserted; (iv) after changing the cannula size or type, to check its position using simple fiber-optic tracheoscopy [4].

Mask ventilation is the first option for older children and adult patients presenting with late-onset CCHS. Since some infants with early-onset CCHS have received mask ventilation without ever using tracheotomy, European guidelines state that mask ventilation may be considered in infants and young children with close monitoring [4]. Mask ventilation may be considered as an alternative initial modality for very specific patients, such as babies with milder mutations (20/24, 20/25 PARM mutations) associated with milder hypoventilation and no comorbidities [6].

Mask ventilation requirements are (i) cooperative patient with normal airway and either adequate spontaneous ventilation or phrenic nerve pacing during wakefulness; (ii) high degree of supervision by the carers during sleep, especially for infants and young children as there may be serious consequences of dislocation of the mask or obstruction of the upper airway; and (iii) preventive measures to avoid long-term facial deformities (alternating interfaces, avoiding tight fitting, use of full-face mask, and long-term follow-up by maxillofacial and dental teams) [4].

Transition from tracheostomy to face mask varies and is usually initiated in cooperative children between 5 and 11 years old. There are many reasons to change, such as preventing infections and other complications from the tracheostomy, avoiding daily tracheostomy care, preventing stigma, and improving self-confidence. Before the change, assessment for possible upper airway obstruction should be performed and treated appropriately [4, 9].

Phrenic nerve pacing [4] offers freedom from the ventilator during daytime in patients ventilated 24 h a day, thus increasing their mobility and engagement in activities. Pacing during daylight hours switches to tracheostomy or mask during night time. Also, pacemaker can be used in teenagers or adult patients only with nocturnal ventilation [4–6]. Pacing more than 12–16 h/day is generally not recommended.

Phrenic pacemaker device is composed of external (radio-transmitter, antenna) and internal components (receptor, wires, and bilateral electrodes, placed surgically in the thorax). It electrically stimulates the phrenic nerve, generating the diaphragmatic contraction. When stimulation stops, passive expiration follows. In order to work adequately, the antenna needs to be just above the receptor to receive the signal appropriately. Two phrenic nerve pacing systems are currently commercially available: a monopolar electrode system from Avery® Biomedical Devices Inc. (New York, USA) and a quadripolar electrode system from Atrotech® Ltd. (Tampere, Finland) [4]. A new pacemaker model has been developed that stimulates diaphragm muscles directly.

An experienced center is needed for surgery and follow-up, not available in all countries. Surgical procedure includes a cervical approach, open thoracotomy, or thoracoscopy. After 2–6 weeks of wound healing and resting, the pacing training period of 2–4 months is initiated. First pacing should not last longer than 1–2 h/day, increasing weekly by 30–60 min/day, until full pacing of 12–16 h/day. The aim is to achieve adequate ventilation and oxygenation with a minimum electrical phrenic stimulation. Respiratory pacing is not indicated under 1 year of age. Relative contraindications enclose chronic lung or airway disease, including obstructive sleep apnea (OSA), severe behavioral disorders, and obesity. Patients under 6 years of age also need tracheostomy in order to prevent recurrent OSAs. Between 6 and 12 years old, successful decannulation is feasible with caution and careful observation for airway obstruction which can be managed by increasing the inspiratory time and decreasing the force of inspiration or with mask ventilation. Phrenic nerve pacing requires careful training of the caregivers and the patients, and at least yearly follow-up in a center with expertise in phrenic pacing [4, 5].

Risks are postoperative infection which requires surgical removal and replacement of the implants and phrenic paralysis, usually transient. Over time, pacer malfunction due to defect of the external or internal components may appear and can need surgical replacement [4].

Mode

Patients with CCHS have reduced spontaneous breaths and tidal volume, and they cannot properly trigger the ventilator. Therefore, the selected ventilation mode should ensure total ventilatory support, regardless of whether the patient participates or not. This is achieved with the controlled and assisted/controlled modes. The assisted/support mode can also be used if appropriate parameters are set (optimal minimum inspiratory time, backup rate, and minimal guaranteed volume) [4].

Pressure-Controlled Versus Volume-Controlled

Pressure-controlled ventilation provides better ventilation than volume-controlled in case of variable or large leaks, e.g., with uncuffed tracheostomy cannulas or during mask ventilation [4, 5]. Newly designed home ventilators have mixed ventilation modes, combining a pressure-controlled mode with a minimal guaranteed volume. Such devices may allow more stable PCO_2 values during different sleep states in children [10, 11].

Pressure-controlled ventilation (e.g., pressure control on the ventilators, or timed mode on the bi-level devices or pressure support with optimal minimum inspiratory time, backup rate, and minimal guaranteed tidal/minute volume) is recommended. Inspiratory positive pressure (IPP) and expiratory positive pressure (PEEP) are set independently to provide optimal tidal volume and should be individualized for each patient. IPP-PEEP ≥ 10 cmH_2O is usually needed to achieve it. PEEP commonly set is 5 cm H2O [4]. Respiratory rate and inspiratory time are set according to the patient's age. Pressure support mode (e.g., pressure support on ventilators, spontaneous/timed

(S/T) on some bi-level devices, and spontaneous (S) modes on bi-level devices) and CPAP mode should be avoided because they could provide inadequate ventilation [4].

Home Ventilators [3–5, 12]

Transition to portable ventilator is easy in CCHS patients, who participate very little in ventilation. Availability of brands and models of positive-pressure home ventilators varies between centers and countries. Modern home devices incorporate some technological innovations of PICU devices, in addition to including portability (small sized, light, internal and external battery for several hours, room air as gas source, low-pressure O2 connection) and comfort (quiet or even silent in normal operation). Ventilators should be suitable for the age and weight of the patient (this is critical for infants and small children). Some modern machines deliver 30 ml of minimum tidal volume. According to the author's experience, also a 50 ml minimum tidal volume device can be safety used in CCHS children under 5 kg if pressure-controlled mode is set and an uncuffed cannula or mask ventilation is used. Bi-level devices must include a minimum inspiratory time and a backup rate setting to be used safely in patients with central hypoventilation on mask ventilation. Security alarms must be properly adjusted according to the set ventilation mode and regularly checked. Patients with CCHS should have a second, backup ventilator available, being a life support therapy [3–5].

1.2 Follow-Up [4, 11, 12]

After discharge, a comprehensive follow-up program should be established in an experienced reference center providing regular multidisciplinary reviews. Children under 2 years old should be evaluated every 2–6 months and those over 2, once a year or more frequent if symptoms are present. Respiratory status should be assessed both awake and asleep. Spontaneous breathing is valued with SpO2, Tc, or Et-CO2 while awake. Adjusting of ventilator settings is performed by polysomnography (PSG) or cardiorespiratory recording with oximetry and PCO2 during sleep. Neurodevelopment, growth, and family and educational needs should be evaluated as well. In addition to referral center, there should be close follow-up by a local pulmonologist or pediatrician [12]. As lifelong ventilatory support is required, transition to adult care should be planned.

2 Other Diseases with Central Hypoventilation

Rapid-onset obesity, hypothalamic dysfunction, hypoventilation, and autonomic dysregulation (ROHHAD) is a very rare condition with no known associated mutation that differs from CCHS. Affected subjects most commonly present with dramatic and rapid weight gain and associated hyperphagia during childhood. Other key clinical features develop later and include hypoventilation that can produce sudden cardiorespiratory arrest, endocrinopathies (water-sodium imbalance, early or late puberty, cortisol, prolactin anomalies), autonomic dysregulation (strabismus, disorders of temperature control), and neuroendocrine tumors in a subset of patients. Some children may initially need artificial ventilation during sleep and then progress to 24-h respiratory support [4, 5].

Central hypoventilation may be secondary to drugs and CNS disorders, such as a metabolic disease (carnitine, pyruvate kinase deficiencies); syndromes like Leigh, Moebius, and Prader-Willi; malformation (Arnold-Chiari); asphyxia; tumor; stroke; infection; or trauma [4].

Subjects with Arnold-Chiari malformation may associate central or obstructive hypoventilation, with the latter secondary to vocal cord palsy that can present with sudden and intermittent suffocating events. Neurosurgery (decompressive laminectomy, correction of associated syringomyelia, or hydrocephalus) can stabilize respiratory status and sometimes allow removal of the respiratory support.

Mask or tracheostomy ventilation will be chosen according to each patient diagnosed of central hypoventilation, and the selected ventilation mode should ensure total respiratory support, as noted above [4].

3 Disorders Causing Upper Airway Obstruction

3.1 *Cardiopulmonary No OSA Disorders*

Some congenital or acquired entities (craniofacial syndromes, airway malformations, subglottic stenosis, vocal cord paralysis, laryngomalacia, tracheal stenosis, trachea-bronchomalacia, etc.) can produce significant airway obstruction in infants and children who may benefit from nocturnal home noninvasive CPAP treatment, associated or not with a reparative surgical procedure [13]. In daily care, mask fitting and the CPAP level should be adjusted according to the resolution of respiratory symptoms, a pulse oximetry above 95%, the greatest decrease in heart and respiratory rates, and the best comfort for the child [14]. Optimal setting will be done under polysomnography. A mean pressure of 7.3 cm H2O improved obstruction in infants and children with cardiopulmonary no OSA disorders [13].

However, airway conditions can cause continuous airway obstruction requiring tracheostomy not only if life-threatening, but also if neurodevelopment and growth are involved and NIV has failed or is not indicated, and a surgical technique is not available. Infants with trachea-bronchomalacia (secondary or not to tracheostomy) may require ventilatory support with 24-h CPAP and trach until skeletal maturation during early childhood increases the tone of airway cartilage or, if suitable, until a surgical approach is performed.

3.2 Obstructive Sleep Apnea (OSA)

Obstructive sleep apnea (OSA) is characterized by episodes of complete or partial upper airway obstruction during sleep, often resulting in gas exchange abnormalities and arousals. OSA can occur in predisposed patients (with congenital syndromes, malformations, metabolic disorders, neuromuscular disorders, or obesity) or in otherwise healthy children due to adenotonsil hypertrophy [15–17]. At present, OSA represents one of the most prevalent pediatric conditions of those under long-term MV [1, 2, 18].

Different treatment modalities are often combined depending on the age of the child, severity, and underlying conditions predisposing to OSA (Table 3) [3]. Goals of treatment include improvement of cognitive fitness, behavioral and attentional disturbances, increasing weight, and preventing the development of cardiovascular complications [15, 16].

Positive airway pressure therapy (continuous positive airway pressure [CPAP] or bi-level positive airway pressure [BPAP]) through a mask prevents upper airway obstruction and is indicated for children with moderate or severe OSA and any of the following: minimal adenotonsillar tissue, persistent OSA despite adenotonsillectomy, craniofacial abnormalities (if suitable, until surgical techniques are performed), or if adenotonsillectomy is contraindicated. Also, it should be necessary before adenotonsillectomy if severe symptoms and hypoxemia are present. Generally, nasal

Table 3 Clinical and polysomnographic criteria and respiratory support in pediatric OSA [3]

Obstructive sleep apnea	
Clinical criteria	Sleep disorders: heavy snoring, observed apneas, restlessness during sleep, excessive sweating, mouth breathing, nocturnal enuresis Daytime involvement: excessive sleepiness, inattention/hyperactivity, cognitive deficits and learning difficulties, behavioral disorder Failure to thrive, systemic arterial hypertension, pulmonary hypertension, cor pulmonale
Polysomnographic criteria	Apnea-hypopnea index (AHI): >1–4.9, mild OSA; 5–9.9, moderate OSA; >10, severe OSA End-tidal or transcutaneous CO2 > 50 mmHg for >25% total sleep time (obstructive hypoventilation)
Treatment	Depends on child's age, clinical symptoms, comorbidities, risk factors, and polysomnographic result if performed Important to consider: AHI >5 or AHI >1 and comorbidity End-tidal or transcutaneous CO2 > 50 mmHg for >25% total sleep time Ventilation strategy (CPAP, BPAP): It will be discussed after considering adenotonsillectomy/weight loss/nasal corticosteroid therapy/antileukotriene treatment/orthodontics It may be necessary before adenotonsillectomy if severe symptoms and hypoxemia are present

OSA Obstructive sleep apnea; *AHI* Apnea-hypopnea index; *CPAP* Continuous positive airway pressure; *BPAP* Bi-level positive airway pressure; CO_2 Carbon dioxide interfaces are used although a full-face mask may be necessary in a few patients, such as those with craniofacial abnormalities or complete nasal obstruction [14–16].

Ideally, the equipment fitting and CPAP titration are performed during polysomnography (PSG) in a sleep laboratory with expertise in managing pediatric patients [15], but other easily available and simpler tools (symptoms, comfort, SpO2, Tc CO2, built-in software of home devices) have been successfully used in selected children [19, 20]. CPAP pressures should be started at 4 cmH_2O and progressively increased until snoring and airflow obstruction resolve. Symptoms, signs, and hypopnea index (AHI) improvement has been reported in a series of children under CPAP therapy administered at a mean pressure level of 8 cmH_2O. The "treatment-emergent central sleep apnea" may develop in some patients during a successfully titrating CPAP, due to sudden fall in $PaCO_2$ levels below the threshold for apnea. Excessive CPAP pressure should be avoided to minimize the issue; switching to BPAP may not produce improvement but worsening of central apnea. Problem generally resolves over time [14, 15].

BPAP may be used instead of CPAP in children with OSA if significant pulmonary hypoventilation or clinically significant central apneas are present. Sometimes, BPAP can improve tolerability if higher CPAP pressure is needed [16]; however, asynchronies can appear using BPAP [21].

Auto-CPAP devices automatically adjust CPAP pressure between a set range, based on detection of apnea, hypopnea, flow limitation, snoring, or free-flowing air. Auto-CPAP is effective, well tolerated, and widely used in adult patients, but there is not enough evidence for its generalized recommendation in children. Auto-CPAP has shown safety and efficacy in initiating therapy in older children [22, 23], but lower self-titrated than polysomnographic titrated pressure level has been seen in other reported children's work [24]. According to manufacturers' indications, auto-CPAP can be only used if more than 30 kg.

3.3 *Follow-Up*

Close follow-up should be performed assessing efficacy, side effects (especially skin injury or facial deformity), adherence and weaning attempt to CPAP, and changes in child clinical status. Nocturnal positive airway pressure therapy can be a challenge at the beginning and ongoing therapy, especially in young children because of intolerance to technique or unavailability of a proper interface; therapy requires a motivated family [2, 13]. Adherence can be optimized with proper mask fitting, custom-made interface, optimal positive-pressure titration, warm humidifier adding, or behavioral and family support [14, 18, 25]. High-flow nasal cannula may be an alternative for children not compliant with continuous positive airway pressure [26], although portable devices provide minimum 15 Lpm flow and are not approved under 30 kg. Most patients, especially infants with respiratory obstruction, can be weaned from CPAP by spontaneous improvement to growth or after orthodontics, surgery, or lost weight. Long-term follow-up is always necessary in children with associated disorders [27].

4 Bronchopulmonary Dysplasia

Bronchopulmonary dysplasia (BPD) is a lung development chronic disease secondary to prematurity. In more severe forms (defined as type 2 severe BPD, sBPD), infants may need prolonged mechanical ventilation beyond 36 weeks' corrected age or at hospital discharge [28, 29]. Preterm infants with sBPD remain intubated or dependent on noninvasive support. Such infants demonstrate tachypnea, increased work of breathing, and air hunger whenever ventilatory support is weaned. Also, they may have repeated hypoxic spells. They develop chronic respiratory insufficiency, as demonstrated by retained carbon dioxide and oxygen dependence, and atelectasis and hyperinflation appear on chest X-ray. More severe patients require tracheostomy. Severe forms of BPD occur in 16% of premature infants younger than 32 weeks of GA. Mortality of infants with tracheostomy-dependent BPD is around 15%. BPD is a heterogeneous disease both among patients and in the same patient, resulting from the simultaneous phenomena of maturation, damage, and lung repair after birth. It can affect the pulmonary parenchyma, pulmonary vessels, or small and large airways. In the same patient, variable anatomical changes appear that may include areas of lung destruction with macrocysts and hyperinflation, microcysts, atelectasis, or fibrosis. Lesions may result in increased dead space, impaired ventilation/perfusion, pulmonary hypertension, or small and large airway collapse (trachea-bronchomalacia) [28, 29]. Concurrent obstructive and restrictive patterns are present. Airway resistance is also highly variable resulting in lung segments with strikingly different respiratory time constant (trs). Functionally, alveoli result in two different simultaneous compartments, slow one (high resistance (R) and low compliance (C)) and fast one (relatively normal R and C), according to their trs, and therefore have diverse ventilatory needs [29].

4.1 *Ventilation Strategy*

Several chronic ventilator dependence predicting factors have been described in extremely preterm babies [30, 31]. Low gestational age and low birth weight are the main predictors, and also pulmonary hypertension, trachea-bronchomalacia, and progressively elevated CO_2 may be related to chronic ventilation. Regarding treatment, high tidal volumes in the first 24 hours of life (early volutrauma) predict chronic ventilator dependence and that together with atelectasis and oxygen toxicity contributes mainly to ventilator-induced lung injury, being a major, potentially modifiable, risk factor of BPD. Such findings have led to the use of the least invasive mode possible that meets the infant's needs, avoiding intubation with early nasal NIV and selective less invasive surfactant administration or early extubating to nasal NIV in acutely preterm infants with respiratory distress syndrome (RDS), in order to prevent lung injury and BPD [32, 33]. Also, a pulmonary protection ventilatory strategy (permissive hypercapnia, permissive hypoxemia with low tidal volume, short inspiratory time, high frequency) is used if intubated [34]. However, persistent use of early protective ventilator approaches in established lung disease leads to worsening of both hyperinflation and atelectasis, impaired gas exchange, predisposition for respiratory spells, and increased work of breathing [34].

4.1.1 Long-Term MV at NICU

Noninvasive Ventilation [32–37]

Noninvasive neonatal ventilation plays a key role in maintaining respiratory function from delivery room until pulmonary maturity is reached. NIV allows infants with BPD to wean from invasive mechanical ventilation and prevents the recurrence of respiratory failure requiring re-intubation. Often, preterm babies spend several months at NICU under NIV. Binasal prongs/nasal mask and different modes of non-invasive neonatal ventilation are used [32–37]:

High-flow nasal cannula (HFNC) is the most used for long respiratory support [35], where heated and humidified air is delivered through specialized nasal prongs at flow rates generally ranging between 2 and 8 L/min.

Nasal continuous positive airway pressure (NCPAP) is also recommended for long respiratory support after RSD to minimize lung injury until respiratory stability [32–36]. NCPAP systems are classified into constant flow (bubble CPAP and ventilator CPAP) and variable flow systems (infant flow), depending on the technique used to control the gas flow to the patient. Bubble CPAP is an affordable and readily available device in low-income countries.

Noninvasive neurally adjusted ventilatory assist (NIV-NAVA): NAVA is another relatively new modality, available both invasively or noninvasively (NIV-NAVA). The ventilator synchronizes with the patient by detecting the electrical activity of the diaphragm using a special nasogastric tube with electrodes and delivers a pressure support proportional to the patient's inspiratory efforts during respiratory rate and inspiratory time, also decided by the patient's inspiratory effort. This ability to synchronization (neural triggering) is not influenced by leaks and allows for decreased work of breathing, improved gas exchange, and earlier extubating [37].

Nasal intermittent positive-pressure ventilation (NIPPV) is a pressure-controlled, time-cycled mode. It can be synchronized (SNIPPV) with the patient's inspiratory effort through flow triggering, which has shown the greatest effectiveness in acute RSD.

Invasive Ventilation [34–36, 38–43]

When anatomical changes appear (usually after 36 weeks of GA), change to a chronic ventilatory strategy for intubated infants with severe BPD is recommend by experts [34–36, 38–43]. However, it is not an evidence-based recommendation, but rather a recommendation based on the heterogeneity of disease. Actually, different strategies are used [36]. The following settings are advisable, based on expert recommendations:

Mode: The most physiologically appropriate chronic ventilation mode may be the combined mode of volume-guaranteed synchronized intermittent mandatory ventilation (SIMV+VG) and pressure support ventilation (PSV). With the SIMV+VG mode, slow compartments of the lung with high R and low C can be adequately ventilated, while fast compartments having relatively normal R and C can be ventilated well with the pressure support mode. Also, volume-control SIMV mode can be used. Controlled or assisted/controlled modes (both with invariable inspiratory time) can cause severe air trapping in case of tachypnea, so they are generally not recommended.

Settings:

Regional heterogeneity: High Vt (10–15 mL/kg), due to the increase in the dead space; slow rate (12–20/bpm); and long Ti (0.5–1 seconds), to allow proper filling and emptying of slow compartment. The IPP achieved is usually high (30–40 cm H20 or higher) due to low compliance and high resistance in sBPD. PS (6–18 cmH2O, as needed), in order to ventilate rapid compartments, and spontaneous breathing are supported with adequate PS and shorter Ti. PS should not exceed the inspiratory pressure of the set breaths.

Airway collapse: High PEEP levels (7–12 cmH_2O) [36]. PEEP level should be individualized in each patient. Generally, PEEP elevated levels are required to avoid atelectasis and overcome expiratory collapse of both small airway (which generates intrinsic PEEP) and large airway (if associated trachea-bronchomalacia). A minimum 6–8 cm H_2O is usually necessary, and until 15 cm H_2O has been described. High PEEP must be associated with low mandatory rate strategy; otherwise, there is high risk of gas trapping. Higher PEEP may improve synchrony and reduce breathing work when significant trachea-bronchomalacia is present.

NAVA invasive**:** NAVA is an emerging ventilator strategy, alternative to conventional flow-triggered ventilation, which may improve outcomes for infants with evolving or established sBPD. A retrospective study in infants with sBPD placed under NAVA at PMA 40 +/− 5 weeks showed that NAVA can be used safely and effectively, allowing both extubating to noninvasive positive-pressure ventilation (avoiding tracheostomy) or support with a home ventilator in some selective sBPD infants [35, 37].

Target [32–44]

Assessment of adequate respiratory support goes beyond monitoring oxygenation status (O2 sat 92–95% to prevent pulmonary hypertension) and ventilation (permissive hypercapnia, to facilitate weaning). In addition, goals should be aimed at prioritizing respiratory stability by supporting breathing and relieving respiratory distress, keeping the infant calm without sedation, weaning with patience and caution, and surveillance and support of somatic and neurodevelopmental growth to promote lung damage healing. Careful attention should be paid to the negative impact of weaning on these goals [32, 44].

When to Perform Tracheostomy [40, 41, 44–46]

Tracheostomy decisions and determining the optimal tracheostomy time are challenging in infants with severe BPD, both intubated or on noninvasive support [40, 45]. Tracheostomy for chronic ventilation is a difficult and complex decision in which ethical and social considerations are raised. An interdisciplinary medical team and the child's family will share decision-making, considering advantages and disadvantages [46]. Tracheostomy should not be viewed as a method for rapid weaning of respiratory support but, despite its risks, rather as a means of reducing respiratory distress and providing respiratory stability to enhance growth and developmental outcomes, facilitating rehabilitation, participation in daily living, and developmental activities, and also allowing NICU discharge to transitional care unit or at home. There are no guidelines or consensus on tracheostomy decision on sBPD. A recent analysis survey with 31 NICUs of the USA participating showed that tracheostomy was strongly considered when airway malacia or pulmonary hypertension was present, $PCO2 \geq 76–85$ mmHg, $FiO2 \geq 0.60$, PEEP $\geq 9–11$ cm H2O, respiratory rate $\geq 61–70$ breaths/min, PMA ≥ 44 weeks, and weight $< 10\%$ at 44 weeks PMA. They were generally less likely to agree on offering tracheostomy if the infant was demonstrating weaning of respiratory support and was on noninvasive ventilation (NIV), FiO2 was lower than 0.4, or PMA was <44 weeks or PMA was up to 52 weeks if on NIV [45].

The decision of tracheostomy in NIV-dependent children is much more difficult and, according to the mentioned survey, it arises later than in intubated [45]. Another question to consider is whether the child could continue with NIV support outside the NICU or even at home. Several aspects should be considered in this debate regarding (i) the patient, such as the level of respiratory autonomy, clinical stability, and ensuring adequate physical growth and neurodevelopment; (ii) the institution/country, by checking if healthcare facility and health authorities are provided or not of NIV approach for infants; BiPAP and CPAP are not FDA-approved modalities for outpatient treatment in infants, but they are used in Europe and Australia; and (iii) the family, knowing its involvement in the patient's care.

Home Ventilator [34]

Successful transition to home ventilators can be difficult and challenging due to the light weight of recently tracheostomized preterm infants. Sometimes, it is necessary to wait for their growing, often weeks or months, to get optimal ventilation and infant's comfort with home devices. Home ventilators on SIMV volume-controlled mode may be unable to generate the low flows needed to deliver the set volume in a longer inspiratory time, according to the chronic ventilation strategy shown above.

In addition, preterm infants may be unable to trigger ventilator inspiration, resulting in asynchronies. However, inspiratory time may be lengthened using SIMV pressure-controlled mode, though unexpected changes in compliance or resistance can lead to significant changes in ventilation. Also, mixed ventilation modes (combining a pressure-controlled mode with a minimal guaranteed volume) permit longer inspiratory times with smaller targeted tidal volumes. As indicated above, NAVA has also shown efficacy during the transition to home ventilator [37].

Controlled or assisted/controlled modes (both with invariable inspiratory time) can cause severe air trapping in case of tachypnea, so they are generally not recommended for these patients.

Pressure support or CPAP modes may suffice in some patients.

Pressure support mode (also called S mode—spontaneous—in BLPAP ventilators): Respiratory rate is decided by the patient and ideally also the inspiratory time. The ventilator detects the patient's effort and, over a constant expiratory pressure (PEEP, EPAP), supports it with an inspiratory pressure (PIP, IPAP) until expiratory trigger (inspiratory cycle off sensitivity) is activated. The duration of the inspiratory time will depend on the patient's inspiratory effort, the programmed cycling flow rate percentage—expiratory trigger—leakages, and minimum and maximum inspiratory times set. Inspiratory trigger and expiratory cycle off sensitivity can be set or are automatically fixed, depending on devices. Also, an inspiratory rise time (or slope), that regulates the higher or lower flow rate at inspiratory onset, can be set for optimizing the patient's comfort. Pressure support is a physiological mode and improves patient's comfort and patient-ventilator synchrony.

CPAP: The ventilator delivers a constant pressure (CPAP, EPAP, PEEP) throughout the respiratory cycle and, over pressure, the patient is breathing spontaneously. It is the most comfortable mode, and patient-ventilator synchrony is 100%.

New home devices can deliver 30 ml minimum tidal volume and allow to set several scenarios simultaneously (night, day, exacerbation, exercise, etc.), combining several modes, which enable their use for more kinds of patients or for the same patient in different clinical conditions.

4.1.2 Out-of-ICU Long-Term Ventilation

Currently, invasive ventilation remains a common treatment for children with BPD requiring long-term ventilatory support [47–50]. Discharge home, usually from transitional care units, is a long and complex process; available data report a mean hospital stay between 6.9 and 12.9 months for BPD tracheostomized patients [50]. Coordination of multiple issues required for discharge (patient's medical condition, devices, assistance at home, family support, follow-up after discharge) will be optimized by a home ventilation program [50].

Long-term home NIV [13, 14, 51–54]: Data for patients with BPD are quite sparse in studies evaluating patients using long-term NIV or they are limited to a few reported individual cases, out of North America. BLPAP and CPAP are not FDA-approved modalities for outpatient treatment in infants, but they are being used in Europe, Australia, and South America. Sometimes, sBPD infants are discharged home with no ventilation, and NIV is then begun at follow-up in order to enhance gas exchange and reduce work of breathing. Use of home NIV CPAP and BPAP and AVAPS modes have been reported, usually during sleeping. The most frequent interface used is a nasal mask. Titrating CPAP value is recommended, and need of high levels (a mean of 8 cmH_2O) has been reported [13, 14].

4.2 Follow-Up

Outpatient follow-up care with regular reviews is clearly important, although specific guidelines have not been elaborated. Comprehensive and coordinated care by the general physician and subspecialist is recommended [2, 12]. Regular surveillance and support of both physical and neurodevelopmental growth are critical, as well as vigilance for pulmonary hypertension.

Successful decannulation is the end target of any tracheostomy for BPD. Release from mechanical ventilation and decannulation will be successful in most survivor patients with sBPD, as a result of the continuous and physiological process of lung maturation. Decreased dependence on mechanical ventilation is the earliest indicator of readiness for decannulation. The patient can be decannulated even if oxygen therapy is still needed. Decannulation may also be considered if the child tolerates noninvasive procedures (e.g., nasal cannula or CPAP). Liberation from MV took place before age 5 (median age of 2 years) and decannulation before age 6 (median age of 3 years) in a retrospective study of 83 surviving sBPD children [47].

5 Cystic Fibrosis

Cystic fibrosis (CF) is an autosomal recessive disease, usually caused by a mutation in the CFTR (CF transmembrane conductance regulator) gene, which affects mucus- and sweat-producing cells. Many vital organs are involved, especially the lung, the primary cause of morbidity and mortality in patients with CF, despite optimized care. The thick and sticky mucus obstructs the airway since infancy, leading to recurrent and serious infections. Chronic inflammation causes bronchiectasis and progressive destruction of pulmonary tissue, followed by a progressive deterioration in lung function with low compliance, which leads to respiratory muscle load and increased total work of breathing. Patients with mild-moderate CF lung disease may develop hypoventilation during sleep, exercise, or acute respiratory exacerbations. Different respiratory mechanics are involved in sleep hypoventilation: alveolar hypoventilation, increase in ventilation–perfusion mismatch, increase in airflow resistance, and decrease in functional residual capacity. Severe lung disease is characterized by a rapid shallow breathing pattern, daytime hypercapnia and hypoxia, and pulmonary hypertension, which indicates poor prognosis and prompts referral for lung transplantation [55–57]

5.1 Noninvasive Ventilation

Chronic Respiratory Failure (CRF) with Hypoxia and Hypercapnia Usually Appears in Adulthood, more Rarely in Adolescence and Seldom in Children [57–59]. In the Coming Years, a Progressive Age Delay of Developing CRF Is Expected, Due to CFTR Modulator Treatment. This Therapy Is Likely to Make the Need for Noninvasive Support Even less Prevalent than at Present, for the CF Pediatric Population, in which a 2011 Survey Showed Only a 0.4% of NIV Use [60]

Physiological effects [54–56]: NIV improves pulmonary and chest compliance; decreases respiratory muscle load, respiratory work, fatigue, and polypnea; and enhances tidal volume, alveolar ventilation, and gas exchange, even if used for a short time (sleep, exercise) in CF.

Outcomes [54–60]: NIV can improve quality of sleep, exercise tolerance, and airway clearance during chest physiotherapy; can prevent invasive ventilation during acute exacerbations; can reduce the number of infectious exacerbations; and can improve hypercapnia and stabilize the decrease in lung function in patients with advanced FC lung disease [57].

5.2 Indications [55–59]

NIV has been used in acute and chronic respiratory failure in children and adults with CF; however, there are no validated criteria for its initiation**.** CF Foundation Consensus Guidelines from 2020 recommend home NIV in patients with advanced FC lung disease with PaCO2 ≥ 55 mmHg or PaCO2 50–54 mmHg and nocturnal hypoxemia, or PaCO2 50–54 mmHg and more than two hospitalizations for hypercapnic respiratory failure in the previous year. Also, several clinical criteria are applied for indicating NIV both in acute and chronic settings: severe respiratory exacerbation and diurnal hypercapnia, prevent or treat severe respiratory exacerbations, patient's wishes for relief of dyspnea, accelerated fall in lung functions, palliative care for end-stage CF lung disease, and postoperative period of transplanted patients. Also, NIV may be added to chest physiotherapy in patients with muscle fatigue, desaturation, and poor tolerance of the physiotherapy or in children admitted due to accelerated fall lung function. However, there is a need for long-term randomized controlled trials to determine the clinical effects of NIV in adults and children with cystic fibrosis. If subpleural bullae are present, NIV must not be performed.

5.3 Mode

Pressure support modes (PS, BPAP S) with nasal masks are the most frequently used because of the most physiological mode and better comfort than fixed mandatory or volume modes [61]. Also, BPAP ST can reduce respiratory effort and tachypnea in some patients [62]. No randomized controlled trials have evaluated the efficacy of novel modes of NIV such as VAPS in hypercapnic CF patients. Ventilatory settings should be adjusted to improve symptoms associated with alveolar hypoventilation. In clinical practice, several noninvasive clinical parameters such as comfort, SpO2, tcCO2, respiratory rate, and tidal volume are used to guide this titration during awake and sleep [63]. Use of polysomnography when initiating NIV in CF patients has not been established [64]. There is no consensus on the ventilatory strategy for chronic CF patients. A possible lower inspiratory pressure peak is recommended to avoid barotrauma. Expiratory pressure (EPAP, PEEP, or CPAP) can be programmed to overcome intrinsic PEEP and bronchial obstruction, or not added PEEP in young stable patients with CF, who generally have minimal intrinsic PEEP [55, 63]. Expiratory trigger between 30 and 50% of peak inspiratory flow and a slow slope (inspiratory rise time) have been used in those young patients. CPAP mode should be used if OSA is present and no adenotonsillar tissue obstruction [65].

Risks [55–60] of NIV that should be avoided in CF patients: (i) gastric hyperinflation: it can worsen respiratory symptoms and increases risk of aspiration; (ii) barotrauma: as low as possible inspiratory pressure peak and optimal synchrony should be assured to prevent it; and (iii) infection from distilled water: daily rigorous and careful cleaning and disinfection of the devices must be carried out to avoid possible infections from the water reservoirs. Sterile water should be used for refilling, because distilled water has the risk of CF pathogen contamination.

5.4 Follow-Up [2, 55–60]

Low adherence to the highly chronic therapy burden is a common problem in CF patients, and NIV failure is common in the sparse pediatric population users [60]. Individual education on disease progress and the need for therapy, and family and social support, can improve patient adherence. Regular clinical screening for respiratory symptoms, sleep quality, and NIV side effects can detect issues early and promote compliance. Pulse oximetry is one of the most used methods for follow-up respiratory evaluation, and also periodic recordings of transcutaneous PCO_2 are recommended [60]. The new home ventilators can provide useful information on built-in software (adherence, leaks, efficacy of ventilation) for telemonitoring ventilation [20]. Long-term NIV outcome, especially in a better survival and quality of life, is insufficient and should be assessed in the future.

6 Conclusion

LTV strategy (technique, mode, parameters, devices, place, etc.) should be individualized for each patient taking into account the underlying pathology, clinical status, and patient/family wishes (if possible), aiming optimal growth and neurodevelopmental outcomes. A comprehensive and multidisciplinary follow-up program should be established for also monitoring adherence, need of changes on ventilation strategy (including possibility of withdrawal or decannulation), and educational and family needs. If lifelong ventilatory support is required, transition to adult care should be planned.

References

1. Castro Codesal ML, Featherstone R, Martínez Carrasco C, et al. Long-term non-invasive ventilation therapies in children: a scoping review protocol. BMJ Open. 2015;5:e008697. https://doi.org/10.1136/bmjopen-2015-008697.
2. Fauroux B, Abel F, Amaddeo A, et al. ERS statement on paediatric long-term noninvasive respiratory support. Eur Respir J. 2022;59:2101404. https://doi.org/10.1183/13993003.01404-2021.
3. García-Teresa MA, Pons-Ódena M, De Lama G, et al. Home mechanical ventilation in paediatrics. In: Medina A, Pilar J, García Cusco M, et al., editors. Handbook of paediatric and neonatal mechanical ventilation. 2nd. ed. Las Palmas de Gran Canaria: Tesela ediciones; 2021. Chapter 24.
4. Trang H, Samuels M, Ceccherini I, et al. Guidelines for diagnosis and management of congenital central hypoventilation syndrome. Orphanet J Rare Dis. 2020;15:252. https://doi.org/10.1186/s13023-020-01460-2.
5. Weese-Mayer DE, Berry-Kravis EM, Ceccherini I, et al. An official ATS clinical policy statement: congenital central hypoventilation syndrome genetic basis, diagnosis, and management. Am J Respir Crit Care Med. 2010;181:626–44. https://doi.org/10.1164/rccm.200807-1069ST.
6. Garcia Teresa MA, Porto Abal R, Rodríguez Torres S, et al. Spanish patients with central hypoventilation syndrome included in the European registry. The 2015 data. An Pediatr (Barc). 2017;86(5):255–63.
7. Lee JH, Smith PB, Quek MB, et al. Risk factors and in-hospital outcomes following tracheostomy in infants. J Pediatr. 2016;173:39–44.
8. Ramesh P, Boit P, Samuels M. Mask ventilation in the early management of congenital central hypoventilation syndrome. Arch Dis Child. 2008;93:F400–3. https://doi.org/10.1136/adc.2008.139931.
9. Paglietti MG, Porcaro F, Sovtic A, et al. Decannulation in children affected by congenital central hypoventilation syndrome: a proposal of an algorithm from two European centers. Pediatr Pulmonol. 2019;54:1663–9. https://doi.org/10.1002/ppul.24448.
10. Khayat A, Medin D, Syed F, et al. Intelligent volume-assured pressure support (iVAPS) for the treatment of congenital central hypoventilation syndrome. Sleep Breath. 2017;21:513–9.
11. Saddi V, Thambipillay G, Martin B, et al. Pediatric average volume assured pressure support. Front. Pediatr. 2022;10:868625. https://doi.org/10.3389/fped.2022.868625.
12. Sterni LM, Collaco JM, Baker CD, et al. An official American Thoracic Society clinical practice guideline: pediatric chronic home invasive ventilation. Am J Respir Crit Care Med. 2016;193:e16–35.
13. Al-Iede M, Kumaran R, Waters K. Home continuous positive airway pressure for cardiopulmonary indications in infants and children. Sleep Med. 2018;48:86–92.
14. Khirani S, Ramírez A, Aloui S, et al. Continuous positive airway pressure titration in infants with severe upper airway obstruction or bronchopulmonary dysplasia. Crit Care. 2013;17:R167. https://doi.org/10.1186/cc12846.
15. Kaditis AG, Alonso Alvarez ML, Boudewyns A, et al. Obstructive sleep disordered breathing in 2- to 18-year-old children: diagnosis and management. Eur Respir J. 2016;47:69–94.

16. Amaddeo A, Moreau J, Frapin A, et al. Long term continuous positive airway pressure (CPAP) and noninvasive ventilation (NIV) in children: initiation criteria in real life. Pediatr Pulmonol. 2016;51:968–74.
17. Verhulst S. Long term continuous positive airway pressure and non-invasive ventilation in obstructive sleep apnea in children with obesity and down syndrome. Front Pediatr. 2020;8:534. https://doi.org/10.3389/fped.2020.00534.
18. Tsang Y-P, To C-Y, Tsui C-K, Leung S-Y, Kwok K-L, Ng DK-K. Feasibility of long-term home noninvasive ventilation program in a general pediatric unit: 21 years' experience in Hong Kong. Pediatr Pulmonol. 2021;56:3349–57. https://doi.org/10.1002/ppul.25593.
19. Amaddeo A, Frapin A, Touil S, et al. Outpatient initiation of long-term continuous positive airway pressure in children. Pediatr Pulmonol. 2018;53:1422–8. https://doi.org/10.1002/ppul.24138.
20. Perrem L, Mehta K, Syed F, Baker A, Amin R. How to use non-invasive positive airway pressure device data reports to guide clinical care. Pediatr Pulmonol. 2020;55:58–67. https://doi.org/10.1002/ppul.24555.
21. Essouri S, Nicot F, Clément A, et al. Noninvasive positive pressure ventilation in infants with upper airway obstruction: comparison of continuous and bilevel positive pressure. Intensive Care Med. 2005;31:574–80. https://doi.org/10.1007/s00134-005-2568-6.
22. Khaytin I, Tapia I, Xanthopoulos M, et al. Auto-titrating CPAP for the treatment of obstructive sleep apnea in children. J Clin Sleep Med. 2020;16:871–8. https://doi.org/10.5664/jcsm.8348.
23. Palombini L, Pelayo R, Guilleminault C. Efficacy of automated continuous positive airway pressure in children with sleep-related breathing disorders in an attended setting. Pediatrics. 2004;113:e412–7. https://doi.org/10.1542/peds.113.5.e412.
24. Mihai R, Vandeleur M, Pecoraro S, et al. Autotitrating CPAP as a tool for CPAP initiation for children. J Clin Sleep Med. 2017;13:713.
25. Watach AJ, Xanthopoulos MS, Afolabi-Brown O, et al. Positive airway pressure adherence in pediatric obstructive sleep apnea: a systematic scoping review. Sleep Med Rev. 2020;51:101273.
26. Amaddeo A, Khirani S, Frapin A, et al. High- flow nasal cannula for children not compliant with continuous positive airway pressure. Sleep Med. 2019;63:24.
27. Mastouri M, Amaddeo A, Griffon L, et al. Weaning from long term continuous positive airway pressure or noninvasive ventilation in children. Pediatr Pulmonol. 2017;52(10):1349–54. https://doi.org/10.1002/ppul.23767.
28. Thébaud B, Goss KN, Laughon M, et al. Bronchopulmonary dysplasia. Nat Rev Dis Primers. 2020;5:78. https://doi.org/10.1038/s41572-019-0127-7.
29. Nelin LD, Abman SH, Panitch HB. A physiology-based approach to the respiratory care of children with severe bronchopulmonary dysplasia. In: Bancalari E, editor. The newborn lung: neonatology questions and controversies. 3rd ed. Philadelphia, PA: Elsevier; 2019. p. 363–85.
30. Ali K, Kagalwalla S, Cockar I, et al. Prediction of prolonged ventilator dependence in preterm infants. Eur J Pediatr. 2019;178:1063–8. https://doi.org/10.1007/s00431-019-03394-9.
31. Yossef L, Shepherd EG, Lynch S, Reber KM, Nelin LD. Factors associated with long-term mechanical ventilation in extremely preterm infants. J Neonatal Perinatal Med. 2018;11:29–35. https://doi.org/10.3233/NPM-181711.
32. Vikramaditya D, Bhandari V. Non-invasive ventilatory strategies to decrease bronchopulmonary dysplasia-where are we in 2021? Children (Basel). 2021;8:132. https://doi.org/10.3390/children8020132.
33. Ho JJ, Subramaniam P, Davis PG. Continuous positive airway pressure (CPAP) for respiratory distress in preterm infants. Cochrane Database Syst Rev. 2020;10(10):CD002271. https://doi.org/10.1002/14651858.CD002271.
34. Baker CD. Chronic respiratory failure in bronchopulmonary dysplasia. Pediatr Pulmonol. 2021;56:3490–8. https://doi.org/10.1002/ppul.25360. PMID: 33666365.
35. McKinney RL, Napolitano N, Levin JJ, et al. Ventilatory strategies in infants with established severe bronchopulmonary dysplasia: a multicenter point prevalence study. J Pediatr. 2022;242:248–52.

36. Gibbs K, Jensen EA, Alexiou S, et al. Ventilation strategies in severe bronchopulmonary dysplasia. NeoReviews. 2020;21:e226. https://doi.org/10.1542/neo.21-4-e226.
37. McKinney RL, Keszler M, Truog WE. Multicenter experience with neurally adjusted ventilatory assist in infants with severe bronchopulmonary dysplasia. Am J Perinatol. 2021;38(Suppl S1):e162–6.
38. O'Connor KL, Davies MW. Ventilation settings in preterm neonates with ventilator-dependant, evolving bronchopulmonary dysplasia. Early Hum Dev. 2021;159:105417.
39. Sindelar R, Shepherd EG, Ågren J, et al. Established severe BPD: is there a way out? Change of ventilatory paradigms. Pediatr Res. 2021;90(6):1139–46.
40. Baker CD. Mechanical ventilation during chronic lung disease. Clin Perinatol. 2021;48(4):881–93.
41. Gupta S, Sinha SK, Donn SM. Ventilatory management and bronchopulmonary dysplasia in preterm infants. Semin Fetal Neonatal Med. 2009;14:367–73.
42. Abman SH, Collaco JM, Shepherd EG, et al. Interdisciplinary care of children with severe bronchopulmonary dysplasia. J Pediatr. 2017;181:12–28. https://doi.org/10.1016/j.jpeds.2016.10.082.
43. Özkan H, Duman N, Tüzün F. Pathophysiologically based ventilatory management of severe bronchopulmonary dysplasia. Turk Arch Pediatr. 2022;57:385–90. https://doi.org/10.5152/TurkArchPediatr.2022.22112.
44. Vento G, Tirone C, Paladini A, et al. Weaning from the ventilator in bronchopulmonary dysplasia. Clin Perinatol. 2021;48:895–906. https://doi.org/10.1016/j.clp.2021.08.005.
45. Yallapragada S, Savani RC, Mūnoz-Blanco S, et al. Qualitative indications for tracheostomy and chronic mechanical ventilation in patients with severe bronchopulmonary dysplasia. J Perinatol. 2021;4:1–7.
46. Fuller C, Wineland AM, Richter GT. Update on pediatric tracheostomy: indications, technique, education, and decannulation. Curr Otorhinolaryngol Rep. 2021;15:1–12.
47. Cristea AI, Carroll AE, Davis SD, et al. Outcomes of children with severe bronchopulmonary dysplasia who were ventilator dependent at home. Pediatrics. 2013;132(3):e727–34. https://doi.org/10.1542/peds.2012-2990. PMID: 23918888.
48. DeMauro SB, D'Agostino JA, Bann C, et al. Developmental outcomes of very preterm infants with tracheostomies. J Pediatr. 2014;164(6):1303–1310.e2. https://doi.org/10.1016/j.jpeds.2013.12.014.
49. Luo J, Shepard S, Nilan K, et al. Improved growth and developmental activity post tracheostomy in preterm infants with severe BPD. Pediatr Pulmonol. 2018;53(9):1237–44. https://doi.org/10.1002/ppul.24087.
50. Morrow CB, McGrath-Morrow SA, Collaco JM. Predictors of length of stay for initial hospitalization in infants with bronchopulmonary dysplasia. J Perinatol. 2018;38(9):1258–65. https://doi.org/10.1038/s41372-018-0142-7.
51. Saddi V, Thambipillay G, Teng A. Non-invasive home ventilation using the average volume assured pressure support feature in an infant with severe bronchopulmonary dysplasia and chronic respiratory failure. Pediatr Investig. 2020;4:222–4. https://doi.org/10.1002/ped4.12221.
52. Chatwin M, Tan HL, Bush A, et al. Long term non-invasive ventilation in children: impact on survival and transition to adult care. PLoS One. 2015;10:e0125839.
53. Graham RJ, Fleegler EW, Robinson WM. Chronic ventilator need in the community: a 2005 pediatric census of Massachusetts. Pediatrics. 2007;119:e1280–7.
54. Atag E, Krivec U, Ersu R. Non-invasive ventilation for children with chronic lung disease. Front Pediatr. 2020;8:561639. https://doi.org/10.3389/fped.2020.561639.
55. Jobanputra A, Jagpal S, Marulanda P, et al. An overview of noninvasive ventilation in cystic fibrosis. Pediatr Pulmonol. 2022;57(Suppl 1):S101–12. https://doi.org/10.1002/ppul.25753.
56. Fauroux B. Why, when and how to propose noninvasive ventilation in cystic fibrosis? Minerva Anestesiol. 2011;77:1108–14.

57. Fauroux B, Le Roux E, Ravilly S, et al. Long-term noninvasive ventilation in patients with cystic fibrosis. Respiration. 2008;76:168–74.
58. Flight WG, Shaw J, Johnson S, et al. Long-term non-invasive ventilation in cystic fibrosis—experience over two decades. J Cyst Fibros. 2012;11(3):187–92. https://doi.org/10.1016/j.jcf.2011.11.006.
59. Archangelidi O, Carr SB, Simmonds NJ, et al. Non-invasive ventilation and clinical out-comes in cystic fibrosis: findings from the UK CF registry. J Cyst Fibros. 2019;18:665–70.
60. Collins N, Gupta A, Wright S, Gauld L, Urquhart D, Bush A. Survey of the use of non-invasive positive pressure ventilation in UK. and Australasian children with cystic fibrosis. Thorax. 2011;66:538–9. https://doi.org/10.1136/thx.2010.139063.
61. Fauroux B, Pigeot J, Polkey MI, et al. In vivo physiologic comparison of two ventilators used for domiciliary ventilation in children with cystic fibrosis. Crit Care Med. 2001;29:2097–105.
62. Fauroux B, Louis B, Hart N, et al. The effect of back-up rate during non-invasive ventilation in young patients with cystic fibrosis. Intensive Care Med. 2004;30(4):673–81. https://doi.org/10.1007/s00134-003-2126-z.
63. Fauroux B, Nicot F, Essouri S, et al. Sctting of noninvasive pressure support in young patients with cystic fibrosis. Eur Respir J. 2004;24:624–30.
64. Macrea M, Oczkowski S, Rochwerg B, et al. Long-term noninvasive ventilation in chronic stable hypercapnic chronic obstructive pulmonary disease. An Official American Thoracic Society Clinical Practice Guideline. Am J Respir Crit Care Med. 2020;202(4):e74–87. https://doi.org/10.1164/rccm.202006-2382ST.
65. Reiter J, Breuer O, Cohen- Cymberknoh M, Forno E, Gileles-Hillel A. Sleep in children with cystic fibrosis: more under the covers. Pediatr Pulmonol. 2022;57:1944–51. https://doi.org/10.1002/ppul.25462.

PMV in Children with Hemato-Oncologic Disease

Marshay N. James, Jason Rains, and Asya Agulnik

1 Introduction

Pediatric hematology-oncology (PHO) patients frequently develop critical illness; approximately every 1 in 3–4 children with cancer will require care in the pediatric intensive care unit (PICU) during the course of cancer-directed therapy [1]. Unfortunately, these patients experience higher mortality than other children with critical illness, ranging from 7 to 30% in high-resource settings [2, 3]. Mortality in resource-limited hospitals is unknown, but expected to be even higher due to challenges delivering critical care in these settings [4, 5].

Critically ill children with cancer with respiratory failure requiring mechanical ventilation (MV) have a particularly high mortality [2, 3], especially post-hematopoietic cell transplantation (HCT) [6–8]. Accordingly, recent international consensus identified understanding the appropriate timing and use of invasive and noninvasive MV a priority to improve outcomes for these patients [9]. The following chapter summarizes what is known regarding risk factors, etiology,

M. N. James
Pediatric Emergency Medicine, Texas Children's Hospital, Houston, USA
e-mail: mxjames4@texaschildrens.org

J. Rains
Division of Critical Care, Department of Pediatrics, St Jude Children's Research Hospital, Memphis, TN, USA

e-mail: jason.rains@stjude.org

A. Agulnik (✉)
Division of Critical Care, Department of Pediatrics, St Jude Children's Research Hospital, Memphis, TN, USA

Department of Global Pediatric Medicine, St Jude Children's Research Hospital, Memphis, TN, USA
e-mail: Asya.agulnik@stjude.org

A. Kawaguchi et al. (eds.), *Prolonged and Long-Term Mechanical Ventilation in Children*, https://doi.org/10.1007/978-981-97-8903-0_13

management considerations, complications, and research priorities in PHO patients requiring prolonged mechanical ventilation (PMV).

2 Risk Factors for Respiratory Failure and PMV in PHO Patients

While PHO patients develop respiratory failure from similar pathologies as non-PHO patients, this patient population has several unique features making them more susceptible to respiratory failure and subsequent prolonged need for MV, including immunosuppression and preexisting organ injury.

2.1 Immunosuppression

Children with cancer and other blood disorders are frequently immunocompromised, either from their underlying disease or its treatment, making them more susceptible to infections. Common causes of respiratory tract infections in these patients include pathogens seen in non-PHO patients (gram-positive bacteria such as *Streptococcus pneumoniae* and viruses such as respiratory syncytial virus) [10], as well as pathogens unique to these patients (e.g., *Pneumocystis pneumonia*) [11–13]. Similarly, cancer-directed therapy can further exacerbate preexisting immunosuppression resulting in a dysregulated pulmonary response to infection [14]. Regardless of the cause of respiratory infection, immunocompromised patients frequently develop a more severe, protracted disease course requiring prolonged respiratory support.

2.2 Preexisting Organ Injury

In addition to immunocompromise, PHO patients frequently have preexisting organ injury and/or dysfunction making them more susceptible to respiratory failure. Preexisting organ injury can result from past cancer-directed therapy or from direct tumor effect. A common complication in children with cancer is cardiomyopathy, both associated with anthracyclines, and from newer agents causing significant inflammation and endothelial dysfunction [15, 16]. Similarly, PHO patients frequently have pulmonary complications from cancer-directed therapy, including chemotherapy and radiation therapy, resulting in chronic lung disease [17]. Symptoms of pulmonary toxicity can begin within 1–3 months post-therapy and progress to fibrotic lung injury, increasing the risk of PMV with any subsequent pulmonary insult [18]. Additionally, prolonged respiratory dysfunction requiring oxygen use prior to development of critical illness is another risk factor for more severe disease and mortality in PHO patients [6, 19].

3 Etiology of Respiratory Failure and PMV in PHO Patients

Respiratory failure is the leading cause of admission to the pediatric intensive care unit (PICU) for PHO patients [7]. If reversibility is feasible in acute respiratory failure, MV is often a part of the treatment course. The average length of ventilator days in PHO PICU patients is 5–6 days [7]. More than 50% of PHO are admitted to the PICU for recovery following scheduled surgery; in this subset of patients, respiratory failure is typically mechanical or iatrogenic due to the operative course, with a short and uncomplicated MV course [2, 3]. The remainder of PHO patients requiring MV for respiratory failure, however, have a more complex etiology and protracted MV course, frequently resulting in PMV. To estimate MV duration in PHO patients, understanding etiology is paramount (Table 1).

3.1 *Tumor Effect*

Oncology patients can have respiratory decompensation specific to their primary malignancy or due to complications of initial treatment. Patients newly diagnosed with lymphoma or acute leukemia may present with mediastinal masses and, due to mass or compressive effect, manifest symptoms of mechanical respiratory failure. Similarly, acute leukemia frequently presents with hyperleukocytosis, which in severe cases can lead to pulmonary leukocytosis, resulting in hypoxemic respiratory failure. Solid tumors and metastatic disease of the thoracoabdominal cavity and central nervous system can also lead to respiratory insufficiency, either through direct airway compression or indirectly through loss of airway reflexes or respiratory drive [20]. While some masses with potential for respiratory failure are rapidly responsive to chemotherapy (e.g., lymphoma or anterior mediastinal masses from leukemia), others require prolonged treatment to see tumor response. In those cases, patients frequently require a surgical airway with or without MV for the duration of cancer-directed therapy.

3.2 *Complications of Cancer-Directed Therapy*

Chemotherapy agents frequently result in complications that can lead to short-term or prolonged respiratory failure. For example, mucositis, a side effect of many chemotherapy agents, can result in airway compromise. Mucositis causes pain, swelling, increased mucous production, and airway bleeding [21]. Inability to mobilize secretions and narrowing of the airway due to swelling can be significant in younger patients. In severe cases, intubation may be required to support the child through convalescence. In addition to general complications from chemotherapy, individual agents may also cause specific toxicities resulting in respiratory failure. For

Table 1 Etiology, expected duration, and treatment for causes of respiratory failure in pediatric hematology-oncology patients

Etiology	Disease/patient population	Examples	Treatment
Tumor effect	Acute leukemia, lymphoma, CNS, and non-CNS solid tumor	Hyperleukocytosis and leukocytosis, mediastinal mass, airway (heme malignancy) compression, loss of airway reflexes (CNS tumor)	Airway protection Supportive care Initiation of cancer-directed therapy
Chemotherapy complications	Acute leukemia (including APML), lymphoma, CNS, and non-CNS solid tumor	Mucositis, serositis, vocal cord paralysis (vincristine), differentiation syndrome, pancreatitis (asparaginase)	Airway protection Supportive care Dexamethasone (differentiation syndrome)
Infection	All immunosuppressed patients	Systemic infection (bacterial, viral fungal), pneumonia	Infection-directed therapy Supportive care
Heart failure	All PHO patients	Cardiomyopathy, pulmonary hypertension, acute on chronic heart failure	Cardiomyopathy management Fluid restriction and supportive care
Post-HCT complications	HCT patients, PHO patients requiring intensive chemotherapy	Engraftment syndrome (ES), thrombotic microangiopathy (TMA), diffuse alveolar hemorrhage (DAH), veno-occlusive disease (VOD), bronchiolitis obliterans syndrome (BOS), cryptogenic organizing pneumonia (COP)	Steroids (ES, DAH, BOS, COP), eculizumab (TMA), defibrotide (VOD), inhaled therapies (DAH), immunosuppression (BOS/COP)
Sickling crisis	Sickle cell disease (HgSS)	Acute chest syndrome	Simple or exchange blood transfusion Supportive care

Abbreviations: *CNS* Central nervous system; *PARDS* Pediatric acute respiratory distress syndrome

example, vinca alkaloids like vincristine are known to cause neuropathy, including occasionally vocal cord palsy requiring mechanical ventilation [20].

Endothelial injury and vascular leak causing non-cardiogenic pulmonary edema and serositis are other early pulmonary toxicities from certain chemotherapeutic agents [22]. Serositis describes a clinical syndrome involving the inflammation of serous tissues resulting in fluid collections in the pericardial, pleural, and peritoneal cavities. Serositis is often considered in the absence of infectious etiology and in the setting of concurrent multiple fluid collections; it may or may not be indicative of underlying graft-versus-host disease (GVHD) or chemotherapy toxicity [22].

Patients undergoing induction therapy for acute promyelocytic leukemia (APML) have a unique risk in the form of differentiation syndrome. Differentiation syndrome occurs in roughly 1 in 4 APML patients during treatment induction [23]. The granulocyte maturation triggered by all-trans retinoic acid (ATRA) in isolation or when combined with the apoptosis of APL cells incited by arsenic trioxide (ATO) is thought to contribute to hyperinflammation [23]. Clinical manifestations are fever, respiratory distress, cardiac involvement, hypotension, and acute renal failure. Specific respiratory sequela can include pulmonary infiltrates, pleural effusion, and respiratory distress [18]. Treatment involves dexamethasone, and, in severe cases, holding ATRA/ATO until symptoms improve.

3.3 Inflammatory and Infection

Infectious and inflammatory insults are a common pathway to PMV in PHO patients. Like other pediatric patients, PHO patients require vigilant monitoring for the development of pediatric acute respiratory distress syndrome (PARDS), with stratification of illness severity to facilitate early and appropriate intervention [18, 24]. Acute lung injury causing PARDS in PHO patients is often connected to infection, inflammation, and/or direct pulmonary toxicity from chemotherapy and/or radiation.

Systemic infection, including bacteremia and other serious infections, is a common cause of PARDS in PHO patients. Of the microorganisms attributed to infectious etiology of acute respiratory failure, the frequent culprit is viral infection (i.e., EBV, CMV, adenovirus); bacterial, fungal, and parasitic infections, however, can also occur [25]. Noninfectious causes of PARDS are also common, including pancreatitis (e.g., from PEG-asparaginase) or hypersensitivity to medication leading to anaphylactoid reaction and acute lung toxicity.

Distinguishing infectious from inflammatory causes of respiratory failure in PHO patients is integral to guide management and predict the likely duration of MV. Respiratory PCR studies can identify pathogenic organisms and guide curative therapies. Specimens can often be obtained via nasal swab or wash. In stable MV patients, bronchoscopy and bronchoalveolar lavage (BAL) specimens may be considered and are often more helpful to guide therapy [18]. Diagnostic imaging such as computerized tomography (CT) of the lungs can also help with diagnosis [18].

Typically, respiratory failure from acute inflammation and systemic infection respond well to supportive care and have a good prognosis without requiring PMV. These processes, however, are confounded by patient comorbidities and can often co-occur with other causes of respiratory failure, resulting in the need for PMV and a more complicated hospital course.

3.4 Heart Failure

Cardiac complications in children undergoing cancer-directed therapy or hematopoietic cell transplantation are increasingly appreciated as a major cause of critical illness and acute respiratory failure. The most common acute manifestations include cardiac dysfunction, pulmonary hypertension, and pericardial effusions [22]. Acute cardiotoxic events happen within the first week of therapy and are usually reversible with dose reduction or discontinuation of the causative chemotherapy agent. Reversibility, however, is not 100%, and there can be progression of left ventricular (LV) dysfunction. Early-onset cardiotoxicity occurs within weeks to months of chemotherapy and can present with restrictive cardiomyopathy and filling defects or dilated cardiomyopathy with LV wall thinning and systolic dysfunction [22]. Late-onset cardiotoxicity is more common, defined by cardiac dysfunction after 1 year of exposure to chemotherapy. Dilated cardiomyopathy can convert to a restrictive cardiomyopathy with diastolic dysfunction, or diastolic dysfunction can be an early marker or future systolic heart failure.

Positive-pressure ventilation lowers the transmural pressure and off-loads the heart. This can also be extremely beneficial in decreasing metabolic demand by decreasing the work of breathing in a decompensated patient. Positive-pressure ventilation should be strongly considered in any patient with increased work of breathing and moderate-to-severe heart failure with worsening perfusion [22]. As a result, patients in acute or progressive heart failure often require MV in addition to cardiomyopathy management during acute resuscitation.

3.5 Post-Hematopoietic Cell Transplantation (HCT) Complications

In addition to the complications listed above, patients who are post-HCT are at risk for multiple specific complications which can result in respiratory failure requiring PMV. While classically observed in post-HCT patients, many of these complications can also occur in other PHO patients exposed to intensive chemotherapy regimens.

Engraftment Syndrome Engraftment syndrome (ES) is characterized by fever, rash, and non-cardiogenic pulmonary edema occurring at the time of neutrophil recovery after HCT [18]. ES may be related to a graft-versus-host response [18]. Corticosteroids can ameliorate ES symptoms, although they should be used in consultation with the HCT team as anti-graft effect may also occur.

Thrombotic Microangiopathy (TMA) TMA presents as "thrombocytopenia, schistocytes on peripheral blood smear, acute kidney injury (AKI), altered mental status, severe pulmonary arterial hypertension (PAH), and dysfunction of other organs," leading to multisystem organ failure [26–28]. Complement activation mediated by high-dose chemotherapy, radiation therapy, GVHD, or infections results in vascular endothelial damage and subsequent organ failure [28]. Respiratory insufficiency in TMA is attributable to either effusive processes impairing vital capacity and therefore ventilation or endothelial injury contributing to pulmonary hypertension. Eculizumab, an inhibitor of complement activation, is an effective treatment for TMA [26, 27].

Diffuse Alveolar Hemorrhage (DAH) DAH occurs in the setting of injury to the pulmonary microvasculature in response to alveolar assault which may be due to chemotherapy, radiation, immune-mediated events, or systemic/pulmonary infection [18]. Persistent, bloody aliquots returned on BAL, rapid opacification on chest radiograph, and profound hypoxemia are common clinical correlates. Management includes application of pressure tamponade (i.e., higher mean airway pressures via invasive MV), inhaled recombinant factor VIIa, and tranexamic acid to achieve alveolar hemostasis [29, 30]. However, despite treatment, mortality is estimated to be as high as 80% [18].

Veno-Occlusive Disease (VOD) VOD results from endothelial injury to the liver leading to hepatic dysfunction, thrombocytopenia, ascites, and fluid overload [31–33]. Treatment includes meticulous fluid management and defibrotide [33]. Frequently, abdominal competition from massive ascites can lead to mechanical respiratory failure requiring MV; this complication is typically responsive to peritoneal drainage [31]. Pulmonary veno-occlusive disease (PVOD) is a rare complication resulting in pulmonary hypertension and increasing dyspnea [22]. CXR findings include cardiomegaly and pulmonary edema, while an echocardiogram shows pulmonary hypertension [22]. If a biopsy is performed, characteristic findings are fibrosis of the small pulmonary veins and venules, while the larger pulmonary veins are normal [34, 35]. Lung biopsy had been the gold standard; however, it carries a high risk of complications and is not commonly used in practice [22].

BOS/COP and cGVHD Bronchiolitis obliterans syndrome (BOS) and cryptogenic organizing pneumonia (COP) are late-onset noninfectious pulmonary complications of HSCT often requiring chest computed tomography (CT) or lung biopsy for diagnosis [36]. BOS is a progressive obstructive disease with an onset of 3–24 months posttransplant. Patients typically present with wheezing and dyspnea. Chest CT may demonstrate air trapping, centrilobular nodules, or bronchiectasis [18]. COP is a restrictive lung disease with an onset of 2–12 months posttransplant with acute-onset fever, cough, and dyspnea. Chest CT may demonstrate patchy airspace disease or nodular opacities. Both BOS and COP are related to T-cell-mediated injury to lung epithelium [18]. Both etiologies are long-term complications of chronic GVHD and managed with a combination of immunosuppression and supportive care. Even with management, patients with these pulmonary complications frequently require PMV, at times leading to pulmonary transplant.

3.6 Special Considerations in Hematology Patients

Hemoglobin SS or sickle cell disease (HgbSS/SCD) patients represent most hospitalized nonmalignant hematology patients. In the context of MV, the leading indication for admission is acute chest syndrome (ACS). Extensive lobar infection, pulmonary hypertension, asthma, and restrictive lung disease contribute to poor prognosis in this subpopulation [37]. While SCD patients represent only 2% of all PICU admissions, 13% of patients with ACS will require MV, with mortality as high as 44% [38]. Timely admission to the ICU and timely interventions, such as simple or exchange transfusion, lead to improved outcomes and shortened course of MV in these patients.

4 Ventilatory Management Considerations in PHO Patients

Children with cancer and other blood disorders have several unique features requiring special consideration if they develop respiratory failure. The following describes ventilatory management considerations in these patients, including special considerations during intubation and MV.

4.1 Timing of Intubation

Recognition of the signs of respiratory distress combined with early intervention is important to improve outcomes in children with cancer. Intubation and invasive MV (IMV) should not be delayed once the patient shows signs of respiratory failure [7, 39]. High-flow nasal cannula (HFNC)/noninvasive positive-pressure ventilation (NPPV) are useful early interventions to prevent progression to respiratory failure, but careful monitoring of the level of support is required. If the FiO2 begins to trend higher, or the level of pressure required begins to increase, early intubations should be considered. Prolonged NPPV/HFNC before intubation is linked to increased mortality in this population [19, 39]. There is often hesitation to implement IMV due to fears of infection and other complications; however, there is no strong evidence for a higher risk of ventilator-associated pneumonia in these patients [40, 41]. As such, intubation should occur before signs of respiratory failure to improve outcomes in PHO patients [42].

4.2 Considerations During Intubation

When the determination has been made to implement IMV, there are several considerations unique to children with cancer. This patient population has an increased likelihood for difficult intubation due to anatomical abnormalities, tumors, mediastinal masses, and mucositis. An institutional standard of practice for difficult airway management and the availability of fiber-optic video bronchoscopy are imperative to prevent complications during intubation in these patients. Important considerations during intubation in PHO patients include positioning, airway and medication selection, anticipating obstructed view during laryngoscopy, and manual ventilation.

Positioning Children with cancer may have conditions which prevent positioning in the standard supine and classic sniffing position for intubation. Ascites, blood, or tumors in the abdomen can push up on the diaphragm and lungs causing increases in transpulmonary pressures and difficulty breathing or manually ventilating while lying flat. There is also the potential for tumors or masses in the thoracic cavity to cause difficulty ventilating the patient in prone position. These positional difficulties can often be diagnosed by observing the breathing pattern and self-positioning of the patient. Careful consideration of the disease process should be taken with each individual patient to anticipate potential problems with positioning during intubation.

Airway Selection Children with cancer are more likely to need high initial pressures during mechanical ventilation for respiratory failure [6]. For this reason, cuffed endotracheal tubes should be considered for all patient sizes and ages.

Medication Considerations The treatment for cancer can cause chronic lung conditions in patients, particularly those with a prolonged history of cancer-directed therapy or HCT. These patients may have chronic respiratory insufficiency with baseline increased respiratory rate, use of accessory muscles, and shortness of breath on exertion. The loss of spontaneous respiratory effort during intubation in these patients may result in greater than anticipated ventilatory failure. Similarly, patients with anterior mediastinal masses are at risk for airway compression and respiratory catastrophe during intubation, particularly with the use of paralytics. As such, medication selection for intubation in these patients must consider individual risk factors.

Obstruction of View Children with cancer may have conditions which affect the ability to visualize the vocal cords during intubation. The most common condition is mucositis causing thick secretions which cover the area over the epiglottis. These secretions may need to be suctioned several times before a clear view of the trachea is obtained. There is risk of agitating the inflamed mucosal lining during direct laryngoscopy or suctioning, which may further obstruct the view with blood or saliva. A tumor or mass located in the mouth or oropharynx may also obstruct the view for intubation. The use of a video laryngoscope or the availability of video bronchoscopy can be helpful in these situations to prevent emergency complications.

Manual Ventilation Children with cancer may have conditions which make it difficult to manually ventilate the patient using a standard bag-valve-mask. Conditions to evaluate include any anatomical abnormality to the face or jaw which could hinder the ability to get a good seal on the mask during manual ventilation. Children with cancer may have received long-term regimen of high-dose steroids as treatment, resulting in cushingoid facies with cheek swelling, also making the mask seal difficult to obtain.

4.3 Strategies for Management During Invasive Mechanical Ventilation

While typical ventilatory management best practices apply to PHO with respiratory failure, several considerations are unique to these patients, including requirements for higher level of support, prolonged course of mechanical ventilation, airway clearance, and decisions around weaning support.

Ventilator Management Ventilatory management for PHO patients with acute respiratory failure is similar for other pediatric patients, including mode selection and ventilation strategies [24]. PHO patients, however, are more likely to require higher initial pressures to appropriately ventilate due to complications of prior cancer-directed therapy and fluid overload. To prevent lung injury, permissive hypercapnia should be considered [6]. Early consideration should be given to optimal PEEP/FiO2 [6, 43], as high FiO2/low PEEP strategies have been linked to higher mortality [43]. High PEEP settings >15cmH2O should not be avoided, with the goal to use PEEP sufficient to require >60% FiO2 [24] with an SpO2 target of >97% [6]. When conventional mechanical ventilation fails to achieve goal ventilation and oxygenation without settings resulting in lung injury, high-frequency oscillatory ventilation (HFOV) may be attempted; however, data in HCT patients suggests that late initiation of HFOV is associated with very poor outcomes in these patients [7].

Fluid Management Fluid balance is a key concept and metric in the care of critically ill PHO patients. Prevalent comorbid conditions in this population including endothelial injury, acute kidney injury, and cardiac dysfunction make achieving euvolemia challenging. As a result, fluid overload (i.e., fluid volume intake more than output by the admission weight x 100%, with accounting for insensible losses) is common. A direct relationship exists between fluid overload and respiratory morbidity [44]. With protracted fluid overload, PHO patients on MV demonstrate a longer time to extubation, more ventilator days, poorer oxygenation index, and higher mortality, with the highest mortality observed in patients with a cumulative fluid overload of 10–20% [44]. As a result, careful fluid management and early intervention to prevent fluid overload are recommend to improve outcomes.

Anticipating a Prolonged Ventilation Course PHO patients with respiratory failure frequently require a prolonged course of mechanical ventilation. To avoid complications, excellent oral hygiene is critical to reduce VAP in children with cancer [45]. Anticipating a prolonged duration of IMV, a supportive care [46] and sedation strategy should be chosen that minimizes the risk of delirium [47], which is already elevated in these patients [48].

Airway Clearance Considerations Airway clearance techniques (ACTs) can be an important adjunct therapy in PHO patients requiring PMV. PMV can result in an increased volume and viscosity of pulmonary secretions due to the prolonged presence of the endotracheal tube, the lack of humidity from inspired medical gas, as well as the underlying disease process (e.g., mucositis) [49]. The presence of an endotracheal tube decreases the physiologic function of mucociliary clearance, requiring frequent suctioning of the airway. Patients with obstructive pulmonary secretions, or a compromised ability to clear thick secretions, may benefit from ACT. A team approach consisting of nursing care, appropriate sedation, frequent repositioning of the patient, adequate heat and humidity of medical gases, and early mobilization can help to minimize the occurrence of obstructive pulmonary secretions in PMV [49]. ACT should not be considered a routine order for PMV patients [50]; each patient should be assessed for the possibility of benefit from ACT [49, 50]. As ACT is heavily precautioned or contraindicated by many conditions common to children with cancer (DAH, thrombocytopenia, cardiac instability, pulmonary hypertension), the use of ACT should be carefully evaluated with each case [49, 51, 52].

Weaning Respiratory Support Decisions of when to remove respiratory support and wean ventilation must consider both the acute cause of respiratory failure (e.g., infection) and underlying conditions that may result in failure of extubation (e.g., airway anomaly or ongoing mucositis). As a result, weaning from respiratory support should not occur until the underlying cause resulting in respiratory failure is resolved, which may require waiting for effects from cancer-directed therapy and require a prolonged course of MV.

4.4 Unique Considerations for Tracheostomy in PHO Patients

Along with typical medical and ethical considerations around surgical tracheostomy in children requiring PMV [53], PHO patients have several additional concerns. Medical considerations include weighing the potential risks of surgical infection and bleeding in the setting of severe immune suppression and thrombocytopenia during active cancer-directed therapy [54]. Additional medical concerns include the impact of poor nutrition and mucositis on healing following a surgical procedure.

Beyond risks of medical complications, several timing and ethical concerns must be considered in PHO patients requiring PMV. Importantly, a patient's future need for chemotherapy (and subsequent cytopenia) and radiation therapy (and potential impacts on wound healing) must be considered when planning the timing of any surgical procedure, including tracheostomy. Additionally, tracheotomy procedures may be delayed due to the need for prolonged use of higher pressures during mechanical ventilation in these patients. Finally, a patient's overall prognosis, both in the setting of respiratory failure requiring PMV and due to the underlying oncologic process, must be considered when weighing the risks and benefits of surgical tracheostomy. These complex decisions should be made jointly by the multidisciplinary team with close collaboration with the patient and family to reflect patient-centered, goal-based care.

5 Complications of PMV in PHO Patients

5.1 Myopathy

Despite the significant advancements in supportive PICU care, the idea of illness means stillness still abides. PMV is often associated with prolonged periods of continuous sedation and occasional neuromuscular blockade, catabolism, suboptimal nutrition, and confinement to a hospital bed, resulting in significant muscle loss and dysfunction [55]. In PHO patients requiring PMV, muscle wasting and generalized weakness are even further exacerbated by the frequent use of steroids. As a result, PMV patients often contend with critical illness myopathy. While PMV is defined as MV duration greater than 14 days, one-third of MV patients begin to experience generalized paralysis of the extremities and trunk as soon as 5 days into immobility [55]. Early mobility and rehabilitative therapies can help mitigate myopathy; many ICU liberation initiatives view early mobilization as an equal part of the standard of care as classic heroic efforts [46, 56].

5.2 Delirium and Withdrawal

Therapies such as PMV are often accompanied by significant side effects with great physical and psychosocial tolls on patients. One sequela that occurs in pediatric, including PHO, patients receiving critical care is delirium. Delirium is an acute, reversible disruption of a patient's consciousness and cognition; this may be manifested as "a reduced ability to focus, shift, or maintain attention, memory deficit, disorientation, language disturbances, or hallucinations" [57]. Precipitants to delirium can include "an illness itself (e.g., serious infection or neoplasm), by-products of illness (e.g., metabolic or endocrine dysfunction), or side effects of treatment (e.g., sedative drugs or drug withdrawal)" [58]

Flaigle, Ascenzi, and Kudchadkar [59] assert that delirium in the PICU setting is often unrecognized and undertreated. The paucity of delirium screening is juxtaposed against a delirium incidence rate of 20–30% amongst critically ill children and adolescents [58, 60]. Unfortunately, delirium is likely even more prevalent in PHO and post-HCT patients [48]. Even with significant symptomology, providers miss delirium 75–95% of the time [59, 61]. The immediate outcomes that await children in the absence of screening include increased morbidity and mortality, increased length of mechanical ventilation, increased length of stay, and neurocognitive affects [59, 61–63].

A tangential consideration to delirium is drug withdrawal. As PMV often requires long-term use of multidrug sedative regimens, cessation or rapid weaning can lead to significant physiologic symptoms [64]. Prudent use of sedatives requires thoughtful use and structured, proactive abatement strategies. Clinician teams should have transparent, shared goals with regard to each patient's targeted sedation, with frequent reassessment and goal resetting [65]. During use of continuous sedation, the Richmond Agitation Sedation Scale (RASS) can be helpful in providing clinicians with a metric by which to set sedation targets [66]. Though not an intended effect in delirium screening, the concern for level of sedation aligns with the use of RASS in creating sedation weans or holidays in the PICU setting. As a precursor to many delirium screens, nurses are prompted to alert providers when patients are too deeply sedated (i.e., RASS −4 or − 5) to screen. When the time to gradually remove sedative agents arises, tools such as the Withdrawal Assessment Tool-1 (WAT-1) can help providers detect abstinence symptomology [67].

6 PMV Research Priorities in PHO Patients

While much is known regarding the causes and management of respiratory failure in PHO patients, including challenges regarding PMV, there remains several impor tant knowledge gaps that must be addressed in future research. Recently, an international consensus panel identified establishing the ideal timing of advanced therapies, including noninvasive and invasive mechanical ventilation, and extracorporeal support as key research priorities to improve outcomes for children with cancer [9]. Similarly, ideal timing and management of advanced support are important questions for children post-HCT [68–70]. More research is also needed to understand the pathophysiology of and develop management strategies for complications resulting in PMV in PHO patients, including DAH and endothelial dysfunction [71]. Similarly, long-term (community-based) PMV in children with a history of cancer and other blood disorders, including their epidemiology, resource utilization, and outcomes, must be described and is likely evolving over time. Finally, treatment approaches to maximize not only survival but also quality of life and functional status following critical illness for PHO patients, including following PMV, are urgently needed [29, 72, 73]. Addressing these urgent research priorities is integral to improving outcomes for these high-risk patients.

References

1. Demaret P, Pettersen G, Hubert P, Teira P, Emeriaud G. The critically-ill pediatric hemato-oncology patient: epidemiology, management, and strategy of transfer to the pediatric intensive care unit. Ann Intensive Care. 2012;2(1):14.
2. Zinter MS, DuBois SG, Spicer A, Matthay K, Sapru A. Pediatric cancer type predicts infection rate, need for critical care intervention, and mortality in the pediatric intensive care unit. Intensive Care Med. 2014;40(10):1536–44.
3. Wosten-van Asperen RM, van Gestel JPJ, van Grotel M, et al. PICU mortality of children with cancer admitted to pediatric intensive care unit a systematic review and meta-analysis. Crit Rev Oncol Hematol. 2019;142:153–63.
4. Agulnik A, Cárdenas A, Carrillo AK, et al. Clinical and organizational risk factors for mortality during deterioration events among pediatric oncology patients in Latin America: a multicenter prospective cohort. Cancer. 2021;127(10):1668–78.
5. Muttalib F, González-Dambrauskas S, Lee JH, et al. Pediatric emergency and critical care resources and infrastructure in resource-limited settings: a multicountry survey. Crit Care Med. 2021;49(4):671–81.
6. Rowan CM, McArthur J, Hsing DD, et al. Acute respiratory failure in pediatric hematopoietic cell transplantation: a multicenter study*. Crit Care Med. 2018;46(10):e967–e74.
7. Rowan CM, Gertz SJ, McArthur J, et al. Invasive mechanical ventilation and mortality in pediatric hematopoietic stem cell transplantation: a multicenter study*. Pediatr Crit Care Med. 2016;17(4):294–302.
8. Lindell RB, Gertz SJ, Rowan CM, et al. High levels of morbidity and mortality among pediatric hematopoietic cell transplant recipients with severe sepsis: insights from the sepsis PRevalence, OUtcomes, and therapies international point prevalence study. Pediatr Crit Care Med. 2017;18(12):1114–25.
9. Soeteman M, Potratz J, Nielsen JSA, et al. Research priorities in pediatric onco-critical care: an international Delphi consensus study. Intensive Care Med. 2019;45(11):1681–3.
10. Rowan CM, Gertz SJ, Zinter MS, et al. A multicenter investigation of respiratory syncytial viral infection in children with hematopoietic cell transplantation. Transpl Infect Dis. 2018;20(3):e12882.
11. Gertz SJ, McArthur J, Hsing DD, et al. Respiratory pathogens associated with intubated pediatric patients following hematopoietic cell transplant. Transpl Infect Dis. 2020;22(4):e13297.
12. Zinter MS, Dvorak CC, Mayday MY, et al. Pulmonary metagenomic sequencing suggests missed infections in immunocompromised children. Clin Infect Dis. 2019;68(11):1847–55.
13. Zinter MS, Levy ER, Gertz SJ. A review of pathogens causing lower respiratory tract infection in the pediatric hematopoietic stem cell transplant recipient. J Pediatr Intensive Care. 2014;3(3):115–32.
14. Zinter MS, Hume JR. Effects of hematopoietic cell transplantation on the pulmonary immune response to infection. Front Pediatr. 2021;9:634566.
15. Elbahlawan L, Morrison R, Li Y, et al. Outcome of acute respiratory failure secondary to engraftment in children after hematopoietic stem cell transplant. Front Oncol. 2020;10:584269.
16. Baumeister SHC, Mohan GS, Elhaddad A, Lehmann L. Cytokine release syndrome and associated acute toxicities in pediatric patients undergoing immune effector cell therapy or hematopoietic cell transplantation. Front Oncol. 2022;12:841117.
17. Fitch T, Myers KC, Dewan M, Towe C, Dandoy C. Pulmonary complications after pediatric stem cell transplant. Front Oncol. 2021;11:755878.
18. Rajapreyar P, Kopp W, Randolph A. Chapter 11: Acute respiratory failure and management. In: Duncan CN, Talano JM, McArthur JA, editors. Critical care of the pediatric immunocompromised hematology/oncology patient: an evidence-based guide. Springer; 2019.
19. Lindell RB, Fitzgerald JC, Rowan CM, et al. The use and duration of preintubation respiratory support is associated with increased mortality in immunocompromised children with acute respiratory failure. Crit Care Med. 2022;50(7):1127–37.

20. Capsomidis A, Hall A, Daya H, Round J, Lancaster D, Bate J. Vocal cord palsy in children with cancer: a 10-year analysis of UK pediatric intensive care admissions. J Pediatr Hematol Oncol. 2017;39(4):293–5.
21. Leary B, Cuccovia B, Nixon C. Chapter 19: Nursing considerations. In: Duncan CN, Talano JM, McArthur JA, editors. Critical care of the pediatric immunocompromised hematology/oncology patient: an evidence-based guide. Springer; 2019.
22. Ghafoor S, James M, Goldberg J, McArthur J. Chapter 12: Cardiac dysfunction in hematology oncology and hematopoietic cell transplant patients. In: Duncan CN, Talano JM, McArthur JA, editors. Critical care of the pediatric immunocompromised hematology/oncology patient: an evidence-based guide. Springer; 2019.
23. Rego EM, De Santis GC. Differentiation syndrome in promyelocytic leukemia: clinical presentation, pathogenesis and treatment. Mediterr J Hematol Infect Dis. 2011;3(1):e2011048.
24. Pediatric acute respiratory distress syndrome: consensus recommendations from the pediatric acute lung injury consensus conference. Pediatr Crit Care Med. 2015;16(5):428–39.
25. Khandaker MH, Espinosa RE, Nishimura RA, et al. Pericardial disease: diagnosis and management. Mayo Clin Proc. 2010;85(6):572–93.
26. Jodele S, Davies SM, Lane A, et al. Diagnostic and risk criteria for HSCT-associated thrombotic microangiopathy: a study in children and young adults. Blood. 2014;124(4):645–53.
27. Dandoy CE, Rotz S, Alonso PB, et al. A pragmatic multi-institutional approach to understanding transplant-associated thrombotic microangiopathy after stem cell transplant. Blood Adv. 2021;5(1):1–11.
28. Dhakal P, Giri S, Pathak R, Bhatt VR. Eculizumab in transplant-associated thrombotic Microangiopathy. Clin Appl Thromb Hemost. 2017;23(2):175–80.
29. Fan K, McArthur J, Morrison RR, Ghafoor S. Diffuse alveolar hemorrhage after pediatric hematopoietic stem cell transplantation. Front Oncol. 2020;10:1757.
30. Fan K, Hurley C, McNeil MJ, et al. Case report: management approach and use of extracorporeal membrane oxygenation for diffuse alveolar hemorrhage after pediatric hematopoietic cell transplant. Front Pediatr. 2020;8:587601.
31. Mahadeo KM, McArthur J, Adams RH, et al. Consensus report by the pediatric acute lung injury and sepsis investigators and pediatric blood and marrow transplant consortium joint working committees on supportive care guidelines for management of veno-occlusive disease in children and adolescents: part 2-focus on ascites, fluid and electrolytes, renal, and transfusion issues. Biol Blood Marrow Transplant. 2017;23(12):2023–33.
32. Ovchinsky N, Frazier W, Auletta JJ, et al. Consensus report by the pediatric acute lung injury and sepsis investigators and pediatric blood and marrow transplantation consortium joint working committees on supportive care guidelines for management of veno-occlusive disease in children and adolescents, part 3: focus on cardiorespiratory dysfunction, infections, liver dysfunction, and delirium. Biol Blood Marrow Transplant. 2018;24(2):207–18.
33. Bajwa RPS, Mahadeo KM, Taragin BH, et al. Consensus report by pediatric acute lung injury and sepsis investigators and pediatric blood and marrow transplantation consortium joint working committees: supportive care guidelines for management of veno-occlusive disease in children and adolescents, part 1: focus on investigations, prophylaxis, and specific treatment. Biol Blood Marrow Transplant. 2017;23(11):1817–25.
34. Bunte MC, Patnaik MM, Pritzker MR, Burns LJ. Pulmonary veno-occlusive disease following hematopoietic stem cell transplantation: a rare model of endothelial dysfunction. Bone Marrow Transplant. 2008;41(8):677–86.
35. Trobaugh-Lotrario AD, Greffe B, Deterding R, Deutsch G, Quinones R. Pulmonary veno-occlusive disease after autologous bone marrow transplant in a child with stage IV neuroblastoma: case report and literature review. J Pediatr Hematol Oncol. 2003;25(5):405–9.
36. Fuhrmann BPZJ. Chapter 38: Critical illness involving children undergoing hematopoietic progenitor cell transplantation. In: Pediatric critical care. 5th ed. Elsevier; 2016. p. 1325–42.

37. Rosanwo T, McArthur J, Archer N. Chapter 6: Care of the critically ill pediatric sickle cell patient. In: Duncan CN, Talano JM, McArthur JA, editors. Critical care of the pediatric immunocompromised hematology/oncology patient: an evidence-based. Guide: Springer; 2019.
38. Vichinsky EP, Neumayr LD, Earles AN, et al. Causes and outcomes of the acute chest syndrome in sickle cell disease. National Acute Chest Syndrome Study Group. N Engl J Med. 2000;342(25):1855–65.
39. Rowan CM, Fitzgerald JC, Agulnik A, et al. Risk factors for noninvasive ventilation failure in children post-hematopoietic cell transplant. Front Oncol. 2021;11:653607.
40. Park SA, Cho SS, Kwak GJ. Factors influencing ventilator-associated pneumonia in cancer patients. Asian Pac J Cancer Prev. 2014;15(14):5787–91.
41. Battaglia CC, Hale K. Hospital-acquired infections in critically ill patients with cancer. J Intensive Care Med. 2019;34(7):523–36.
42. Hurley C, Zinter MS. Should we intubate pediatric hematopoietic cell transplant patients with respiratory failure sooner? Crit Care Med. 2022;50(7):1163–7.
43. Khemani RG, Parvathaneni K, Yehya N, Bhalla AK, Thomas NJ, Newth CJL. Positive end-expiratory pressure lower than the ARDS network protocol is associated with higher pediatric acute respiratory distress syndrome mortality. Am J Respir Crit Care Med. 2018;198(1):77–89.
44. Arikan AA, Zappitelli M, Goldstein SL, Naipaul A, Jefferson LS, Loftis LL. Fluid overload is associated with impaired oxygenation and morbidity in critically ill children. Pediatr Crit Care Med. 2012;13(3):253–8.
45. Zhao T, Wu X, Zhang Q, Li C, Worthington HV, Hua F. Oral hygiene care for critically ill patients to prevent ventilator-associated pneumonia. Cochrane Database Syst Rev. 2020;12(12):Cd008367.
46. Ghafoor S, Fan K, Williams S, et al. Beginning restorative activities very early: implementation of an early mobility initiative in a pediatric onco-critical care unit. Front Oncol. 2021;11:645716.
47. Rosenberg L, Traube C. Sedation strategies in children with pediatric acute respiratory distress syndrome (PARDS). Ann Transl Med. 2019;7(19):509.
48. Traube C, Gerber LM, Mauer EA, et al. Delirium in children undergoing hematopoietic cell transplantation: a multi-institutional point prevalence study. Front Oncol. 2021;11:627726.
49. Morrow BM. Chest physiotherapy in the pediatric intensive care unit. J Pediatr Intensive Care. 2015;4(4):174–81.
50. Spapen HD, De Regt J, Honoré PM. Chest physiotherapy in mechanically ventilated patients without pneumonia-a narrative review. J Thorac Dis. 2017;9(1):E44–E9.
51. Wang TH, Wu CP, Wang LY. Chest physiotherapy with early mobilization may improve extubation outcome in critically ill patients in the intensive care units. Clin Respir J. 2018;12(11):2613–21.
52. Morrow BM. Airway clearance therapy in acute paediatric respiratory illness: a state-of-the-art review. S Afr J Physiother. 2019;75(1):1295.
53. Wakeham MK, Kuhn EM, Lee KJ, McCrory MC, Scanlon MC. Use of tracheostomy in the PICU among patients requiring prolonged mechanical ventilation. Intensive Care Med. 2014;40(6):863–70.
54. Manna SS, Malik R, Douthwaite A, Vaidya S. Surgical tracheostomy in children with malignancy receiving intensive chemotherapy: a case series and review of literature. Pediatr Blood Cancer. 2020;67(4):e28105.
55. Larsson L, Friedrich O. Critical illness myopathy (CIM) and ventilator-induced diaphragm muscle dysfunction (VIDD): acquired myopathies affecting contractile proteins. Compr Physiol. 2016;7(1):105–12.
56. Morrow BM. Building a culture of early mobilization in the pediatric intensive care unit-a nuts and bolts approach. Transl Pediatr. 2021;10(10):2845–57.
57. Schieveld JN, van Tuijl S, Pikhard T. On nontraumatic brain injury in pediatric critical illness, neuropsychologic short-term outcome, delirium, and resilience. Crit Care Med. 2013;41(4):1160–1.

58. Silver G, Traube C, Kearney J, et al. Detecting pediatric delirium: development of a rapid observational assessment tool. Intensive Care Med. 2012;38(6):1025–31.
59. Flaigle MC, Ascenzi J, Kudchadkar SR. Identifying barriers to delirium screening and prevention in the pediatric ICU: evaluation of PICU staff knowledge. J Pediatr Nurs. 2016;31(1):81–4.
60. Smith HA, Fuchs DC, Pandharipande PP, Barr FE, Ely EW. Delirium: an emerging frontier in the management of critically ill children. Anesthesiol Clin. 2011;29(4):729–50.
61. Schieveld JN, Janssen NJ, van Cauteren YJ. On the Cornell Assessment for Pediatric Delirium and both the diagnostic and statistical manual, 5th edition, and International Classification of Diseases, 11th revision: quo vadis?*. Crit Care Med. 2014;42(3):751–2.
62. Giusti GD, Piergentili F. Knowledge on ICU delirium: the worldwide perspective. Intensive Crit Care Nurs. 2014;30(3):177–8.
63. Schieveld JN, Leroy PL, van Os J, Nicolai J, Vos GD, Leentjens AF. Pediatric delirium in critical illness: phenomenology, clinical correlates and treatment response in 40 cases in the pediatric intensive care unit. Intensive Care Med. 2007;33(6):1033–40.
64. Brummel NE, Ely EW. Sedation level and the prevalence of delirium. Intensive Care Med. 2014,40(1).135.
65. Taran Z, Namadian M, Faghihzadeh S, Naghibi T. The effect of sedation protocol using Richmond agitation-sedation scale (RASS) on some clinical outcomes of mechanically ventilated patients in intensive care units: a randomized clinical trial. J Caring Sci. 2019;8(4):199–206.
66. Kerson AG, DeMaria R, Mauer E, et al. Validity of the Richmond Agitation-Sedation Scale (RASS) in critically ill children. J Intensive Care. 2016;4:65.
67. Franck LS, Harris SK, Soetenga DJ, Amling JK, Curley MA. The Withdrawal Assessment Tool-1 (WAT-1): an assessment instrument for monitoring opioid and benzodiazepine withdrawal symptoms in pediatric patients. Pediatr Crit Care Med. 2008;9(6):573–80.
68. Di Nardo M, Ahmad AH, Merli P, et al. Extracorporeal membrane oxygenation in children receiving haematopoietic cell transplantation and immune effector cell therapy: an international and multidisciplinary consensus statement. Lancet Child Adolesc Health. 2022;6(2):116–28.
69. Zinter MS, McArthur J, Duncan C, et al. Candidacy for extracorporeal life support in children after hematopoietic cell transplantation: a position paper from the pediatric acute lung injury and sepsis investigators network's hematopoietic cell transplant and cancer immunotherapy subgroup. Pediatr Crit Care Med. 2022;23(3):205–13.
70. Ghafoor S, Fan K, Di Nardo M, et al. Extracorporeal membrane oxygenation candidacy in pediatric patients treated with hematopoietic stem cell transplant and chimeric antigen receptor T-cell therapy: an international survey. Front Oncol. 2021;11:798236.
71. Tamburro RF, Cooke KR, Davies SM, et al. Pulmonary complications of pediatric hematopoietic cell transplantation. A National Institutes of Health Workshop Summary. Ann Am Thorac Soc. 2021;18(3):381–94.
72. Zinter MS, Holubkov R, Steurer MA, et al. Pediatric hematopoietic cell transplant patients who survive critical illness frequently have significant but recoverable decline in functional status. Biol Blood Marrow Transplant. 2018;24(2):330–6.
73. Crocco M, d'Annunzio G, La Valle A, et al. Endothelial dysfunction in childhood cancer survivors: a narrative review. Life (Basel). 2021;12(1):45.

PMV in Resource-Poor Settings

José Colleti

1 Introduction

Children with prolonged mechanical ventilation (PMV) dependence are a diverse group of children with special healthcare needs [1]. PMV has become an important challenge in pediatric intensive care units (PICUs) around the world. These patients represent a select cohort with significant morbidity, mortality, and resource use. Medical oversight, equipment management, and hospital resources vary widely depending on the country [1, 2].

Long-term mechanical ventilation significantly alters the quality of life in most children with chronic respiratory failure. The prolonged use of life support equipment in the institution or at home, even on an intermittent basis, greatly stresses family structure and psychodynamics, also involving costs [1–4].

There is also a dilemma in pediatrics concerning the initiation and/or maintenance of assisted ventilation that creates a multidimensional problem affecting patients, their families, healthcare providers in many fields, funding sources, and government agencies [5].

Pediatricians often find these issues to be confusing, frustrating, and overwhelming as they arrive at therapeutic decisions they, and the family, are comfortable with implementing. It is particularly challenging to face a decision that must be made on an urgent basis regarding the initiation of potentially long-term mechanical ventilation, particularly in poor resource settings [6].

There are also financial stresses inherent in alternative healthcare delivery systems, such as health maintenance organizations, that reward physicians for providing less care [3, 7].

Given the increasing number of pediatric patients who are surviving intensive care with chronic respiratory failure, or who otherwise become candidates for

J. Colleti (✉)
PICU, Hospital Israelita Albert Einstein, São Paulo, Brazil

A. Kawaguchi et al. (eds.), *Prolonged and Long-Term Mechanical Ventilation in Children*, https://doi.org/10.1007/978-981-97-8903-0_14

prolonged mechanical ventilation, the demands of taking care of these patients stress the system for a lack of resources and healthcare providers, particularly in low- and middle-income countries (LMICs).

2 Prolonged Mechanical Ventilation and Mechanical Ventilators

The COVID-19 pandemic transiently raised the need for greater intensive care mechanical ventilation capacity around the world. While ICUs were under immense pressure globally, several high-income countries (HICs) did not, ultimately, require novel prototype ventilators, as standard ventilator supplies were sufficient to meet demand. In contrast, mechanical ventilation capacity and provision of disposable components were, and largely remain, insufficient in most LMICs, limiting access to critical care [8].

Standard ventilators used in HIC hospitals are unaffordable and unsustainable for hospitals with limited resources in LMICs. However, some companies are developing hospital turbine-based ventilators skipping the need of compressed air like it happens in most of the home ventilators. Inbuilt oxygen blenders are usually available in the new devices, so capable to connect low-flow oxygen sources. Some nongovernmental organizations have specifically begun working on designing ventilators for LMICs. University of São Paulo, through its engineering department, designed a low-cost device to be used during the COVID-19 pandemic [9]. A study by Gallifant et al. identified the key technical requirements for the design of a context-specific and sustainable mechanical ventilator for use across LMICs [10]. They performed a cross-sectional survey providing an overview of mechanical ventilation capacity and infrastructure in LMICs. Results of this study showed that the loss of electricity was found to occur daily 19% (9/48), weekly 25% (12/48), or less frequently 48% (23/48), or it did not occur 8% (4/48). Most of these outages (72% [31/44]) lasted <2 h, with backup power from external fossil fuel generators and batteries reported to be supplied within 1 h in 91% (40/44). This electricity availability was like that reported in a survey of ten hospitals in Tanzania. The access to electricity varies within most LMICs, where larger hospitals typically have a more reliable supply. The design of a context-specific mechanical ventilator should include a battery to supply electricity, which could only be needed for a few hours (Table 1), limiting the cost for this relatively expensive component [10].

Compressed air was always available in 35% of hospitals, either piped 68% (19/28) or via cylinders 29% (8/28). Oxygen was reported as always available in 74% of hospitals, at high pressure either piped 44% (20/46) or via cylinders 46% (21/46), or at low pressure via concentrators 11% (5/46). This oxygen availability was lower than observed in 99 Sri Lankan ICUs, where piped oxygen was available, and lower than in 10 hospitals in Tanzania. The result on oxygen availability matches a survey of 97 clinicians from public districts and provincial hospitals in urban and rural areas in 19 countries throughout Africa, Asia, and South America, where 75%

Table 1 Overview of key requirements for the design of a mechanical ventilator usable and sustainable in low- and middle-income countries. Bold text, requirements identified by this survey; italic text, requirements based on prior work, expert opinion, and authors' baseline experience of known needs

Parameter	Requirement
Electricity supply	AC: 100–240 V; 50/60 Hz; DC: 12–30 V; battery operation >2 h[a,b]
Compressed air	Air compressor[a]
Oxygen supply	Oxygen concentrator to deliver >10 L min^{-1}[a] or green-labeled gas cylinder to support 2 h of operation
Electricity and gas supply	Match the national infrastructure (e.g., gas connectors, compatible gas pressures, electricity voltage and frequency, plugs, and sockets[a])
Operating temperature	15–35 °C
Operating humidity	20–70%
Patient monitoring[c,d]	Pulse oximetry, noninvasive BP, electrocardiography, airway oxygen, pressure and flow, end-tidal carbon dioxide, and suction
Internet connectivity	Network access for remote device monitoring (location, usage, self-calibration,[e] and self-testing reports) and firmware updates
Consumable costs	<US$ 50 per patient per day
Support: Technical and training	*Local or in country as a priority, long-term contract for remote support, built-in self-calibration system, product life cycle*
Manufacture, assembly, and testing	*In country as a priority, bench testing to meet regulatory standards; continuous operation > 14 days for critical care applications; built-in self-testing system*[e]
Regulatory standards	*CE marked or FDA approved (or similar)*
Modes of ventilation	*Pressure and/or volume control; spontaneous breathing support if ventilation is required for > 1 day*
Fraction of inspired oxygen	*Up to at least 80%*
Ventilatory frequency	*10–50 bpm; increments of 1 or 2*[f]
PEEP	*5–20 cm H2O, in 5 cm H2O steps or less*[f]
Inspired-to-expired ratio	*1:1 to 1:3*
Tidal volume	*50*[g]*–700 mL, in steps of 50 mL or less*
Inspiratory pressure limits	*15–40 cm H2O, in 5 cm H2O steps or less*
Alarms	*Gas or electricity supply failure, switched off, tidal volumes and pressures exceeded or not reached*
Filtering and humidification	*Bacterial/viral filter; heat and moisture exchanger*
Display and ventilation monitoring	*Set and delivered inspiratory pressure, tidal volume, ventilatory frequency, PEEP, fraction of inspired oxygen, and ventilation mode*

[a]For electricity international standards, see International Electrotechnical Commission guidelines: https://www.iec.ch/world-plugs; [b]98% (135/137) LMICs have either 220 or 230 V, AC, and 84% (115/137) LMICs have a frequency of 50 Hz; [c]listed in order from highest perceived importance from our survey (see Supplementary Fig. S6 for details); [d]apart from suction, all these monitoring priorities match the recent recommended standards of monitoring during anesthesia and recovery; [e]calibration and testing systems need to consider environmental conversion factors (e.g., high altitude); [f]tolerance error < 10%; [g]30 ml for ventilation in neonates. *AC* alternating current; *CE* Conformité Européenne; *DC* direct current; *FDA* US Food and Drug Administration; *LMICs* low- and middle-income countries; *PEEP* positive end-expiratory pressure

Courtesy of Prof. Federico Formenti, Wadham College, University of Oxford [10]

reported that oxygen was available most or all of the time and is similar to that reported by 97 Ugandan anesthetists, where 63% always had access to oxygen [10].

Considered together with evidence from the literature, the results on compressed air and oxygen availability suggest that the design of a mechanical ventilator for hospitals with limited resources must include an air compressor and either a gas cylinder or an oxygen concentrator [10].

Table 1 summarizes the key features to be considered when designing a mechanical ventilator to be useful and usable in LMICs. The requirements listed in this table will not apply fully to a very wide variety of LMIC sites. However, there will be similarities in resource-poor settings applicable to many sites. The trade-off between cost and sophistication is obvious, where in-country manufacture (or at least assembly) is needed for the design to be sustainable [10].

3 Children with Complex Chronic Conditions

The prevalence of children with complex chronic conditions (CCCs) is increasing in LMIC [11]. PMV in CCC is challenging in LMIC due to poor resources and a lack of specialized providers, and it also imposes high costs on the public health system. This cohort of children displays wide ranges of neurodevelopment with a majority experiencing substantial delays in motor, communicative, and adaptive functioning [11].

Studies are scarce regarding the costs of patients receiving PMV in LMIC. A study conducted in a tertiary hospital in Ribeirão Preto, São Paulo, Brazil, shows an increase in the number of hospitalized children with CCC requiring MV from 2006 to 2016. It was associated with a higher proportion of CCC-neurological (NE) patients with increasing complexity, higher technological dependency, and greater use of health resources [12]. It was also observed that hospital mortality rose almost 2.5 times from 2006 to 2016 in patients with CCC, an increase possibly related to the progressively greater complexity of these patients. Moreover, the increase in CCC-NE patient admissions contributed to rising total hospitalization costs over time. The data corroborate the findings of other studies and reinforce the need for reflection on the current care model and its growing impact on hospital costs. This study found that 16.9% of admissions to a pediatric ward of a tertiary referral university hospital consisted of patients with CCC. The proportion of hospitalized CCC patients reported in the literature varies from approximately 10% in studies involving various types of hospitals to almost 80% in studies carried out in pediatric hospitals or specialized reference centers (12). To reduce these rates, we should not only discharge these patients, but also learn to keep them stable at home providing better follow-up and support at home.

Reif LK et al. addressed models of lifelong care for children and adolescents with chronic conditions in LMIC [13]. They discussed three categories of model types and the challenges of dealing with patients with CCC in poor resource settings, including those on PVM:

(a) Care components: involving the patient and family education and involvement; comprehensive care; multisectoral linkages; and mental health and psychosocial support.
(b) Service delivery: including decentralizing services and task shifting; flexible, simplified, and proactive patient care; and differentiated care in LMIC.
(c) Resources invested: comprising health worker training; physical space; and information systems and technology.

The discussion of these topics and models extrapolates the objective of this chapter.

4 Healthcare Resource Use for Children Requiring Prolonged Mechanical Ventilation via Tracheostomy

An increasing number of children with complex medical conditions survive their critical illness with the support of PMV via tracheostomy tubes [1, 3, 4]. In many countries, these patients are utilizing, for months or even years, PICU beds, which represent a limited and expensive resource. The development of home ventilators has improved the safety and effectiveness of managing these patients, either at home or in long-term healthcare facilities [14]. Some studies have reported that patients who require PMV have a high rate of complications and hospital readmissions, and the financial costs associated with caring for them can be a large burden to the healthcare system, especially in LMICs [1, 3, 12, 15]. There are scarce data of financial costs in LMICs; however, a survey of financial burden of families in the USA with children using home mechanical ventilation showed that "families of children who are chronically tracheostomy dependent are often high healthcare users. In the first 2 years following pediatric tracheostomy, median total healthcare spending per child is over \$25,000 and may exceed \$100,000 per child, with over \$1000 in ventilation-related out-of-pocket expenses per month. Among families caring for ventilation-dependent children, 50% have reported difficulty paying for food, 44% have reported difficulty paying for housing, and 33% have reported borrowing money from family/friends" [16].

There are insufficient data describing the healthcare usage of pediatric patients requiring PMV in LMIC. The natural history includes a long initial ICU admission followed by considerable additional hospital time dedicated to the training of the caregivers to safely care for patients at home.

For many patients, despite prolonged hospitalizations and the utilization of large amounts of healthcare resources, readmissions are a frequent occurrence and long-term outcomes are often poor. Some studies show a difference in both costs and outcomes associated with different underlying conditions leading to the need for PMV, but a comparison between these subjects has been described in only a few studies [7, 10, 14]. Data are scarce concerning the differences between HIC and LMIC.

5 Common Barriers for Discharge in LMIC

There are many issues involving the discharge of patients with PMV in LMIC. Although it is not published, discussions are going on regarding these barriers. Some are listed below:

(a) Ventilator availability, oxygen supply, and disposable material due to lack of resourses.
(b) Poor home environment (electricity supply stability, elevator, etc.)
(c) Difficulties in training the family and the healthcare staff.
(d) Shortage of healthcare professionals in LMIC.
(e) Lack of social service support.
(f) Challenges in the follow-up of the patient.

Many of these barriers could be surpassed implementing government policies and education and training. Overall, the barriers are numerous and relevant, but the details are out of the scope of this chapter.

6 Conclusion

Managing patients requiring PMV in poor resource settings is a challenging task due to the lack of resources and other peculiarities. Studies should be encouraged in LMIC to show the patient's necessities, build specific protocols, and support public policies designed to improve these patient's care and outcomes.

Reaching the goal of delivering high-quality respiratory care is lofty, but very possible with a systematic approach to funding, education, and research. Primarily, educational initiatives would be needed to address several issues; not only would physicians and nurses need training on the appropriate care of the ventilated patient, but staff would also need to be trained on the care and maintenance of these machines. Education, in general, is not expensive and delivers good results. Families should be encouraged to participate in training that the government should provide.

Systems would need to be in place to create protocols for complex processes to provide consistent evidence-based care to patients—checklists have been proven very successful in this regard. Several protocols from developed countries will likely need to be modified to best meet the needs and resources of developing countries. Government systems would need to be in place to assure consistent power and oxygen for the machines. Greater education needs to be provided to donors that critical care and mechanical ventilation can be cost-effective and that most evidence-based critical care interventions tend to be inexpensive.

Research should be performed in resource-poor settings to focus on needs assessment, education, implementation, and cost-effectiveness.

While the necessary actions above seem complex, they must be addressed.

References

1. Sauthier M, Rose L, Jouvet P. Pediatric prolonged mechanical ventilation: considerations for definitional criteria. Respir Care. 2017;62(1):49–53.
2. Rose L, Fowler RA, Fan E, Fraser I, Leasa D, Mawdsley C, Pedersen C, Rubenfeld G, CANuVENT group. Prolonged mechanical ventilation in Canadian intensive care units: a national survey. J Crit Care. 2015;30(1):25–31.
3. Lone NI, Walsh TS. Prolonged mechanical ventilation in critically ill patients: epidemiology, outcomes and modelling the potential cost consequences of establishing a regional weaning unit. Crit Care. 2011;15(2):R102.
4. Trudzinski FC, Neetz B, Bornitz F, Müller M, Weis A, Kronsteiner D, Herth FJF, Sturm N, Gassmann V, Frerk T, Neurohr C, Ghiani A, Joves B, Schneider A, Szecsenyi J, von Schumann S, Meis J. Risk factors for prolonged mechanical ventilation and weaning failure: a systematic review. Respiration. 2022;101(10):959–69.
5. Farrell PM, Fost NC. Long-term mechanical ventilation in pediatric respiratory failure: medical and ethical considerations. Am Rev Respir Dis. 1989;140(2 Pt 2):S36–40.
6. Scheinhorn DJ, Chao DC, Stearn-Hassenpflug M. Liberation from prolonged mechanical ventilation. Crit Care Clin. 2002;18(3):569–95.
7. Cox CE, Carson SS, Govert JA, Chelluri L, Sanders GD. An economic evaluation of prolonged mechanical ventilation. Crit Care Med. 2007;35(8):1918–27.
8. Dar M, Swamy L, Gavin D, Theodore A. Mechanical-ventilation supply and options for the COVID-19 pandemic. Leveraging all available resources for a limited resource in a crisis. Ann Am Thorac Soc. 2021 Mar;18(3):408–16.
9. Available at: https://www.poli.usp.br/inspire#:~:text=O%20INSPIRE%20%C3%A9%20um%20equipamento,da%20Escola%20Polit%C3%A9cnica%20da%20USP.
10. Gallifant J, Sharell D, Hashmi M, Riviello ED, Schultz MJ, Ulisubisya MM, Formenti F. Mechanical ventilators for low- and middle-income countries: informing a context-specific and sustainable design. Br J Anaesth. 2022;128(4):e279–81.
11. Junior CJ, Prata-Barbosa A, Lima-Setta F, de Araujo OR, Horigoshi NK, Cesar RG, Souza AAF, Foronda FAK, de Almeida CG, Torreão LA, Crestani F, Carlotti APCP, Garcia PCR. Brazilian Research in Intensive Care (BRICnet). Prevalence and functional status of children with complex chronic conditions in Brazilian PICUs during the COVID-19 pandemic. J Pediatr. 2022,98(5).484–9.
12. Mattiello RMA, Pazin-Filho A, Aragon DC, Cupo P, Carlotti APCP. Impact of children with complex chronic conditions on costs in a tertiary referral hospital. Rev Saude Publica. 2022;17(56):89.
13. Reif LK, van Olmen J, McNairy ML, et al. Models of lifelong care for children and adolescents with chronic conditions in low-income and middle-income countries: a scoping review. BMJ Glob Health. 2022;7:e007863.
14. Kwak S. Home mechanical ventilation in children with chronic respiratory failure: a narrative review. J Yeungnam Med Sci. 2022;40(2):123–35.
15. de Araujo OR, Azevedo RT, de Oliveira FRC, Colleti JJ. Tracheostomy practices in children on mechanical ventilation: a systematic review and meta-analysis. J Pediatr. 2022;98(2):126–35.
16. Baddour K, Mady LJ, Schwarzbach HL, Sabik LM, Thomas TH, McCoy JL, Tobey A. Exploring caregiver burden and financial toxicity in caregivers of tracheostomy-dependent children. Int J Pediatr Otorhinolaryngol. 2021;145:110713.

Evaluation of Respiratory Function of PMVed Children

Vicky MacBean

Accurate assessment of respiratory function is an essential component of respiratory disease management in any population. In the PMVed child, objective assessment techniques can give insight into disease progression or resolution, and responses to changes in ventilation strategies. Respiratory function testing may be used to evaluate changes in the child's physiological state over varying periods of time: from immediate responses to adjustment of ventilator settings, such as the manipulation of PEEP, to the changes associated with physical growth or achievement of developmental milestones. In this complex population, it is not only changes in the structure and function of the respiratory system that will influence pulmonary function; results of any assessments must thus be viewed holistically.

A wealth of testing approaches exists, and the selection of appropriate evaluation techniques for a given child at any one time requires consideration of a range of factors. This chapter outlines key methods for the evaluation of respiratory function in this population. Technical and methodological aspects will not be described in detail (for such information, the reader is directed to more appropriate sources such as technical standards and original publications describing the techniques). Greater emphasis will be placed on what information each technique is able to provide, and what clinical value this may offer, along with practical considerations for implementing specific assessment modalities in the clinical setting. A summary of the testing modalities discussed in this chapter is shown in Table 1.

V. MacBean (✉)
Department of Health Sciences, College of Health, Medicine and Life Sciences, Brunel University London, London, UK
e-mail: Vicky.macbean@brunel.ac.uk

A. Kawaguchi et al. (eds.), *Prolonged and Long-Term Mechanical Ventilation in Children*, https://doi.org/10.1007/978-981-97-8903-0_15

Table 1 Overview of methods for evaluation of respiratory function in PMVed children

	Information provided	Availability of reference data	Equipment required	Specific requirements of patient	Evidence of clinical benefit
Routine clinical data capture	Cardiovascular parameters, oxygen saturations, blood gas partial pressures, CO_2 clearance in exhaled gas, respiratory rate and timing	Yes, robust	Standard clinical equipment only	Passive data collection; feasible in all patients	Established component of clinical practice
Volumetric capnography	Anatomical and physiological dead space	Yes, robust	Dedicated device required	Passive data collection; feasible in all patients	Potential benefit in titrating PEEP and predicting extubation outcome; not well established
Ventilator waveforms	Various, including intrinsic PEEP, lung compliance, patient-ventilator asynchrony, and expiratory flow limitation	Not applicable—Qualitative data analysis	Standard clinical equipment only	Passive data collection; feasible in all patients Waveforms will be influenced by spontaneous breathing and type of airway	Established component of clinical practice
Respiratory mechanics	Compliance (respiratory system as a whole, as well as chest wall and lung in isolation) and resistance	Yes	Respiratory system compliance and resistance can be measured using standard ventilator technology; chest wall and lung compliance require placement of an oesophageal catheter and associated specialised equipment	Spontaneous breathing may need to be inhibited for some measurements; oesophageal catheter placement is uncomfortable	Limited data

	Information provided	Availability of reference data	Equipment required	Specific requirements of patient	Evidence of clinical benefit
Measurement of functional residual capacity	End-expiratory lung volume	Yes, though positional differences must be considered	Technique-dependent, but all methods require equipment beyond that routinely available in the critical care unit (devices for simultaneous measurement of gas concentrations and flows, or CT scanner)	Radiation burden associated with CT-based measures A closed system (cuffed, leak-free airway) and a stable breathing pattern are required for gas dilution techniques	Limited data
Forced oscillation technique	Airway resistance and reactance, and subdivisions of these parameters	No, not for mechanically ventilated children	Dedicated equipment required; commercial devices are available	Tidal breathing only; stable breathing pattern is preferred	Limited data
Electrical impedance tomography	Relative aeration of lung segments	Not applicable—Evaluates intraindividual differences only	Dedicated equipment required	Passive data collection; feasible in all patients	Very limited

(continued)

Table 1 (continued)

	Information provided	Availability of reference data	Equipment required	Specific requirements of patient	Evidence of clinical benefit
Forced deflation techniques	Expired lung volumes and maximal expiratory flows	Can use standard spirometry reference values, though with caution for some parameters that may be affected by the presence of an artificial airway (expiratory flows at higher percentages of vital capacity)	Dedicated equipment required	Passive cooperation is required—Spontaneously breathing children who 'fight' the measurements will not provide accurate data. Cuffed airway required	Very limited
Chest wall measurements	Thoracoabdominal asynchrony; relative motion of chest wall segments	Extremely limited	Dedicated equipment required	Passive data collection, but most modern equipment (structured light plethysmography, optoelectronic plethysmography) unfeasible due to technical requirements of the test	No
$P_{0.1}$	Respiratory drive	Yes (ages 4 and upward)	Available in most modern ventilators	Passive cooperation only; cuffed airway required	May be useful in titrating PEEP and pressure support

	Information provided	Availability of reference data	Equipment required	Specific requirements of patient	Evidence of clinical benefit
Maximal inspiratory pressures	Inspiratory muscle strength	Yes, though with poor coverage for some age groups	Available in most modern ventilators	Degree of cooperation required depends on child age and cognitive function; can be challenging to obtain high-quality results Temporary interruption of ventilation is required, though this is generally well tolerated	Limited data
Maximal expiratory pressure	Expiratory muscle strength	Yes, though with poor coverage for some age groups	Dedicated equipment required	Degree of cooperation required depends on child age and cognitive function; can be challenging to obtain high-quality results Temporary interruption of ventilation is required, though this is generally well tolerated	Very limited data
Invasive measures of respiratory muscle function	Inspiratory and expiratory muscle strength, including specific diaphragm function	Limited	Dedicated, specialist equipment required	Depends on exact testing technique but generally only passive cooperation	Limited data

(continued)

Table 1 (continued)

	Information provided	Availability of reference data	Equipment required	Specific requirements of patient	Evidence of clinical benefit
Respiratory muscle electromyography	Activation of respiratory muscles (mainly diaphragm)	No	Dedicated, specialist equipment required (though available as part of some ventilators)	Passive cooperation only	May be of use in assessing for patient-ventilator asynchrony and titrating ventilator support, but data are limited
Peak cough flow	Cough effectiveness	Yes, but not for mechanically ventilated children	Measurement may be available within ventilator; simple equipment (spirometers, peak flow meters) are not accurate for this purpose	Active cooperation required; suitable for older children Cuffed airway required	Very limited data
Lung ultrasound	Presence/absence of imaging findings consistent with specific pathologies	Not applicable—Qualitative, visual data interpretation only	Equipment available on almost all modern critical care units	Passive cooperation only	Diagnostic merit established; limited data on management of ventilation
Ultrasound imaging of diaphragm function	Size and activation of diaphragm	Yes, robust	Equipment available on almost all modern critical care units	Passive cooperation only	Limited data; focus tends to be on extubation prediction
Energy expenditure	Resting energy expenditure; when measured during manipulation of ventilator settings, changes in metabolic oxygen consumption/CO_2 production of the respiratory muscles can be inferred	Available, but not appropriate to extrapolate data from healthy populations to PMVed children	Incorporated into some ventilators, otherwise dedicated equipment required	Passive cooperation only; cuffed airway required	No

1 Factors Influencing Selection of Testing Technique

Children receiving PMV are a phenotypically diverse group. As such, no single technique will ever be 'the best' for all PMVed children. There are many factors to consider when selecting appropriate assessment tools to be used with an individual child.

- The age and developmental stage of the patient(s): a technique requiring volitional manoeuvres will not be suited for routine use in children under the age of approximately 4–5 years, or for those who have significant cognitive or receptive communication deficits. Similarly, major motor impairments may impede a child's cooperation with volitional manoeuvres.
- Physiological stability and dependence on ventilator breaths: Certain techniques require interruption of normal ventilation, meaning that they may be poorly suited to more dependent patients or those with more labile cardiorespiratory behaviour.
- Intrinsic respiratory drive: patients requiring time-cycled modes of ventilation may be unable to participate in assessment methods that require spontaneous respiratory effort.
- Presence and type of artificial airway: uncuffed tracheostomy tubes will lead to inaccurate data in assessment techniques requiring accurate values for flow, pressure or gas concentration, as gas will enter/exit via the oronasopharynx. Achieving a tight seal via a facemask in children dependent on non-invasive ventilation is entirely possible, but patient cooperation and tolerance may be poor if the test interface is very different to their usual mask. The focus throughout this chapter is predominantly on children undergoing invasive mechanical ventilation.
- Secretion burden: Some techniques require accurate measurement of respiratory flow. Very high secretion loads with resultant flow artefacts may result in inaccurate flow data, rendering measurements inaccurate. Similarly, a child requiring frequent suction may not be able to undergo a lengthy period of uninterrupted respiratory measurement.

A clinical service considering investment in respiratory monitoring technology must bear the above in mind, thinking about the overall case mix within the centre. A service where the majority of PMVed children are over the age of 5 could focus more on techniques requiring active cooperation from the patient, whereas an NICU with a large number of PMVed infants would need to make different decisions. There is also the question of cost-benefit analysis: Can investment in an expensive piece of equipment that provides fascinating insight into a child's physiology, but does not allow the clinician to make changes to care delivery that will actually improve the child's clinical status, be justified? The staffing and expertise required for performing detailed and potentially complex measurements should also be considered, including skill maintenance and succession planning. Decisions in smaller centres with lower patient numbers will be different to those in specialist centres with possibly greater recourse to funds along with the need to assess more complex presentations. Lower resource settings are likely to want to prioritise the use of routinely-captured clinical data; despite many of the devices being described in the literature as 'inexpensive', individuals from different backgrounds may debate the precise definition of this word.

2 A Note on Reference Values

For many of the techniques described in this chapter, there is a dearth of normative data in the target population, meaning that assessment findings often cannot be reliably interpreted against expected values for healthy children. This is potentially problematic. Interpreting a single result without reliable reference data is very difficult—Is the child working at one-third of normal capacity, or are they close to healthy? Longitudinal changes over shorter time periods may be easier to interpret, as any substantial improvement or decline in test results can be temporaly (if not necessarily causatively) associated with any relevant changes in clinical care. Longer term changes are, however, also challenging to interpret without normative values against which to compare. This issue is particularly significant in paediatrics, and even more so in younger children and infants, as changes will naturally occur due to physical growth, and extrapolating the relative impacts of development from those due to changes in disease status and/or ventilation adjustments is difficult. Clinicians are encouraged to take a critical view when evaluating respiratory function using techniques without robust reference data and consider the results of individual tests in the context of the overall clinical picture. Where normative data exist, results should ideally be reported as standardised residuals ('z-scores'), rather than percentage of predicted; this is a more mathematically robust approach that accounts for different distributions of normal values that frequently occurs across the age range encountered in paediatric medicine.

3 Measurement techniques

3.1 Routine Clinical Data Capture

Children undergoing PMV will inevitably have continuous physiological monitoring in place to some extent. At minimum, this is likely to include pulse oximetry, giving a continuous measure of peripheral capillary oxygen saturation and pulse rate. These parameters should be observed for both abrupt changes as well as gradual trends. Pulse rate or heart rate is poorly specific to respiratory function, but can be an early indicator of physiological stress relating to deteriorating respiratory function. Blood pressure can also provide similarly useful information.

Respiratory rate is of course an important variable. A respiratory frequency that is moving (further) out of normal limits may indicate worsening respiratory distress. The respiratory duty cycle (the fraction of the total respiratory time spent in inspiration) is also a useful indicator of respiratory effort. Together with the magnitude of pressure generation of the respiratory muscles, duty cycle is a reliable predictor of the tolerability of respiratory effort [5]. In the PMVed child in whom a reduction in pressure support is implemented as part of a weaning programme (thus increasing the required pressure generation from the respiratory muscles), the duty cycle can be monitored. A substantial increase in duty cycle may suggest that the change in ventilator support will not be tolerated.

Continuous carbon dioxide monitoring can be highly informative. Most accurate is end-tidal CO_2, which has the added benefit of providing qualitative information through evaluation of the shape of the $ETCO_2$ waveform as well as the value itself. A longer rise time and/or loss of the plateau suggests airway obstruction. Transcutaneous CO_2 ($TCCO_2$) monitoring is useful in determining trends in gas exchange, but is less informative with regard to acute changes. $TCCO_2$ also requires careful attention to calibration processes and skin care. Arterial and arterialised capillary blood gases are of course highly informative.

A major advantage of using data measured routinely is that there is no additional cost or care burden associated with obtaining such measurements. Care burden is a key consideration in PMVed children, as these individuals and their families already carry an extraordinary load. Using routine data may also be useful in settings where resources are more limited, including those where provision of PMV may be an evolving specialism.

3.2 Volumetric Capnography

Volumetric capnography is essentially an extension of conventional time-based $ETCO_2$ monitoring and plots exhaled CO_2 against exhaled volume. It is sometimes termed the single-breath test of CO_2. This provides a marker of anatomical and physiological dead space and effectiveness of ventilation [35]. It is based on the principle first described by Ward Fowler in the 1940s, in which nitrogen washout following inhalation of 100% oxygen was used to differentiate physiological dead space from effective tidal volume. As the exhaled CO_2 trace follows the same pattern as that of the exhaled nitrogen curve, dead space can be calculated without the need for interruption of normal ventilation. Qualitative inspection of the waveforms also allows the experienced clinician to identify patterns characteristic of specific pathophysiologies. Volumetric capnography has been shown to be predictive of extubation outcome in the paediatric population [17]. It has also been used for PEEP titration and assessment of lung recruitment manoeuvres, suggesting that there is value in using this technique in clinical evaluation. Dedicated equipment is required to process the breath-by-breath data required for volumetric capnography.

3.3 Ventilator Waveforms

A wealth of data can be extracted from modern ventilators. For a comprehensive overview, the reader is directed to Elizabeth Emrath's clear and informative review paper [12]. Key information that can be gleaned from most ventilators in routine clinical use includes the detection of intrinsic PEEP (PEEPi) resulting from gas trapping, assessment of lung compliance, detection of patient-ventilator asynchrony (PVA), and detection of expiratory flow limitation. Available waveforms include pressure, flow and volume plotted against time, pressure-volume loops and flow-volume loops. PEEPi is present when flow does not return to zero at the end of expiration; this can be seen on a flow-time, volume-time or flow-volume plot. Of note, persistent end-expiratory flow may also indicate a system leak, which is particularly common in PMVed children where uncuffed airways are frequently used.

Many ventilators will quantify lung compliance (see below), but waveform data can be informative too. More rapid expiratory airflow and greater hysteresis (shown as the difference between the inspiratory and expiratory limbs of the pressure-volume curve) are hallmarks of decreased lung compliance. Pressure-time plots can also be used (in patients on volume-controlled ventilation modes) to determine the 'stress index'—a marker of lung compliance.

Increased expiratory airflow resistance will manifest as reduced peak expiratory flow, prolonged expiratory time and a shallower gradient in the expiratory portion of a flow-time or flow-volume plot, comparable to the 'scooping' observed on flow-volume loops obtained during spirometry. The presence of expiratory airflow limitation can be determined by applying manual pressure on the patient's chest or abdomen during expiration and looking for an increase in expiratory flow. No further increase is indicative of expiratory flow limitation.

Poor patient-ventilator interaction has been associated with a number of adverse outcomes in adult critical care populations. Although asynchrony has been shown to affect as many as one-third of all breaths in mechanically ventilated children [7, 27], the association with outcomes is not as clear [20]. Certainly, asynchrony increases work of breathing [27], and its avoidance may therefore arguably aid weight gain (or, at least, nutritional management) in PMVed children. Not all asynchronies can be viewed as measures of respiratory function, but ineffective triggering may occur due to PEEPi and therefore may indicate the presence of, for example, inadequately managed airflow obstruction.

As mentioned above with regard to the use of routine physiological data, using the data already provided by the ventilator has the advantage of imposing no additional time or cost burden on the patient or care provider and is therefore a highly efficient method for assessment of the PMVed child.

3.4 Respiratory Mechanics

Respiratory mechanics refers to the evaluation of pulmonary function through the measurement of respiratory flow and pressure. These can be plotted as described above, and for further quantitative assessment of the patient's respiratory status, specific indices, such as compliance and resistance, can be calculated.

Respiratory system compliance (C_{RS}) is calculated as the tidal volume achieved divided by the pressure required to achieve that tidal volume. It reflects both the compliance of the lungs and the chest wall. In mechanically ventilated patients, the required pressure is determined by plateau pressure minus PEEP, i.e. driving pressure. Plateau pressure is measured during an end-inspiratory hold, allowing proximal airway pressure to equilibrate with alveolar pressure. This technique is only valid in the absence of spontaneous respiratory muscle activity, which is unlikely to be the case in many PMVed children. The Hering-Breuer reflex can be harnessed to inhibit inspiratory muscle activity in spontaneously breathing children [14], though note that performing the required deep inspirations may have an impact on C_{RS}. Other adapted methods are available for determination of the plateau pressure in spontaneously breathing individuals [2]. C_{RS} may be helpful in determining optimal levels of PEEP. Manoeuvres that do not require abolition (albeit temporary) of the child's own respiratory drive would generally be preferable for use in an outpatient setting, though individual clinicians must decide on the level of risk accepted in their centre.

Measurement of chest wall and lung compliance individually requires an index of pleural pressure (derived clinically using intra-oesophageal pressure measurement; see below). Chest wall compliance is calculated by tidal volume divided by change in pleural pressure during a passive inflation. As above, consideration may need to be given to inhibiting spontaneous respiratory muscle activity in some PMVed children to accomplish the required manoeuvres. Chest wall compliance can be affected by pathologies and/or muscle activity affecting the ribcage or the abdominal compartment. In the PMVed child, these may include obesity, altered muscle tone (muscular tone demonstrating an inverse relationship with chest wall compliance) and skeletal deformities, though it should be noted that something as apparently innocuous as faecal constipation may impact chest wall compliance.

Lung compliance is calculated as tidal volume divided by the change in transpulmonary pressure (calculated as the difference between airway and pleural pressure, measured under conditions of zero flow). Lung compliance is impacted by any pathology affecting the lung parenchyma or pleural space, but also by overdistension resulting from excessive ventilator pressures.

Airway resistance is derived again from measurements of inspired pressures and flows and can be divided into inspiratory and expiratory values. Inspiratory resistance is calculated as peak inspiratory pressure minus plateau pressure, divided by end-inspiratory flow ($(PIP—P_{plat})/V'_I$). Expiratory resistance is plateau pressure minus PEEP, divided by peak expiratory flow ($(P_{plat}—PEEP)/V'_E$). Elevated respiratory resistance values may indicate the presence of bronchospasm or retained secretions.

For an extremely detailed and comprehensive description of respiratory mechanics in mechanically ventilated individuals, the reader is referred to Dean Hess's excellent review article [16].

3.5 Measurement of Functional Residual Capacity

Functional residual capacity, defined as the volume of gas remaining in the lungs after a relaxed expiration, can be measured via a number of routes in mechanically ventilated individuals and may be a useful tool for assessing lung recruitment [4]. Computed tomography (CT) scanning is generally viewed as the gold standard method and has the benefit of providing further information regarding structural aspects of the lungs, airways and other intrathoracic structures. Although modern scanning protocols and the use of paediatric-specific settings minimise the effective dose [28], radiation exposure remains a concern. Helical (volumetric) chest CT scans involve the same effective radiation dose as 29–169 chest X-rays, depending on the child's age [36], and are therefore not a suitable method for frequent assessment of FRC.

Body plethysmography is the gold standard technique for measurement of intrathoracic gas volumes in ambulatory populations. This technique has been used in intubated, mechanically ventilated infants [10] but is complex, and at present, there is no commercially available respiratory plethysmography device suitable for use in the PMVed population.

Measurement of FRC by gas dilution uses inert (nitrogen, sulphur hexafluoride) or biologically active (oxygen) gases to determine relevant lung volumes through helium dilution, gas washout or wash-in techniques. Such measurements simply require tidal breathing and so are suitable for use in paediatric populations—perhaps even more so in PMVed children who are familiar with respiratory apparatus and manipulation of their ventilator tubing, and in whom (for those invasively ventilated at least) no facemask is required. Reference values are available for this technique, and the measurements can be performed in an outpatient setting. The influence of posture should not be neglected (the supine position reduces FRC); healthy reference data beyond infancy will have been obtained in the seated position, and PMVed children undergoing FRC measurements should be positioned comparably to the reference cohort wherever possible. The presence of significant gas trapping can however render FRC measurements using this technique inaccurate, so its use requires careful consideration in light of the patient's underlying pathology. Patients with a more chaotic breathing pattern may not produce technically acceptable results, so close attention must be paid to data quality prior to using FRC values to inform clinical decision-making.

3.6 Forced Oscillation Technique

The forced oscillation technique (FOT) involves the application of a small oscillating pressure signal at the airway opening and recording the resultant pressure and flow. By applying this oscillation at a frequency significantly above the patient's natural respiratory frequency, there is no contribution from the patient's own respiratory efforts, meaning that an accurate picture of the mechanical behaviour of the patient's respiratory system can be obtained. Critically, this is a passive assessment technique, not requiring any active cooperation from the patient. The lack of interruption to normal breathing means the tool is well suited to outpatient monitoring of PMVed children. FOT provides a measure of respiratory system impedance, comprising resistance (primarily determined by airway calibre) and reactance. Reactance itself incorporates elastance (the reciprocal of compliance) and inertance and represents the 'stiffness' of the entire respiratory system (tissue and gas) and the opposition to acceleration of the gas column throughout the bronchial tree.

The pressure signal itself comprises multiple frequencies, and the resultant resistance and reactance values can be evaluated at these different frequencies. The 'frequency dependence' of these values (i.e. the extent to which the values vary with frequency) is more pronounced in children and tends to increase with disease. The clinical implications of measures of frequency dependence are as yet unclear.

Oscillometry is ideally suited to settings where conventional pulmonary function testing is more challenging, including paediatrics and intensive care. Commercially-available and bespoke devices have been used in the literature. The potential role of oscillometry in optimising mechanical ventilation has been demonstrated, though this area of research is not well developed. Readers are directed to the European Respiratory Society's technical standard document for respiratory oscillometry for further information [19]. It seems likely that oscillometry will become an increasingly widely used technique in respiratory medicine broadly in coming years. Clinical services where PMVed children are supported may therefore choose to invest in an oscillometry system suitable for use via artificial airways.

3.7 Electrical Impedance Tomography

Electrical impedance tomography (EIT) has received extensive and widespread interest in recent years. It offers clear potential as a non-invasive and non-ionising method for real-time, dynamic assessment of lung aeration and perfusion that can be performed at the bedside. EIT relies on the differing impedances to electrical current offered by different bodily tissues (as well as gas). EIT involves an electrode array (anything from 8 to 64 electrodes) placed around the circumference of the chest wall around the level of the fifth intercostal space at the parasternal line. Each pair of electrodes in turn emits a medium-frequency current, and the remaining electrodes measure the surface potential differences. An impedance 'map' is thus generated, producing a transverse image in which pixels of different colours represent different degrees of lung aeration. It is important to note that EIT does not allow quantification of pulmonary abnormalities, merely comparison between different areas and conditions. Its use is likely to be better suited to inpatient monitoring where ventilator settings or other aspects of care are being manipulated, rather than an outpatient 'snapshot' of respiratory function.

This map allows comparison between different lung segments, adding a clear advantage over global measures that view the respiratory system as a whole. This may be more informative in guiding manipulation of ventilator settings; for example, if increases in PEEP affect anterior lung segments alone, the clinician may not wish to pursue this approach for fear of localised overdistension. EIT has been shown to be responsive to respiratory physiotherapy interventions, changes in positioning, and manipulations of ventilator settings, as well as the presence of pneumothorax, atelectasis, pleural effusion, misplaced artificial airways and pulmonary embolism.

As is frequently the case, much of the research into EIT to date has concentrated on the adult population. The literature base in paediatrics is growing, helped by the availability of dedicated paediatric electrode belts. There are some practical barriers to use in children: the smaller chest size means that EIT measurements may be more likely to encounter interference due to other chest wall apparatus (dressings, metallic implants), and movement artefact is more likely. EIT holds promise in the management of acute respiratory failure, where regional atelectasis and overdistension raise concerns over ventilator-induced lung injury worsening an already severe respiratory failure. It could be argued however that PMVed children should be an area in which the evidence base for EIT warrants expansion; optimal management of respiratory function in this population could help to minimise further lung damage and increase the likelihood of eventual ventilator liberation.

3.8 *Forced Deflation Techniques*

This is the nearest equivalent of spirometry for use in the mechanically ventilated child. The procedure involves lung inflation to total lung capacity, using a positive pressure of 40cmH_2O, an inspiratory hold of 3 s, followed by rapid deflation to residual volume through the application of -40cmH_2O pressure. Measures comparable to conventional spirometry can be obtained, including forced vital capacity (FVC) and maximal expiratory flows at specific lung volumes (conventionally 50%, 25% and 10% of FVC). These values can provide important insight into airway function and its response to treatment, though they do not provide any information on factors such as operating lung volumes, pulmonary compliance or gas exchange. Reduced maximal expiratory flows will however indicate airflow obstruction and hence elevated work of breathing, which will be of clinical relevance in titrating ventilator support.

An animal study showed that the diameter of the artificial airway can have a significant impact on the measured flow at higher lung volumes (50% FVC), though it does not affect the lower flow values at lower lung volumes [15]. Clinicians should use these tests with some caution in patients with lungs more sensitive to such high inflation pressures; repeated use in neonates, for example, may not be appropriate.

3.9 Chest Wall Measurements

These can incorporate a range of techniques, all of which infer volume change by measuring displacement of the external chest wall. The use of such techniques to estimate tidal volume is clearly unnecessary in the PMVed child, in whom accurate measurements of respiratory flow and volume are easily obtained via the ventilator. However, the assessment of relative motion of different segments of the chest and abdomen may be of benefit.

The most well-known technique is respiratory inductive plethysmography (RIP), in which two bands containing coils carrying a weak electrical current are placed around the chest and abdomen, and changes in inductance allow inferences of changes in cross-sectional area. Calibration of RIP systems for accurate volume measurements is time-consuming, but a semi-quantitative approach can be used to examine thoracoabdominal (a)synchrony. Thoracoabdominal asynchrony (TAA), where the motions of the ribcage and abdomen are not in parallel, or are even in complete opposition, may be indicative of airflow obstruction, respiratory muscle dysfunction or inadequate ventilatory support. Semi-quantitative RIP measurements can easily be made in an outpatient setting, though it would be hoped that none of the above issues would be present in a stable, adequately managed PMVed child.

Newer systems for measurement of TAA include structured light plethysmography (SLP) and optoelectronic plethysmography (OEP). SLP involves the projection of a 'chequerboard' of light onto the patient's torso while wearing a tightly fitting white garment. Movement other than tidal breathing must be avoided. Relative motion of chest wall and abdominal segments is quantified by the SLP device. There is evidence to support the use of SLP in assessing paediatric asthma, with limited data available in post-operative, neuromuscular and dysfunctional breathing populations [22]. In theory, it has a role in assessing TAA in the PMVed child, but it is not difficult to see the major barrier to success—dressing the child in a close-fitting T-shirt (and, to a lesser extent in some children, encouraging them to lie still) is likely to be problematic in a large proportion of this population.

OEP uses the same motion-capture technology as is used in the film industry. It requires the placement of multiple light-reflective sensors on the chest and torso. The displacement of these sensors is captured by an array of cameras at specific located angles and distances around the patient. A detailed picture of relative displacement of various ribcage and abdominal segments can be obtained, which can provide an in-depth insight into respiratory biomechanics. However, the sensors must be placed on specific anatomic landmarks on the anterior, posterior and lateral chest wall, and the patient seated upright with arms held away from the torso—this is clearly not a feasible routine measure of pulmonary function in the PMVed child. It seems unlikely that SLP or OEP will gain traction in the critical care setting, nor indeed in paediatric respiratory medicine more broadly. These measures are nevertheless included in this chapter to highlight the weaknesses of these technologies, in the face of occasional enthusiasm from members of the research community to extend such measures into unsuitable settings. There remains of course the possibility that further technical developments may render SLP and/or OEP suitable for use in PMVed children.

3.10 Occlusion Pressures

3.10.1 P0.1

The pressures generated by the respiratory muscles against an airway occlusion can provide valuable information regarding respiratory drive and respiratory muscle function. $P_{0.1}$, or P_{100ms}, is the pressure generated in the first 100 milliseconds of an occluded breath, measured at the airway opening (proximal end of endotracheal or tracheostomy tube in the ventilated individual). This time period is too brief for the patient to detect the occlusion; hence, the pressure generation is the same as that during an unoccluded breath. $P_{0.1}$ is a marker of inspiratory neural drive, and an elevated $P_{0.1}$ may indicate inadequate respiratory support in a ventilated individual. $P_{0.1}$ will be lower in individuals ventilated due to respiratory muscle weakness and should be interpreted in light of the patient's inspiratory muscle strength. Reference values for $P_{0.1}$ in children over the age of 4 are available [13]. The brevity and simplicity of these measurements render them suitable for outpatient monitoring of PMVed children.

$P_{0.1}$ demonstrates a relatively high variability (~50%); hence, it is recommended that several measurements are made and an average value is calculated. $P_{0.1}$ is influenced by operating lung volumes, meaning that high respiratory drive may be masked in patients with significant hyperinflation. The presence of intrinsic PEEP may also render measurement of $P_{0.1}$ inaccurate. Many ventilators will have an in-built $P_{0.1}$ function, though it should be noted that the precise algorithm may vary between manufacturers and models. If sequential measurements are made in an individual patient, these should be undertaken on the same ventilator model.

$P_{0.1}$ may be useful as an indicator of respiratory effort and could help guide decisions about increasing or decreasing a patient's ventilator support to maintain an adequate but sustainable level of inspiratory assistance. $P_{0.1}$ may also be valuable in PEEP titration. Telias et al. provide a brief but useful overview of the value of $P_{0.1}$ during mechanical ventilation [33].

3.10.2 Maximal Inspiratory Pressure

Inspiratory muscle strength can be quantified by measurement of maximal pressure generation against an occluded inspiration, termed maximal inspiratory pressure (MIP or PI_{max}). This is again measured at the airway opening. The use of a one-way valve allows expiration down to residual volume and hence maximises the pressure-generating capacity of the diaphragm. Many ventilators allow measurement of PI_{max}, generally termed negative inspiratory force (NIF).

In younger individuals or those unable to comply with instructions, the testing protocol relies on autonomic respiratory drive alone—the occlusion prevents any inspired volume or gas exchange, and respiratory drive therefore increases over subsequent inspiratory efforts until a maximum effort is obtained (usually five to seven breaths). In older, co-operative individuals, a volitional testing approach can be used, whereby the patient is encouraged to perform a maximum, sustained inspiratory effort against the occlusion. In children aged between approximately 2 and 5 years of age (or those with equivalent cognitive function), a pragmatic, hybrid approach must be used—that of maintaining the occlusion during repeated inspiratory efforts while strong verbal encouragement is used. The testing in this age group may be of variable technical quality; the values obtained must therefore be considered in light of the tester's opinion of the success of the test. It is essential to note that high values unequivocally demonstrate preserved respiratory muscle force-generating capacity, whereas low values may or may not indicate weakness. If the operator is satisfied that maximum (or at least near-maximum) effort was induced, then the PI_{max} value can be viewed as reliable. If there is uncertainty as to the technical quality of the test, results should be used alongside other measurements to reach an overall clinical impression of the patient's respiratory muscle strength.

Many clinicians (and of course parents) are hesitant about imposing a deliberate airway obstruction on PMVed children, who are of course by definition more fragile and physiologically unstable than their spontaneously breathing counterparts. Adverse physiological effects of respiratory muscle strength assessments are very rare and generally are transient if observed at all. These measurements are safe in an outpatient setting. The potential psychological distress associated with such testing should not, however, be overlooked. Some children and families may find these tests very upsetting; the clinical benefit gained from the test results must therefore be balanced carefully against any damage to the therapeutic alliance.

Reference values for PI_{max} in older children (aged 4 and upwards) and infants are available [8, 31, 34], but are currently somewhat lacking in the intermediary age range. Work is currently in progress by the author to remedy this data gap.

Although international guidelines make specific recommendations for the technical specifications of equipment for respiratory muscle strength testing [3, 23], low-resource settings could consider undertaking these measurements using a simple manometer to evaluate the peak pressures achieved.

3.10.3 Maximal Expiratory Pressure

Expiratory muscle function can be evaluated using a similar method to PI_{max}. In testing the expiratory muscles (MEP or PE_{max}), an airway occlusion is applied that permits inhalation but not exhalation, allowing the patient to inspire to total lung capacity and therefore maximise expiratory pressure generation (aided somewhat by chest wall and lung recoil). The same practical considerations apply as for measurement of PI_{max} with regard to patient co-operation, patient distress and equipment requirements, though expiratory muscle strength testing is generally better tolerated than inspiratory muscle assessments. Reference values are available for PE_{max} [8, 34], with the same age representation (or lack thereof) as for PI_{max}. While PE_{max} may not be as immediately relevant with regard to maintaining independent ventilation, intact expiratory muscle function is key for cough and airway clearance and is therefore potentially worthy of assessment. It may be of particular interest to respiratory therapists and physiotherapists and should be considered as a relevant clinical outcome measure if secretion management presents a barrier to effective ventilation and/or weaning.

3.11 Invasive Measures of Respiratory Muscle Function

More detailed measurements of respiratory muscle function can be made through the use of intrathoracic and intra-abdominal pressure sensors mounted on specialised oro- or naso-gastric catheters. These sensors may take the form of liquid- or air-filled balloons or solid-state sensors. Pressure measured in the lower third of the oesophagus (Poes) is equivalent to pleural pressure, and gastric pressure (Pgas) is representative of abdominal pressure. Poes can be used alone as a measure of the pressure generation from the summed activity of all inspiratory muscles, though in practice it has little benefit in invasively ventilated individuals over measuring pressure at the airway opening as described above. Pgas may be measured as a marker of expiratory muscle strength, though again it has little additional value in the ventilated patient.

Subtracting Poes from Pgas gives the pressure gradient across the diaphragm (transdiaphragmatic pressure, or Pdi), providing a direct index of the function of the principal inspiratory muscle. Pdi measurements may be particularly useful if there is a question of phrenic nerve injury (occurring following cardiac or liver surgery, or central venous catheter insertion for example) or diaphragm dysfunction (due to anatomical defects or ventilator-induced diaphragmatic dysfunction). Measurements of Pdi can be made during spontaneous breathing, during inspiratory occlusion manoeuvres as described above for PI_{max} or during direct phrenic nerve stimulation. Pdi responses to unilateral phrenic nerve stimulation can be used to investigate the function of each hemidiaphragm in isolation. Phrenic nerve stimulation and invasive respiratory pressure measurement do however both require extensive technical expertise and specialist equipment, which is unlikely to be an effective use of resources in the majority of clinical settings. A commercially available, combined, self-contained system for the measurement of intrathoracic pressures (with or without phrenic nerve stimulation) does not currently exist. For more complete descriptions of various evaluations of respiratory muscle function, including invasive measurements and stimulation techniques, the reader is directed to the relevant American Thoracic Society and European Respiratory Society Statements [3, 23].

3.12 Respiratory Muscle Electromyography

Previously the preserve of respiratory physiology researchers with specialised equipment, boundless reserves of patience and questionable sanity, respiratory EMG is now a feasible clinical tool thanks to the advent of neurally adjusted ventilatory assist (NAVA) technology. NAVA uses a specialised nasogastric feeding tube equipped with a fine-wire electrode array to measure the electrical activity of the diaphragm (termed EAdi). Proprietary filtering algorithms allow removal of the ECG signal which contaminates diaphragm EMG obtained using conventional approaches.

The EAdi signal is representative of the brainstem output to the diaphragm and therefore of the balance between the load on the respiratory system and the capacity of the respiratory muscles. While NAVA is designed to titrate ventilatory support to match the patient's own physiological requirements (both in terms of timing and magnitude of supported inspiration), the EAdi signal can be used as an assessment tool to guide clinical decision-making (though investment in a NAVA ventilator purely for assessment purposes is unlikely to be warranted). Small increases in EAdi in response to a manipulation of ventilator settings may be appropriate (particularly if the goal is to wean the patient), but substantial increases are likely to be intolerable. It is as yet unknown what constitutes a 'tolerable' level of EAdi. The EAdi signal can also be interrogated for evidence of patient-ventilator asynchrony, including ineffective triggering and post-inspiratory inspiratory activity.

Diaphragm EMG coupled with measures of respiratory muscle function is useful in determining the underlying aetiology of any respiratory muscle dysfunction. Preserved electrical activity in the presence of weakness suggests a myopathic process, whereas reductions in both force generation and electrical activity are likely to be of neurological origin (either neuropathic or resulting from inadequate output from brainstem respiratory centres).

Non-invasive forms of respiratory muscle EMG are also available, but these must be obtained using conventional EMG technology and are therefore far less user-friendly and resource-efficient. Parasternal intercostal EMG has been used in the paediatric intensive care unit [25] but is not currently suitable for routine clinical use due to the manual signal analysis required.

3.13 Peak Cough Flow

Measurements of peak expiratory flow during a cough manoeuvre can provide valuable information about the patient's ability to adequately protect their airway. Peak cough flow (PCF) is likely to be of greater value as a patient approaches extubation, as endotracheal suction will be required to some extent as long as the patient has an artificial airway in situ. PCF has been shown to be predictive of extubation outcome in adult patients [9], but its utility in the paediatric setting is not established. There are some important considerations when measuring PCF. Firstly, it is a composite index of expiratory muscle strength and airway calibre, and as such it is important to ascertain the root cause of any reduction in PCF. Secondly, most commercially available devices are not designed for the very rapid changes in flow (very short rise time) that can be encountered during a true physiological cough and may over- or under-measure [21]. This may be less of a concern in mechanically ventilated patients, given their inability to close the glottis and generate a true physiological cough (compressive followed by expulsive phase), but the suitability of measuring devices must still be considered. Simple peak flow meters (such as those used for home or primary care monitoring of asthma) have been used for the measurement of PCF in ventilated individuals, but these are certainly inadequate for use in PMVed children (both due to the poor response time and the device inertia providing resistance to the lower flows generated by young children with lung, airway and/or respiratory muscle dysfunction).

3.14 Lung Ultrasound

Ultrasonography was, until relatively recently, viewed as a tool poorly suited to imaging of lung tissue. Ultrasound waves penetrate the gas-filled lung poorly, and the air-tissue-liquid interface creates artefacts, hence the dismissal of this technique for assessment of the pulmonary system. Its use was confined to the assessment of masses and pleural effusions. The use of lung ultrasound (LUS) has expanded enormously in recent years however, with the recognition that the artefacts encountered when the lung is imaged, rather than being a barrier to the use of the technique, actually provide valuable clinical information. Ultrasound imaging has clear advantages for both patient and clinician, with the most important being a lack of ionising radiation and the ability to complete rapid and repeated bedside assessments. Ultrasound technology is now ubiquitous on modern critical care units, meaning that no additional equipment need to be purchased. Paediatric patients are particularly well suited to the assessment with LUS, due to the incomplete ossification of the chest wall bony structures as well as generally thinner layers of adipose tissue. Despite this, and as is frequently the case, research in the paediatric field still lags behind that in adult populations.

LUS commonly uses a 10 MHz linear transducer or in older patients a 5 MHz convex probe. Anterior, lateral and (if the patient can be turned prone) posterior lung segments can be imaged, with the thorax divided into upper and lower zones. There are three principal LUS findings [6]:

- Lung sliding: This is created by the movement of the visceral and parietal pleurae against one another. It has been described as a 'shimmering' or (less appealingly) like 'ants marching'. The presence of lung sliding implies the presence of lung tissue at the pleural interface and respiratory activity (whether spontaneous or passive).

- A lines: Hyperechoic (bright white) lines parallel to the pleural line. These are reverberations of the ultrasound waves from the pleural line caused by the interface with aerated lung tissue. The distance between A lines corresponds to the distance between the skin surface and pleurae. A combination of lung sliding and A lines is characteristic of normal lungs.
- B lines: Hyperechoic lines occurring perpendicular to the pleurae. These move with lung sliding. These most commonly represent interstitial fluid, though it may be seen in health in the first 48 h after birth.

Consolidated lung tissue is dense and appears like solid tissue. For this reason, it is termed 'hepatisation'. It may be possible to see small, branching, hyperechoic 'air bronchograms' within the consolidated tissue, which will vary in appearance with the respiratory cycle. Atelectasis, in contrast, will show static air bronchograms, and a 'lung pulse' will be present, where lung tissue moves in synchrony with the cardiac cycle. A pleural effusion will show separation of the visceral and parietal pleurae, with anechoic (black) fluid in between. The presence of anterior B lines with preserved lung sliding has been shown to be diagnostic of cardiogenic pulmonary oedema. A diagnostic algorithm has been developed—the bedside LUS in emergency (BLUE) protocol—which can reliably identify the aetiology of respiratory failure in less than 5 min [24].

Weaknesses of LUS include its inability to visualise the entire thorax, particularly with increasing age of the child. Inter-operator reproducibility of findings can be poor, and training requirements are substantial. When evaluating PMVed children, diagnostics may be less of a focus as the underlying aetiology of the child's condition is likely to be well understood. Nevertheless, ventilator-acquired pneumonias and atelectasis are not uncommon complications of PMV, and indeed other complications such as pulmonary oedema may well be encountered, meaning that LUS may offer an option for the assessment of pulmonary function in both inpatient and outpatient settings.

3.15 Ultrasound Imaging of Diaphragm Function

Activity of the diaphragm may also be investigated using ultrasound imaging, and this is again an area that has received research attention in recent years. As discussed above in the section on respiratory muscle testing, diaphragm dysfunction is not uncommon in paediatric critical care and PMVed children. In the absence of, or alongside, pressure-based measurements of respiratory muscle strength, diaphragm imaging using ultrasound may be of benefit. Fluoroscopy has been used in the past, but this carries risk associated with radiation exposure as well as transport to a radiology department; hence, ultrasound is preferred.

A linear transducer is used, placed perpendicular to the chest wall between the eighth and tenth intercostal spaces between the anterior and midaxillary lines, in order to image the zone of apposition. It is also possible to view both hemidiaphragms simultaneously using a curved array probe placed below the xiphoid process, though the image quality will suffer due to increased distance between probe and muscle. A curved transducer may also be placed over the anterior chest wall subcostally, between the midclavicular and anterior axillary lines (right) or anterior and midaxillary lines (left), and directed cranially, allowing visualisation of the dome of the hemidiaphragm. With unilateral imaging, the right hemidiaphragm tends to be easier to visualise than the left, due to the spleen narrowing the acoustic window and the possible presence of gas in the bowel.

Imaging the zone of apposition allows measurement of thickness of the diaphragm, both at end-expiration and end-inspiration. Expiratory diaphragm thickness alone can provide an indication of diaphragm atrophy. By measuring thickness at both points, the thickening fraction of the diaphragm may also be calculated (defined as the percentage change in thickness from expiration to inspiration). Careful attention must be paid to consistency with the use of measurement landmarks: there is currently no consensus in published literature as to whether the visceral pleura and the peritoneum should be included or excluded in the measurement, or whether their midpoints should be used as anchors. Clinicians undertaking diaphragm ultrasound must be consistent in their approach, and careful documentation of choices is advised.

Diaphragm excursion can be quantified by imaging the domes of the hemidiaphragms and measuring the degree to which they descend during inspiration. The excursion of the two sides can be compared if there is suspicion of unilateral dysfunction. It must be noted that positive-pressure ventilation can provide a misleading impression of active diaphragm movement, so for the most reliable results, measurements should be undertaken without inspiratory support from a ventilator (though this may or may not be possible, depending on the child's clinical status). Paradoxical diaphragm motion (i.e. cranial displacement during inspiration) suggests diaphragm paralysis. Absent motion may indicate partial or complete paralysis, though it may also be seen in cases of severe hyperinflation or very reduced abdominal compliance with preserved force-generating capacity of the diaphragm.

Reference data for diaphragm thickness, excursion and thickening fraction are available, covering over 500 individuals from preterm infants up to 16 years of age [1, 11, 29, 30]. Such data facilitate single-occasion and longitudinal assessment of diaphragm in the PMVed child, which can again be performed in both inpatient and outpatient environments.

3.16 Respiratory Muscle Energy Expenditure

Quantification of energy expenditure via measurements of oxygen consumption ($V'O_2$) and carbon dioxide production ($V'CO_2$) can be used in a number of ways within the paediatric critical care setting. Such measurements clearly have benefit in titrating nutritional provision, but may also be of use in decisions relating to ventilator support. $V'O_2$ and $V'CO_2$ may be measured using stand-alone monitors or devices integrated into the ventilator. Regardless of the device used, accurate flow and gas concentration data must be obtained, meaning that cuffed airways must be used. The device must also be able to accommodate the higher fraction of inspired oxygen encountered in many PMVed children; hence, a standard system designed for the evaluation of exercise performance in healthy (or at least self-ventilating) subjects is unlikely to be suitable.

Reference data are difficult to apply to the PMVed population: energy expenditure would be expected to be very different due to the vastly altered physiology, so comparison with healthy children may be of little value. More useful perhaps is the assessment of $V'O_2$ and $V'CO_2$ in response to changes in ventilator support. Although no significant changes were observed in $V'O_2$ between supported ventilation and a spontaneous breathing trial in 20 children deemed ready for extubation [26], individual patients may demonstrate changes that could indicate tolerance or otherwise of changes in ventilatory support. Data from the author's own laboratory [18] indicate that $V'O_2$ increases significantly when mechanically ventilated adults are exposed to even low levels of inspiratory muscle training, lending support to the idea that $V'O_2$ measurements are sensitive to change in respiratory load. If sequential measurements are to be used in an individual child, it must be noted that $V'O_2$ and $V'CO_2$, even when normalised to body weight, are inversely and non-linearly related to child height and age [32].

4 Summary

Modern critical care and respiratory physiology offer a large and diverse range of options for assessing pulmonary function in the PMVed child. Many of these techniques are visually and scientifically appealing, but their ability to directly influence clinical outcomes is uncertain. Absence of evidence is not, of course, evidence of absence; it is rarely disadvantageous to have more detailed information on a patient's physiology and response to adjustments in therapy, and it is likely that at least some of the techniques described above will in time show clinical benefit as the evidence base evolves. Many of the techniques described above will also provide a more complete understanding of the patient's underlying pathophysiology, which can help the clinician make reasoned judgements about treatment choices. The question that should be in the forefront of a clinician's mind when choosing which measures may be useful in their own clinical practice is 'how will I use the information provided by this test?' If no definitive answer can be provided to this question, then it will be difficult to justify the expenditure of a new piece of apparatus, not to mention the time and inconvenience for staff and patient in performing the measurements. While new equipment may be very appealing, there is a wealth of information contained within the routine data captured in the modern critical care setting; such data should always be the starting point for a thorough evaluation of the PMVed child.

References

1. Alonso-Ojembarrena A, Ruiz-González E, Estepa-Pedregosa L, Armenteros-López AI, Segado-Arenas A, Lubián-López SP. Reproducibility and reference values of diaphragmatic shortening fraction for term and premature infants. Pediatr Pulmonol. 2020;55(8):1963–8. https://doi.org/10.1002/ppul.24866.
2. Al-Rawas N, Banner MJ, Euliano NR, Tams CG, Brown J, Martin AD, Gabrielli A. Expiratory time constant for determinations of plateau pressure, respiratory system compliance, and total resistance. Crit Care. 2013;17(1):R23. https://doi.org/10.1186/cc12500.
3. American Thoracic Society/European Respiratory Society. ATS/ERS statement on respiratory muscle testing. Am J Respir Crit Care Med. 2002;166(4):518–624. https://doi.org/10.1164/rccm.166.4.518.
4. Bellani G, Patroniti N, Pesenti A. Measurement of functional residual capacity during mechanical ventilation. In: Vincent JL, editor. Yearbook of intensive care and emergency medicine 2010. Springer; 2010. https://doi.org/10.1007/978-3-642-10286-8_14.
5. Bellemare F, Grassino A. Effect of pressure and timing of contraction on human diaphragm fatigue. J Appl Physiol Respir Environ Exerc Physiol. 1982;53(5):1190–5. https://doi.org/10.1152/jappl.1982.53.5.1190.
6. Bhalla D, Naranje P, Jana M, Bhalla AS. Pediatric lung ultrasonography: current perspectives. Pediatr Radiol. 2022;52:2038–50. https://link.springer.com/article/10.1007/s00247-022-05412-9
7. Blokpoel RGT, Burgerhof JGM, Markhorst DG, Kneyber MCJ. Patient-ventilator asynchrony during assisted ventilation in children. Pediatr Crit Care Med. 2016;17(5):204. https://doi.org/10.1097/PCC.0000000000000669.
8. Dimitriou G, Greenoug A, Dyke H, Rafferty GF. Maximal airway pressures during crying in healthy preterm and term neonates. Early Hum Dev. 2000;57(2):149–56. https://doi.org/10.1016/s0378-3782(99)00075-4.
9. Duan J, Zhang X, Song J. Predictive power of extubation failure diagnosed by cough strength: a systematic review and meta-analysis. Crit Care. 2021;25:357. https://ccforum.biomedcentral.com/articles/10.1186/s13054-021-03781-5#citeas.
10. Edberg KE, Sandberg K, Silberberg A, Sjoqvist BA, Ekstrom-Jodal B, Hjalmarson O. A plethysmographic method for assessment of lung function in mechanically ventilated very low birth weight infants. Pediatr Res. 1991;30(5):501–4.
11. El-Halaby H, Abdel-Hady H, Alsawah G, Abdelrahman A, El-Tahan H. Sonographic evaluation of diaphragmatic excursion and thickness in healthy infants and children. J Ultrasound Med. 2016;35(1):167–75. https://doi.org/10.7863/ultra.15.01082.
12. Emrath E. The basics of ventilator waveforms. Curr Pediatr Rep. 2021;9(1):11–9. https://doi.org/10.1007/s40124-020-00235-4.
13. Gaultier C, Perret L, Boule M, Buvry A, Girard F. Occlusion pressure and breathing pattern in healthy children. Respir Physiol. 1981;46(1):71–80. https://doi.org/10.1016/0034-5687(81)90069-4.
14. Giffin F, Greenough A, Naik S. The Hering-Breuer reflex in ventilated children. Respir Med. 1996;90(8):463–6. https://doi.org/10.1016/s0954-6111(96)90172-9.
15. Hammer J, Newth CJ. Influence of endotracheal tube diameter on forced deflation flow-volume curves in rhesus monkeys. Eur Respir J. 1997;10:1870–3. https://erj.ersjournals.com/content/10/8/1870.
16. Hess D. Respiratory mechanics in mechanically ventilated patients. Respir Care. 2014;59(11):1773–94. https://rc.rcjournal.com/content/59/11/1773.
17. Hubble CL, Gentile MA, Tripp DS, Craig DM, Meliones JN, Cheifetz IM. Deadspace to tidal volume ratio predicts successful extubation in infants and children. Crit Care Med. 2000;28(6):2034–40. https://doi.org/10.1097/00003246-200006000-00059.

18. Jenkins TO, MacBean V, Poulsen MK, Karbing DS, Rees SE, Patel BV, Polkey MI. The metabolic cost of inspiratory muscle training in mechanically ventilated patients in critical care. Intensive Care Med Exp. 2023;11(1):41. https://doi.org/10.1186/s40635-023-00522-6. PMID: 37415048; PMCID: PMC10326210.
19. King GG, Bates J, Berger KI, Calverley P, De Melo PL, Dellacà RL, Farré R, Hall GL, Ioan I, Irvin CG, Kaczka DW, Kaminsky DA, Kurosawa H, Lombardi E, Maksym GN, Marchal F, Oppenheimer BW, Simpson SJ, Thamrin C, et al. Technical standards for respiratory oscillometry. Eur Respir J. 2020;55(2):1900753. https://doi.org/10.1183/13993003.00753-2019.
20. Kneyber MCJ, de Luca D, Calderini E, Jarreau P, Javouhey E, Lopez-Herce J, Hammer J, Macrae D, Markhorst DG, Medina A, Pons-Odena M, Racca F, Wolf G, Biban P, Brierley J, Rimensberger PC. Recommendations for mechanical ventilation of critically ill children from the Paediatric Mechanical Ventilation Consensus Conference (PEMVECC). Intensive Care Med. 2017;43(12):1764–80. https://doi.org/10.1007/s00134-017-4920-z.
21. Kulnik ST, MacBean V, Birring SS, Moxham J, Rafferty GF, Kalra L. Accuracy of portable devices in measuring peak cough flow. Physiol Meas. 2015;36(2):243–57. https://doi.org/10.1088/0967-3334/36/2/243.
22. Lauhkonen E, Cooper BG, Iles R. Mini review shows that structured light plethysmography provides a non-contact method for evaluating breathing patterns in children. Acta Paediatr. 2019;108(8):1398–405. https://onlinelibrary.wiley.com/doi/10.1111/apa.14769.
23. Laveneziana P, Albuquerque A, Aliverti A, Babb T, Barreiro E, Dres M, Dubé B, Fauroux B, Gea J, Guenette JA, Hudson AL, Kabitz H, Laghi F, Langer D, Luo Y, Neder JA, O'Donnell D, Polkey MI, et al. ERS statement on respiratory muscle testing at rest and during exercise. Eur Respir J. 2019;53(6):1801214. https://doi.org/10.1183/13993003.01214-2018.
24. Lichtenstein DA, Mauriat P. Lung ultrasound in the critically ill neonate. Curr Pediatr Rev. 2012;8(3):217–23. https://doi.org/10.2174/157339612802139389.
25. MacBean V, Jolley CJ, Sutton TG, Deep A, Greenough A, Moxham J, Rafferty GF. Parasternal intercostal electromyography: a novel tool to assess respiratory load in children. Pediatr Res. 2016;80(3):407–14. https://doi.org/10.1038/pr.2016.89.
26. Mortamet G, Nardi N, Groleau V, Essouri S, Fauroux B, Jouvet P, Emeriaud G. Impact of spontaneous breathing trial on work of breathing indices derived from esophageal pressure, electrical activity of the diaphragm, and oxygen consumption in children. Respir Care. 2019;64(5):509–18. https://rc.rcjournal.com/content/64/5/509.full.
27. Mortamet G, Larouche A, Ducharme-Crevier L, Fléchelles O, Constantin G, Essouri S, Pellerin Leblanc A, Beck J, Sinderby C, Jouvet P, Emeriaud G. Patient-ventilator asynchrony during conventional mechanical ventilation in children. Ann Intensive Care. 2017;7(1):122. https://doi.org/10.1186/s13613-017-0344-8.
28. National Cancer Institute. Radiation Risks and Pediatric Computed Tomography (CT): A Guide for Health Care Providers; 2018. Retrieved 15th July 2022, from https://www.cancer.gov/about-cancer/causes-prevention/risk/radiation/pediatric-ct-scans.
29. Rehan VK, McCool FD. Diaphragm dimensions of the healthy term infant. Acta Paediatrica (Oslo, Norway: 1992). 2003;92(9):1062–7.
30. Rehan VK, Laiprasert J, Wallach M, Rubin LP, McCool FD. Diaphragm dimensions of the healthy preterm infant. Pediatrics. 2001;108(5):e91. https://doi.org/10.1542/peds.108.5.e91.
31. Shardonofsky FR, Perez-Chada D, Milic-Emili J. Airway pressures during crying: an index of respiratory muscle strength in infants with neuromuscular disease. Pediatr Pulmonol. 1991;10(3):172–7. https://doi.org/10.1002/ppul.1950100307.
32. Smallwood CD, Walsh BK, Bechard LJ, Mehta NM. Carbon dioxide elimination and oxygen consumption in mechanically ventilated children. Respir Care. 2015;60(5):718–23. https://rc.rcjournal.com/content/60/5/718.
33. Telias I, Damiani F, Brochard L. The airway occlusion pressure (P0.1) to monitor respiratory drive during mechanical ventilation: increasing awareness of a not-so-new problem. Intensive Care Med. 2018;44:1532–5.

34. Verma R, Chiang J, Qian H, Amin R. Maximal static respiratory and sniff pressures in healthy children. A systematic review and meta-analysis. Ann Am Thorac Soc. 2019;16(4):478–87. https://doi.org/10.1513/AnnalsATS.201808-506OC.
35. Verscheure S, Massion PB, Verschuren F, Damas P, Magder S. Volumetric capnography: lessons from the past and current clinical applications. Crit Care. 2016;20(1):184. https://doi.org/10.1186/s13054-016-1377-3.
36. Ward R, Carroll WD, Cunningham P, Ho S, Jones M, Lenney W, Thompson D, Gilchrist FJ. Radiation dose from common radiological investigations and cumulative exposure in children with cystic fibrosis: an observational study from a single UK centre. BMJ Open. 2017;7:e017548.

Management and Strategy of Tracheostomy

Karen Watters

1 Pediatric Tracheostomy

"Tracheostomy" is the physical opening between the skin and the trachea. The first successful pediatric tracheostomy was performed in the sixteenth century on a child who had tracheal compression secondary to swallowed coins impacted in the esophagus [1]. Nowadays, tracheostomy placement is a common procedure in adult intensive care units (ICUs) after a period of prolonged ventilation [2]. In comparison, tracheostomy is much less commonly performed in pediatric patients in the ICU setting. Despite this, the incidence of pediatric tracheostomy has been increasing over the last two decades associated with the improved survival of extremely premature infants and children with complex medical conditions. The majority of pediatric tracheostomies are placed in the first year of life, with approximately 50% of them being placed in infants under 6 months of age [3]. In a multi-site NICU study of almost half a million infants of birth weight < 1.5 kg (VLBW), less than 1% received a tracheostomy [4]. However, the infants who received tracheostomy had twice the risk of mortality and nearly four times the initial length of stay of those without tracheostomy. Chronic lung disease and congenital anomalies were the strongest predictors of tracheostomy placement and mortality [4]. Such data can help guide discussions with caregivers on the decision-making process for tracheostomy placement.

The decision to place a tracheostomy in a child requires multidisciplinary team input. The medical complexity of the child, future prognosis, long-term care needs, and caregiver supports are important factors to consider in the decision-making process. Approximately 50% of infants/children who undergo tracheostomy placement

K. Watters (✉)
Department of Otolarynology and Communication Enhancement, Boston Children's Hospital, Boston, MA, USA
e-mail: karen.watters@childrens.harvard.edu

A. Kawaguchi et al. (eds.), *Prolonged and Long-Term Mechanical Ventilation in Children*, https://doi.org/10.1007/978-981-97-8903-0_16

will be decannulated within 2 years, with a significant number of children requiring the tracheostomy for years and often a lifetime [5–7]. Children with complex medical conditions who undergo tracheostomy placement for chronic ventilatory support may require long-term hospital care or intensive homecare after discharge. The demands of caring for a child with a tracheostomy should be outlined to caregivers preoperatively. All caregivers will require appropriate training to care for their child with tracheostomy. Often, meeting a family who has a child with a long-term tracheostomy can help provide families with a better understanding of the care involved. In children with shortened life expectancies, ethical team input may be necessary to help guide the decision-making process.

2 Indications for Tracheostomy

In the past, tracheostomy was an emergency procedure to relieve upper airway obstruction primarily in children with infectious processes such as diphtheria and epiglottitis, with the expectation that the tube would be removed once the infection had been treated. Nowadays, the indications for tracheostomy in children have changed significantly, with the procedure being primarily performed in children with complex medical conditions including those with chromosomal abnormalities and neurological impairment [7].

The three primary indications for tracheostomy in children include upper airway obstruction (40%), prolonged ventilatory support (60%), and pulmonary toilet or a combination of these [3].

1. **Airway obstruction**: This can be congenital or acquired. Congenital lesions include structural laryngotracheal anomalies such as laryngeal atresia, glottic webs, subglottic stenosis, vocal cord immobility, tracheobronchomalacia, or congenital neoplasms (vascular anomalies, teratomas, neurofibromas) (Fig. 1). The most common acquired upper airway lesion is subglottic stenosis primarily from prolonged intubation in preterm infants. It is important that the child's airway has been completely evaluated for any treatable structural causes of airway obstruction prior to tracheostomy placement. A complete evaluation in the form of a direct laryngobronchoscopy should be performed under general anesthesia.
2. **Failure to Extubate/Ventilator Dependence**: The increased survival of premature infants has led to a small group of infants necessitating tracheostomy for long-term ventilator support for chronic respiratory failure. Approximately 39% of infants born less than 28 weeks gestation develop some degree of bronchopulmonary dysplasia or chronic lung disease of prematurity [8]. Duration of endotracheal intubation prior to tracheostomy in infants is not clearly defined with no consensus regarding the timing of tracheostomy placement in an infant. Premature infants are often intubated for up to 3 months or longer before a tracheostomy is considered [9].

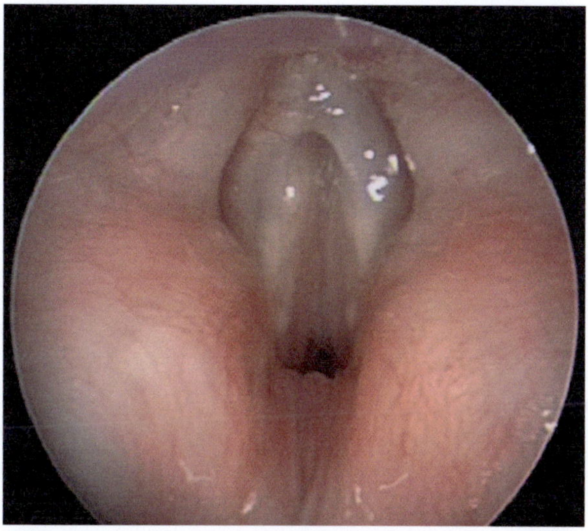

Fig. 1 Congenital grade 3 subglottic stenosis in a newborn requiring emergency tracheostomy following birth

3. **Pulmonary Toilet**: Children with chronic neurological impairment and chronic lung disease may require tracheostomy to facilitate airway clearance and pulmonary hygiene [3].

3 Preoperative Assessment

Pediatric tracheostomy should be performed by an experienced team in pediatric airway management in an institution with pediatric critical care. Preoperative assessment should be performed by the anesthesia team. Comorbid conditions including congenital heart disease, congenital anomalies of the upper airway craniofacial syndromes, and genetic disorders may significantly increase the complexity and risks of the procedure. If the tracheostomy is being placed for upper airway obstruction in the setting of a laryngeal or tracheal anomaly, the surgeon should be aware of the child's airway anatomy to prevent inadvertent airway injury.

4 Anatomy

The pediatric larynx has a number of anatomical differences to that of the adult which the surgical team needs to consider prior to tracheostomy placement [10, 11]. The infant larynx is one-third the size of the adult larynx and sits higher and more anterior in the neck. The neck is shorter, and the airway cartilage is more pliable and softer making anatomical landmarks difficult to identify. In addition, the hyoid bone overlies the thyroid cartilage. It is important to ensure that the cricoid and tracheal rings are clearly identified prior to entry in the airway. If the airway is entered too high at the level of the cricoid, the vocal cords may be damaged. An emergency airway through the cricothyroid membrane, which is very short in an infant, is not recommended in an infant for the same reason. It is important to be aware of the presence of a high-riding innominate artery in an infant which may sit over the upper trachea. The lung apices may also extend into the cervical paratracheal space increasing the risk of pneumomediastinum. Cervical extension of the thymus gland may also impede access to the trachea.

5 Surgical Technique

Pediatric tracheostomies are typically performed by open surgical technique. Percutaneous tracheostomy is not recommended in infants and is infrequently performed in children. There are reports in older children and adolescents [12, 13].

The pertinent anatomical landmarks are first marked on the child's neck. A horizontal midline skin incision is made between the sternal notch and cricoid cartilage. This is followed by dissection through the subcutaneous fat and strap muscles. The thyroid gland may need to be divided or pushed superiorly. Care is taken to stay midline on the trachea to prevent inadvertent injury to the great vessels and nerves. In preparation for a vertical incision in the trachea, lateral stay sutures are placed vertically on either side of the intended incision. These stay sutures are important to assist with replacement of the tracheostomy in the event

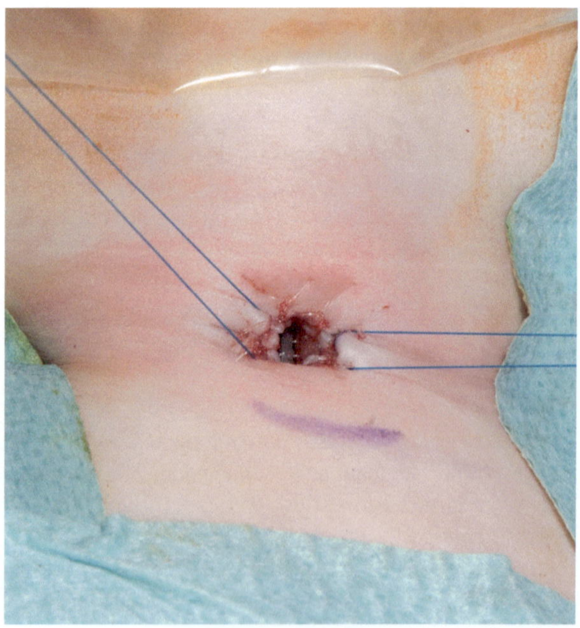

Fig. 2 Intraoperative image of tracheal stay sutures placed at the time of tracheostomy in an infant

of accidental decannulation and are kept in place until after the first tracheostomy tube change [14] (Fig. 2). Direct communication with the anesthesia team is paramount at this time. A midline vertical incision is then made in the trachea between tracheal rings two and four. The endotracheal tube is visualized in the airway. The surgeon then instructs the anesthesiologist to slowly withdraw the endotracheal tube to just below the vocal cords as the surgeon directly visualizes the tube being withdrawn. An appropriately sized tracheostomy tube is then inserted into the trachea and connected to the ventilator tubing. Correct tube position is confirmed with the anesthesia team. Once the patient is adequately ventilated, the endotracheal tube is completely withdrawn though the oral cavity. A flexible scope is passed through the tracheostomy tube to ensure that the length of the tube is correct and it is sitting appropriately above the carina. The tube is then secured with Velcro ties around the neck. The stay sutures are marked "left" and "right" and taped down on the child's chest for easy access.

6 Tracheostomy Tube Types

Tracheostomy tube type and size need to be selected prior to the procedure. Pediatric tracheostomy tubes are made of polyvinylchloride or silicone. Bivona ™ tubes are silicone and have a softer shaft and flange. Shiley ™ tubes are made of polyvinyl chloride and are more rigid. Pediatric tracheostomy tubes do not have an inner cannula.

Tube size is selected according to the age and weight of the child, but importantly, the indication for tracheostomy and the medical condition of the child also need to be taken into consideration when selecting the tube. Tube size is based on the expected endotracheal tube size for the patient's age or the size of the endotracheal tube if the patient is intubated. Pediatric tracheostomy tubes range in size from 2.5 to 5.5. There are two lengths—neonatal and pediatric. Neonatal tubes (30–36 mm) are shorter and are primarily used in infants <4 kg. Pediatric length tubes are longer with lengths starting at 38 mm. Longer length tubes "Pedi Plus" (Bivona ™)) are also made by some manufacturers in tube sizes of 4.0–5.5.

Adjustable length tracheostomy tubes are available in pediatric sizes but are not desired, due to the concern for patient movement causing an inadvertent change in the length of the tube. Custom tubes can be ordered specific to the patient's airway anatomy. Customizations include tube length, cuff type and position, shaft angle, and flange angle and shape. Custom length tubes are frequently used in infants with severe tracheomalacia to assist in stenting the distal airway. Bivona "Flex-tend" ™ tubes have a longer external connector to the flange and are frequently used in infants who have short necks [15].

Cuffed and uncuffed pediatric tracheostomy tubes are available. Cuffed tubes are typically only indicated in children who require mechanical ventilation [15]. Bivona tubes have a tight to shaft (TTS) cuff and are inflated with sterile water. Shiley tubes, with a high-volume low-pressure cuff, are inflated with air. Cuff pressures need to be closely monitored to avoid overinflation, with subsequent formation of granulation tissue, ulceration, or tracheal stenosis. Prolonged overinflation of a cuff can lead to tracheal dilatation and result in difficulties with ventilation [16]. Minimal leak technique is recommended to minimize cuff pressures.

7 Postoperative Management

Following tracheostomy placement, children should be managed in an ICU setting. A chest radiograph should be performed if there is any concern for respiratory distress to rule out pneumothorax or pneumomediastinum. Bloody tracheal secretions may be increased in the immediate postoperative period. Regular suctioning of the tracheostomy tube should be performed as needed. Humidification is essential to prevent dryness and crusting of secretions and blood, which could result in plugging of the tube.

The first tracheostomy tube changed is typically performed on postoperative day 5 by the surgical team [15]. Prior to this change, the child's airway should be considered a "critical airway." Should accidental decannulation occur, there may be difficulty replacing the tube when the stoma is not yet fully formed, resulting in the formation of a false tract with subsequent loss of airway and acute respiratory decompensation. The child is thus kept adequately sedated prior to the first tube change to ensure that decannulation does not occur. An airway plan in the event of accidental decannulation should be discussed with the ICU team and documented at the bedside. It is important to document if the tracheostomy is the child's only airway or if the child can be mask ventilated and intubated by standard methods or if special equipment is required.

8 Tracheostomy Complications

Children with tracheostomy are medically complex and at high risk for complications and adverse events, related to the presence of the tracheostomy tube but also related to their underlying medical conditions. Approximately 39% of children experience an in-hospital tracheostomy-related complication in the first 2 years after tracheostomy placement [17]. The in-hospital mortality rate of children in the first 2 years after tracheostomy placement is 9%, with the majority of these deaths being secondary to underlying medical conditions [3]. The mortality rate is higher (2.2–59%) in children with tracheostomy under 1 year of age and in children who require long-term ventilation [18]. It is important to address these risks with caregivers prior to tracheostomy tube placement.

Tracheostomy-related adverse events range from minor to devastating. Early complications include tube obstruction, accidental decannulation, or bleeding. Later complications are typically related to the pressure or irritation the tube can

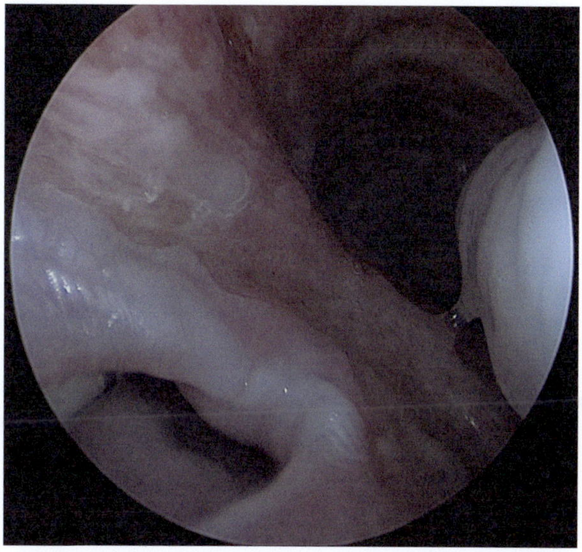

Fig. 3 Endoscopic image of a large tracheoesophageal fistula in a 2-year-old child with tracheotomy dependence secondary to the need for mechanical ventilation. The fistula was caused by excessive tracheostomy tube cuff pressure with resultant erosion of the posterior tracheal wall into the esophagus

cause in the infant's airway and may include tracheostomy-related hemorrhage, stomal issues, suprastomal collapse and granulation, tracheoesophageal fistula, and persistent tracheocutaneous fistula. Ttracheosophageal fistulae can also be caused by over-inflation of the tracheostomy cuff in those children who are ventilator dependent (Fig. 3). The incidence of tracheostomy-related adverse events can be prevented by instituting a comprehensive tracheostomy education program for all providers and caregivers caring for children with tracheostomy.

8.1 Tube Obstruction

Obstruction of a tracheostomy tube in a child is an emergency. It is one of the most common causes of death in a tracheostomy-dependent child. Thick secretions can easily plug the lumen of small neonatal and pediatric tubes and result in acute respiratory distress. Humidification, regular suctioning, and pulmonary hygiene are essential to prevent this occurring. In the event of an obstruction, suctioning and instillation of saline should first be performed. If the mucous plug is not removed with suctioning, the tracheostomy tube should be immediately changed. If the obstruction persists following tube change, bag ventilation through the tube should be performed. If the child continues to deteriorate, emergency services are mobilized and oral mask ventilation is started. Oral endotracheal intubation, if possible, may be necessary. A flexible scope, if available, can be passed through the tracheostomy tube lumen to evaluate tube position and patency. Measures to prevent tube obstruction include upsizing the tube as needed according to the child's growth and provision of humidification which can also be provided via an HME or "trach mist collar" after the child is weaned from the ventilator.

8.2 Accidental Decannulation

Accidental decannulation accounts for a large majority of tracheostomy-related deaths in children [19, 20]. In the immediate postoperative period, accidental decannulation is particularly dangerous as the tracheocutaneous tract is not yet mature and a false passage can easily be created during emergent tube reinsertion. Thus, children should be observed in the intensive care unit during the first tracheostomy tube change at approximately 5 days postoperatively. In the event of an accidental decannulation, the stay sutures should be pulled up to open the trachea and allow replacement of the tube. A spare tracheostomy tube of the same size and one a size smaller should remain at the bedside of every child with a tracheostomy. If the tube cannot be replaced, it is important to remember that the child may be able to be orally masked and intubated from above to secure the airway. Accidental decannulation can also occur in the home setting. Caregivers need to demonstrate competency at both emergency and routine tracheostomy tube care before the child can be discharged.

8.3 Bleeding

Bleeding from the tracheostomy tube can range from minor to life threatening. Self-limited bleeding may frequently occur secondary to suction trauma or tracheal inflammation. Caregivers are educated to avoid suctioning beyond the end of the tracheostomy tube to prevent tracheal trauma. Adequate humidification is essential. Antibiotics may be required if tracheitis is present. An ill-fitting tracheostomy tube may cause tracheal granulation and ulceration, which can lead to erosion of the tube into the esophagus and more persistent bleeding.

Sudden massive hemorrhage from the tracheostomy tube may be caused by a tracheoinnominate artery fistula. This is a result of the tracheostomy tube tip eroding through the anterior tracheal wall into the innominate artery creating a fistula. Although rare, children with tracheostomy experience twice the number of tracheo-innominate hemorrhage events, in comparison to adult patients [21]. Bleeding may be heralded by smaller sentinel bleeds in up to 30% of patients [22]. Innominate arterial bleeding is life-threatening. Digital pressure should be immediately applied through the stoma to tamponade the bleeding followed by placement of a cuffed endotracheal tube through the stoma, inflating the cuff to maximal and retracting it back to the level of the stoma. Tracheoinnominate artery fistula bleeding mortality rate approaches 100%. If the patient survives the bleeding, urgent repair by cardiothoracic team is necessary. Thus, any child with frequent tracheostomy bleeding from an unknown source should undergo full airway endoscopic assessment (direct laryngobronchoscopy) under general anesthesia. Pulsations with mucosal disruption seen on the anterior tracheal in the region of the innominate artery are concerning signs for fistula formation. A computed tomography arteriogram may also be helpful in assessing the position of the innominate artery in relation to the tracheostomy tube.

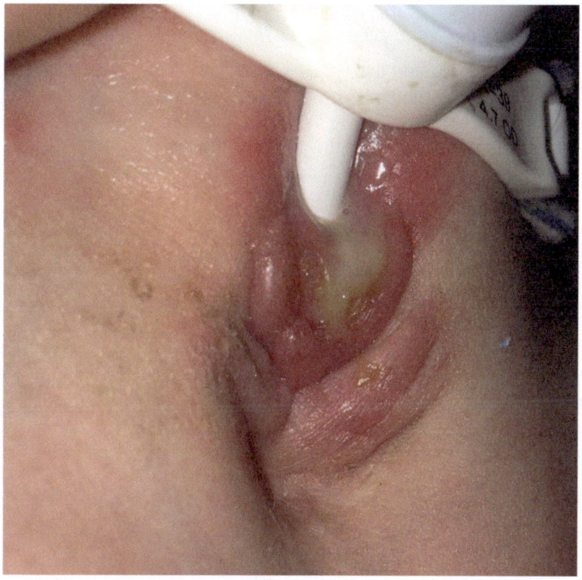

Fig. 4 Peristomal inflammation and granulation tissue in a young child with tracheostomy

8.4 Stomal Problems

Tracheostomal irritation and granulation can occur from tube pressure and wound breakdown from excessive secretions and infection (Fig. 4). Irritation can be managed with daily stomal care, topical antibiotic ointment, and stomal dressings. Granulations can be managed with silver dressings (e.g., Mepilex AG ™), topical steroid ointment, and chemical or surgical cauterization. If granulation interferes with tracheostomy tube changes, surgical stoma revision may be necessary.

8.5 Suprastomal Granulomas and Collapse

Suprastomal granulomas and suprastomal collapse are a common finding in young children with tracheostomy, occurring in up to 30–40% [23]. They usually occur at the intratracheal superior stomal margin where the tube presses against the tracheal cartilage and are more common in children who are ventilator dependent perhaps from the torque of the tubing and movement of the ventilator (Fig. 5). Suprastomal granulomas need to be removed if obstructing the airway, causing bleeding or to assist with decannulation [24] (Fig. 6). Repeated excision of suprastomal granulomas can weaken the suprastomal cartilage and lead to further suprastomal collapse. Depending on the severity of the suprastomal collapse, airway reconstruction may be necessary to enable decannulation.

Granulation tissue may also form within the trachea at the distal tip of the tracheostomy tube. It is often caused by excessive suctioning and bleeds on contact with

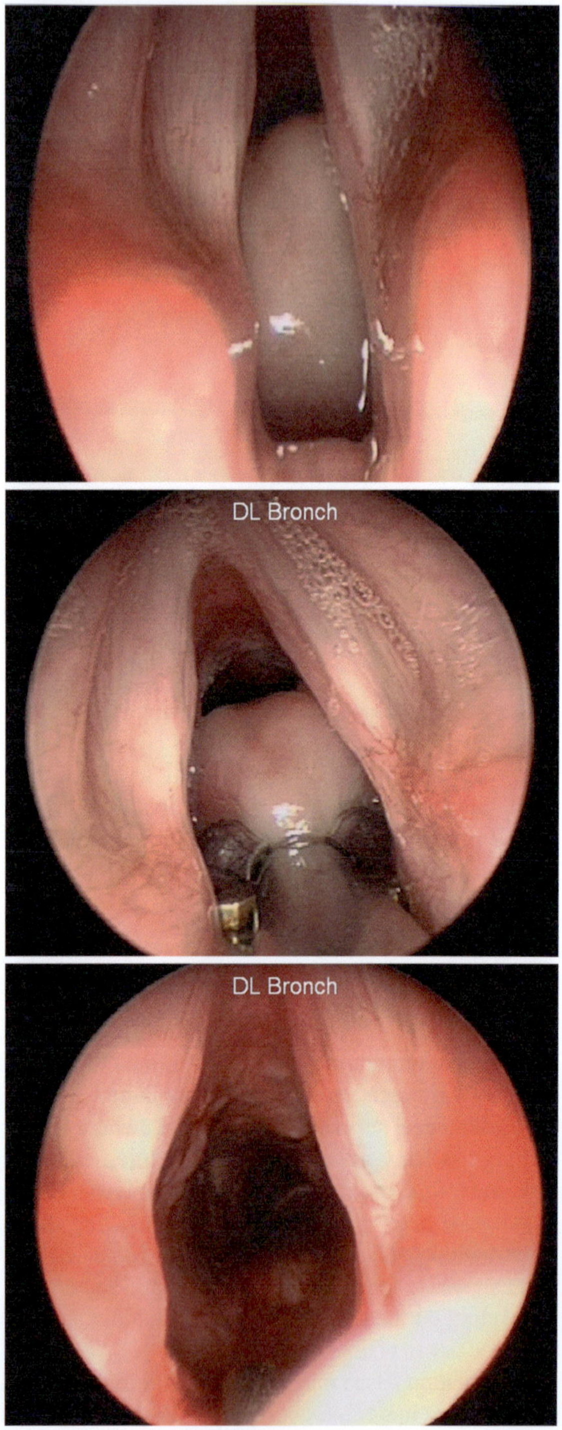

Fig. 5 Endoscopic image of a large suprastomal granuloma occluding the airway. The granuloma is removed with a microlaryngeal forceps under endoscopic guidance. The airway is widely patent following removal

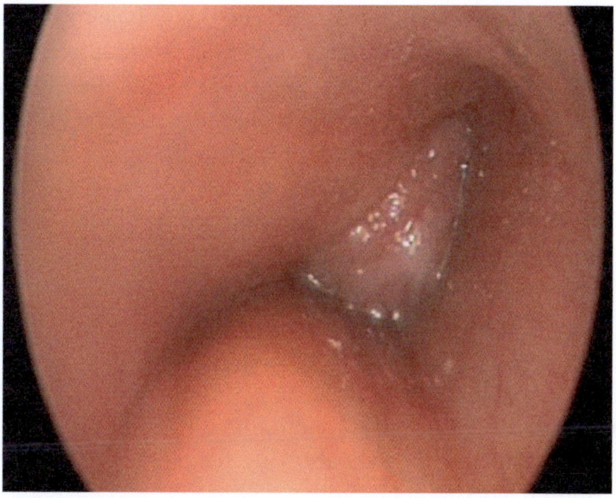

Fig. 6 Endoscopic image of suprastomal granuloma and suprastomal collapse in an infant

the suction catheter. If nonobstructive, topical steroid drops can be applied down the tube. If the tissue is occluding the tube, it can be removed surgically with the use of a microdebrider or microlaryngeal instruments. Modifying the length of the tube may also help to prevent it from reoccurring.

8.6 Tracheocutaneous Fistula

This incidence of persistent tracheocutaneous fistula after decannulation occurs in more than 40% of children [25]. The younger the age at tube placement, the longer the duration of the tube, and the use of stomal maturation techniques is a factor contributing to persistence of the fistula [26]. Management includes excision of the tracheocutaneous tract with primary closure of the trachea and overlying tissue or de-epithelialization of the tract and secondary healing.

9 Swallowing and Speech and Language Development

It is essential to involve the speech-language pathology team early for assessment and intervention related to swallowing and communication in children with tracheostomy.

The presence of a tracheostomy alone is not a contraindication to oral feeding. However, the tracheostomy may produce swallowing and feeding difficulties by inhibition of laryngeal reflexes, laryngeal elevation reduction, strap muscle interruption, and increased hypopharyngeal pressure from an inflated cuff. Tracheostomy may also prevent the generation of adequate subglottic pressure to allow for clearance of secretions through coughing. In addition, underlying medical and neurological comorbidities necessitating the tracheostomy may also lead to motor weakness, reduced reflexes, and oral aversion contributing to oropharyngeal dysphagia. Feeding therapy is very important for children who have the capacity to feed orally [27].

Tracheostomy also affects speech and language development in both children who are neurodevelopmentally normal and in those neurological disorders. Young age at the time of the tracheostomy tube placement and the presence of the tube between the years of critical language development can predispose the child to delayed communication skills [27, 28]. Early speech and language therapy and communication enhancement is essential to allow the child to develop communication skills. A Passy-Muir valve is a one-way speaking valve that permits inspiration through the stoma but on expiration directs air up around the tracheostomy tube and through the vocal cords allowing for phonation. This can help promote speech in children who do not require a cuffed tube and have a patent upper airway.

10 Multidisciplinary Tracheostomy Care

Tracheostomy care is high risk with significant morbidity and mortality, especially in infants. Children with tracheostomy are often followed by multiple medical providers, and caregivers may experience extremely disorganized fragmented care both at home and in hospital settings. It has been demonstrated that care of a child with a tracheostomy can be dramatically improved, and tracheostomy-related adverse events can be radically reduced by implementing multidisciplinary tracheostomy care teams [29–32]. Multidisciplinary teams help to standardize protocols of care, improving consistency of patient care and in turn reducing tracheostomy-related adverse events. All caregivers and medical staff caring for tracheostomy-dependent children both in hospital and home settings should be required to undergo a standardized tracheostomy education program with "hands-on" training.

The keys to safe tracheostomy care include establishing multidisciplinary tracheostomy teams, standardization of care protocols, staff and caregiver education, family and patient involvement, and monitoring outcomes with pediatric tracheostomy quality metrics.

11 Tracheostomy Monitoring

Children with chronic tracheostomy should be evaluated at a multidisciplinary tracheostomy clinic at a minimum of every 6 months. Visits may be more frequent in younger children. At these visits, endoscopic evaluation of the airway can be performed via flexible tracheoscopy to ensure that the tube size is adequate and the distal airway is healthy. Caregiver's emergency supplies can be checked at these visits. Surveillance of the airway may help prevent tracheostomy complications; however, there is no consensus on the timing of routine airway evaluation under anesthesia [33]. Direct laryngobronchoscopy under general anesthesia should be performed if the child is having problems with the tracheostomy, is undergoing anesthesia for another reason, or is being worked up for decannulation. Tracheostomy bleeding or issue with tube changes or granulation tissue may require urgent endoscopy.

12 Conclusion

Children who require tracheostomy are medically complex patients. Factors that need to be considered prior to placement of a tracheostomy in a child include the indication, airway anatomy, associated comorbidities, neurodevelopmental issues including feeding and speech, and long-term needs for patients and caregivers. A multidisciplinary approach is very important in the care of children with tracheostomy. It can help to standardize tracheostomy care protocols, provide education to both staff and caregivers, reduce tracheostomy-related adverse events, and ultimately provide quality-driven care.

References

1. Frost EA. Tracing the tracheostomy. Ann Otol Rhinol Laryngol. 1976;85(5 Pt 1):618–24.
2. Veenith T, Ganeshamoorthy S, Standley T, et al. Intensive care unit tracheostomy: a snapshot of UK practice. Int Arch Med. 2008;1:21.
3. Berry JG, Graham DA, Graham RJ, Zhou J, Putney HL, O'Brien JE, Roberson DW, Goldman DA. Predictors of clinical outcomes and hospital resource use of children after tracheotomy. Pediatrics. 2009;124:563–72.
4. Han SM, Watters KF, Hong CR, Edwards EM, Knell J, Morrow KA, Soll RF, Jaksic T, Horbar JD, Modi BP. Tracheostomy in very low birth weight infants: a prospective multicenter study. Pediatrics. 2020;145(3):e20192371.
5. Mahadevan M, Barber C, Salkeld L, Douglas G, Mills N. Pediatric tracheotomy: 17 year review. Int J Pediatr Otorhinolaryngol. 2007;71:1829–35.
6. de Trey L, Niedermann E, Ghelfi D, Gerber A, Gysin C. Pediatric tracheotomy: a 30-year experience. J Pediatr Surg. 2013;48:1470–5.
7. Carron JD, Derkay CS, Strope GL, Nosonchuk JE, Darrow DH. Pediatric tracheotomies: changing indications and outcomes. Laryngoscope. 2000;110:1099–104.
8. Stoll BJ, et al. Neonatal outcomes of extremely preterm infants from NICHD Neonatal Research Network. Eunice Kennedy Shriver National Institute of Child Health and Human Development Neonatal Research Network. Pediatrics. 2010;126(3):443–56.
9. Lewis CW, Carron JD, Perkins JA, Sie KC, Feudtner C. Tracheotomy in pediatric patients: a national perspective. Arch Otolaryngol Head Neck Surg. 2003;129(5):523–9.
10. Monnier P. Applied surgical anatomy of the larynx and trachea springer. In: Monnier P, editor. Pediatric airway surgery: management of laryngotracheal stenosis in infants and children. Berlin Heidelberg: Springer-Verlag; 2011. p. 7–10.
11. Henick DH, Holinger LD. Laryngeal development. In: Holinger LD, Lusk RP, Green CG, editors. Pediatric laryngology and bronchoesophagoscopy. Philadelphia; New York: Lippincott-Raven; 1997. p. 1–17.
12. Raju A, Joseph DK, Diarra C, Ross SE. Percutaneous versus open tracheostomy in the pediatric trauma population. Am Surg. 2010;76(3):276–8.

13. Gollu G, Ates U, Can OS, Kendirli T, Yagmurlu A, Cakmak M, Aktug T, Dindar H, Bingol-Kologlu M. Percutaneous tracheostomy by Griggs technique under rigid bronchoscopic guidance is feasible in children. J Pediatr Surg. 2016;51(10):1635–9.
14. Ruggiero FP, Carr MM. Infant tracheotomy: results of a survey regarding technique. Arch Otolaryngol Head Neck Surg. 2008;134(3):263–7.
15. Mitchell RB, Hussey HM, Setzen G, et al. Clinical consensus statement: tracheostomy care. Otolaryngol Head Neck Surg. 2013;148(1):6–20.
16. Schroeder JW Jr, Schneider JS, Walner DL. The influence of peak airway pressure and oxygen requirement on infant tracheostomy. Int J Pediatr Otorhinolaryngol. 2012;76(6):869.
17. Watters K, O'Neill M, Zhu H, Graham RJ, Hall M, Berry J. Two-year mortality, complications, and healthcare use in children with medicaid following tracheostomy. Laryngoscope. 2016;126(11):2611–7.
18. Zhu H, Das P, Roberson DW, Jang J, Skinner ML, Paine M, Yuan J, Berry J. Hospitalizations in children with preexisting tracheostomy: a national perspective. Laryngoscope. 2015;125(2):462–8.
19. Tantinikorn W, Alper CM, Bluestone CD, Casselbrant ML. Outcome in pediatric tracheotomy. Am J Otolaryngol. 2003;24(3):131.
20. Wood D, McShane P, Davis P. Tracheostomy in children admitted to paediatric intensive care. Arch Dis Child. 2012;97(10):866–9.
21. Das P, Zhu H, Shah RK, Roberson DW, Berry J, Skinner ML. Tracheotomy-related catastrophic events: results of a national survey. Laryngoscope. 2012;2012(122):30–7.
22. Gelman JJ, Aro M, Weiss SM. Tracheo-innominate artery fistula. J Am Coll Surg. 1994;179(5):626–34.
23. Merritt RM, Bent JP, Smith RJ. Suprastomal granulation tissue and pediatric tracheotomy decannulation. Laryngoscope. 1997;107(7):868–71.
24. Chen C, Bent JP, Parikh SR. Powered debridement of suprastomal granulation tissue to facilitate pediatric tracheotomy decannulation. Int J Pediatr Otorhinolaryngol. 2011;75(12):1558.
25. Kremer B, Botos-Kremer AI, Eckel HE, Schlöndorff G. Indications, complications, and surgical techniques for pediatric tracheostomies – an update. J Pediatr Surg. 2002;37(11):1556–62.
26. Colman KL, Mandell DL, Simons JP. Impact of stoma maturation on pediatric tracheostomy-related complications. Arch Otolaryngol Head Neck Surg. 2010;136(5):471–4.
27. Baumgatener CA, Bewyer E, Bruner D. Management of communication and swallowing in intensive care: the role of the speech pathologist. AACN Adv Crit Care. 2008;19(4):433.
28. Gereau SA, Navarro GC, Cluteria B, et al. Selection of pediatric patients for use of the Passy-Muir valve for speech production. Int J Pediatric Otolaryngol. 1996;35:11–7.
29. Garrubba M, Turner T, Grieveson C. Multidisciplinary care for tracheostomy patients: a systematic review. Crit Care. 2009;13:177.
30. Cetto R, Arora A, Hettige R, et al. Improving tracheostomy care: a prospective study of the multidisciplinary approach. Clin Otolaryngol. 2011;36:482–8.
31. McKeon M, Kohn J, Munhall D, Wells S, Blanchette S, Santiago R, Graham R, Nuss R, Rahbar R, Volk M, Watters K. Association of a multidisciplinary care approach with the quality of care after pediatric tracheostomy. JAMA Otolaryngol Head Neck Surg. 2019;145(11):1035–42.
32. Hettige R, Arora A, Ifeacho S, Narula A. Improving tracheostomy management through design, implementation and prospective audit of a care bundle: how we do it. Clin Otolaryngol. 2008;33:488–91.
33. Kharasch VS, Dumas HM, Haley SM, et al. Bronchoscopy findings in children and young adults with tracheostomy due to congenital anomalies and neurological impairment. J Pediatr Rehabil Med. 2008;1(2):137.

Transfer from Hospital to Home Ventilation (Including NIV and MV): A Medical Point of View

Marti Pons Odena

The progressive improvement in neonatal and pediatric intensive care and the new surgical procedures for complex congenital malformations in the last two decades have increased the patient's survival.

However, some of these patients remain dependent on technology, especially those having chronic respiratory failure with ventilator dependency. According to the British guideline published in 1998 [1], definition of long-term ventilation is considered to be "any child who, when medically stable, continues to require a mechanical aid for breathing, after an acknowledged failure to wean, or a slow wean, three months after the institution of ventilation." The American guidelines published in 2016 stated that "the best place for the well-being of a technology-dependent child is with the family/caregivers in the community, and that all aspects of the medical care should be family-centered, coordinated, and integrated with community services" [2]. However, ventilator dependency is usually a massive limitation for early discharge in many countries, causing a lengthening of the hospital stays in critical care units.

The economic burden associated with the equipment needed for home ventilation is not only about the initial cost of the ventilator; the related equipment, maintenance, and replacement of malfunctioning equipment should also be considered. However, in those countries where the families may have healthcare staff support at home, the most considerable amount of the budget will be spent on this part. The Canadian clinical guidelines [3] strongly recommend a publicly funded system to facilitate patient family-centered care.

M. Pons Odena (✉)
University Hospital Sant Joan de Déu Barcelona, Esplugues de Llobregat, Spain

Home Mechanical Ventilation Program, Barcelona, Spain
e-mail: marti.pons@sjd.es

A. Kawaguchi et al. (eds.), *Prolonged and Long-Term Mechanical Ventilation in Children*, https://doi.org/10.1007/978-981-97-8903-0_17

So, ultimately, the discharging process will be totally different according to the national health resources available in each country to support those families with insufficient funding.

Children requiring home ventilation are typically chronically ill or have complex medical needs. When they are stable enough to leave the hospital, they are often supported by a multidisciplinary team of healthcare professionals who ensure a safe home-care transition. Chapter "Evaluation of the Child with Home Ventilation" (Graham) describes some general considerations for the transfer from hospital to home.

In this chapter, the main focus will be on medical issues and barriers related to mechanical ventilation. The aim is to help future home ventilation teams shorten their learning curve to get these patients safely discharged. The challenge of transferring ventilator-dependent children is entirely different from patients who are dependent on ventilation for life support like tracheostomized and invasively ventilated or patients with noninvasive support more than 16 hours a day compared to those who receive electively noninvasive support for health maintenance and illness prevention [4]. So Sect. 1 relates to children who are dependent on ventilation for life support, and Sect. 2, Part 2, discusses ventilatory support for children in whom CPAP and NIV are appropriate health strategies for health maintenance and illness prevention.

1 Transferring Patients Requiring Ventilatory Life Support to Home

1.1 Transferring Invasively Ventilated Patients

General considerations focused on mechanical ventilation:

The first step, without doubt, is to stabilize the patient adequately on his/her hospital ventilator. This is not a significant problem for the average pediatric patient. Moving to a home ventilator for infants with low weights, inferior to 6 kg, will imply a careful selection of the ventilator and the mode, and it will also require a fine-tuning of the settings. Unfortunately, only a few home devices can ventilate patients below five kilograms. Regarding neonates, before moving to a home ventilator, neonatal literature supports using invasive and noninvasive NAVA mode in preterms to reduce the time on the ventilator, extubation failure, and length of stay [5].

Furthermore, the previous steps before transfer to a home ventilator may be even more challenging, for example, in patients suffering from tracheobronchomalacia. Several options have been described to stabilize these patients, including surgical procedures like Aortopexy, airway stents, or individualized-designed cannula. Combining NAVA mode with PEEP maneuvers to reduce tracheal collapse has also been published [6].

There is no evidence about the best approach to switching children from a PICU ventilator to a home ventilator. According to Agarwal [7], the authors prefer to switch when the patient tolerates the new device altogether 24 hours a day. Alternatively, other authors advocate progressively gaining time on the home ventilator to avoid excessive fatigue.

Asynchrony is a common phenomenon in infants, with inspiratory asynchrony being the most frequent. Missing efforts are clinically relevant and usually will make it difficult to progress. Each ventilator shows different capabilities that can be evaluated and compared by looking at the data provided by the manufacturer. Critical points in inspiratory synchrony are the trigger delay and the 0.3-second area. The trigger delay is measured in milliseconds, and values vary from 40 to 200 milliseconds [8]. Trigger performance is usually improved by the companies offering alternative flow sensors close to the patient's mouth or algorithms dedicated to neonates.

It is common to see ex-preterm patients who are not capable of activating the inspiratory trigger more than 60–80% of the time. To prevent the patient from fatigue, the team returns to the conventional ventilator so the patient remains in the hospital longer.

A similar ventilatory strategy may be used based on the RCT studies in preterm babies [9], showing the superiority of non-synchronized IPPV in front of CPAP to prevent reintubation. So, an assisted pressure control mode may be used, setting a respiratory rate close to the patient's respiratory rate, associated with an appropriate inspiratory time (Ti). We recommend calculating the patient's Ti by dividing the duration of one complete breath by three.

This way, the patient has the chance to get synchronized to the ventilator by receiving a controlled breath very close to the time the patient starts a new breath. Ti duration is important to prevent expiratory asynchrony, which would increase the patient's work of breathing. Regarding flow asynchrony, even though the patient activates the ventilator's trigger properly, if leaks are present, it may affect the ventilator's performance. The capability to pressurize varies from one ventilator to another [10], so flow-asynchrony may be a significant problem. Tracheostomy cannulas with low-pressure balloons are used more frequently to reduce leaks and minimize insufficient leak compensation.

The severity of asynchrony may also change depending on the circuit used. Ventilator algorithms vary if a double arm, single arm with PEEP valve, or single passive circuit is used. As you can observe in the figures, there are significant differences in keeping the PEEP stable in the presence of massive leaks using the same ventilator between a single-arm circuit with a PEEP valve and a passive circuit (Fig. . 1).

Proper tubing selection is crucial when assured volume modes are used. Some authors strongly recommend double tubing to ensure appropriate measurement of delivered volume and avoid the algorithm's misinterpretation of the leaks [11].

Patients who do not have inspiratory asynchrony or leaks may benefit from using pressure support because expiratory asynchrony is also very unlikely.

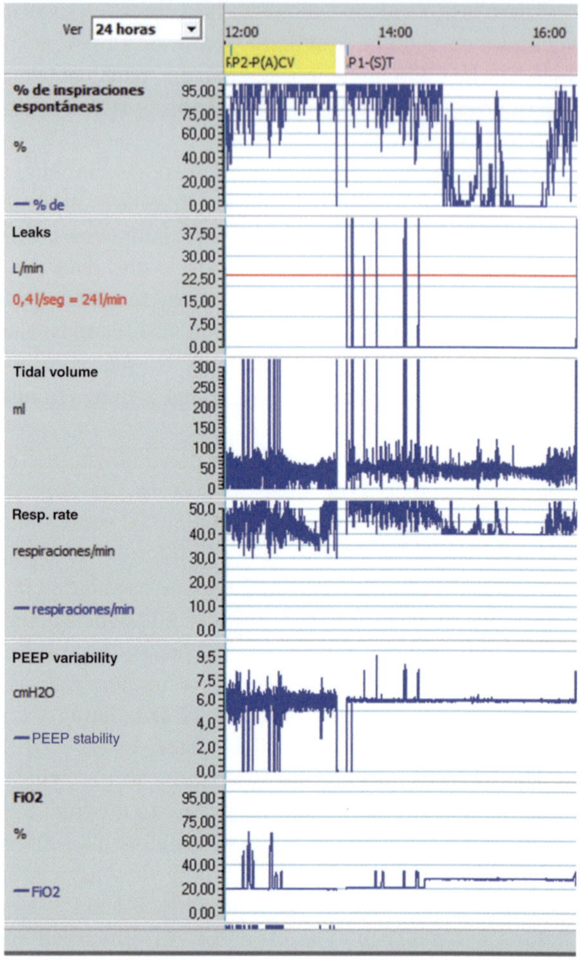

Fig. 1 Single tube with PEEP valve changed to passive circuit

After this first step with the home ventilator is accomplished, the weaning process should start.

Without an expert consensus or a guideline, some authors [12] describe using various ventilator modes throughout the weaning process. SIMV VC/PS was the most common mode used except for at the initiation of inpatient TC trials, which were primarily initiated in CPAP mode. HMV settings decreased during the weaning process, except for tidal volume, which was weight-adjusted.

In our center, Hospital Sant Joan de Déu in Barcelona has used a stepwise approach for long-term weaning.

There are two modes: night and day. In the day mode, the support (pressure gradient and backup respiratory rate) is slightly reduced to promote active breath activation and training of the respiratory muscles. We also encourage periods of complete disconnection according to the patient's capabilities.

At least 10 to 20 minutes of tolerance to disconnection is progressively attempted to reduce the risk of respiratory arrest, for example, in case of failing cannulation after accidental decannulation or obstruction. Usually, many patients progress to six to twelve hours free from the ventilator. In our opinion, this facilitates the neurological development of infants and toddlers and makes families' daily lives much easier.

Last but not least, a rescue program is preset. Parents are trained to activate it in case of a sudden change in the patient's lung compliance due to aspiration or mucus plugs related to viral infections.

1.1.1 Transfer from NICU to Home

A key point in this scenario is that most home ventilators are not prepared to ventilate patients weighing less than five kilograms. Many patients cannot remain stable for different reasons until they achieve this weight, so this limitation only affects a minor percentage of patients.

So, it will depend on the hospital policy about when to transfer these small patients to the PICU. If the NICU takes care of the patient until discharge, the neonatal team and the pulmonologist should be prepared to use hospital ventilators capable of covering the patient's needs and introduce ventilation settings not usual in preterm babies but sometimes required in the PICU.

The main key points will be discussed in Sect. 1.1.3.

1.1.2 Transfer from NICU to PICU

Preterm babies or neonates with severe malformations requiring long postoperative management and prolonged ventilation have spent a long time in the NICU. An emotional bond with the NICU team has been established, making finding the best moment for the transfer challenging.

The NICU and PICU are departments where critical care is performed. Still, even in the same hospital, several differences may be observed in many areas, such as mechanical ventilation, drug management, and nutrition. Additionally, units may have different policies, such as time for visiting, night overstay, and information style. These differences which usually doctors do not perceive as relevant for the patient's evolution may be seen as radical for the families, generating additional stress. In our opinion, pediatric intensivists with expertise in mechanical ventilation should collaborate with neonatologists and pulmonologists during this period to make all the important decisions for the patient's future, like doing a tracheostomy or continuing on noninvasive ventilation.

A multidisciplinary meeting to plan the patient's future should be organized, and later, the conclusions should be explained to the family. If ventilator weaning is an option, a weaning plan with realistic expectations should be shared. The weaning plan will be updated and adapted according to the patient's evolution in the posterior weeks or months. We believe that meeting in advance with the PICU team may help achieve a smoother transfer.

1.1.3 Transfer from PICU to Home

Meanwhile patient stabilization is achieved, the whole team should be working on family caregiver training:

Standards for training and evaluating the competency of family caregivers vary between institutions. Families and their medical teams must agree on the minimum security preparation and the number of responsible people available to help at home. For patients requiring invasive mechanical ventilation, it is recommended that at least two family caregivers be fully trained in all aspects of child care before discharge. In addition to practical bedside training, family caregivers may often require additional educational experiences to address scenarios that may not occur during the child's hospitalization. Simulation sessions can be instrumental in improving the management of situations such as cannula obstruction or aspiration.

Within this family training process, it is crucial to consider a period of hospital stay in units outside the PICU, where the family progressively takes control of the situation under supervision. Such units previously cited are respiratory intermediate care units (RICUs), step-down units, transitional care units, and weaning centers. In our region in Spain, there is only a pediatric intermediate care center called Casa Sofia, which is located a few minutes away from the hospital Sant Joan de Déu [https://www.sjdhospitalbarcelona.org/ca/pacients/guia/instalacions/casa-sofia].

Although pediatric respiratory intermediate care units (RICUs) are not available in many countries, the data obtained from adult studies [13] suggest that they may play a positive role in the weaning and/or discharging process, shortening at least the length of the stay in critical care units. The respiratory intermediate care units (RICUs) or mechanical ventilation weaning centers have demonstrated their effectiveness. In some Western countries, they are already a reality in adults and pediatrics [14]. Its future development and generalization will make it possible to shorten extended stays in the NICU and PICU, prevent admissions in these departments, and potentially shorten hospital stays.

1.2 Transferring Noninvasively Ventilated Patients

General considerations focused on mechanical ventilation:

In this section, there are two main groups of patients for whom ventilation cannot be discontinued, so it should be considered conceptually as vital support.

Severe central hypoventilation disorders and patients using 24 h/day NIV

1.2.1 Severe Central Hypoventilation Disorders

Patients suffering from CCHS may be identified as responders or nonresponders to NIV based on their PHOXb-2 genotype. Patients with 25 PARM copies usually have a better prognosis in this aspect, as the opposite happens to patients with 33 PARM copies or non-PARM patients [15].

Patients who suffer from congenital central hypoventilation syndrome (CCHS) or secondary to brain tumor/trauma should receive a pressure control mode with a programmed safety respiratory rate to compensate for the lack of drive happening in certain phases of sleep. Some authors [16] use the newer modes (assured volume) to address changes to maintain patients' minute volume within a specific range. However, there are some concerns due to the possibility of misinterpretation of moderate-severe leaks as high tidal volume, driving a progressive reduction of the pressure gradient and risky hypoventilation [17].

Sleep monitoring with pulse oximetry is considered mandatory to increase safety in case of ventilator failure.

1.2.2 Patients Using 24 h/day NIV

Patients requiring 24-h respiratory support are currently on invasive ventilation. Most HMV teams consider that patients requiring more than 16 hours per day on a ventilator are not safe or comfortable receiving NIV support [18]. However, patients and HMV teams disagree with this generalized approach and prefer to stay on non-invasive ventilation [19, 20].

Overcoming this challenge requires advanced knowledge, including using interfaces like the pipe or the straw (Fig. 2) and other settings to manage the alarms' different behaviors [21].

Nowadays, some ventilators offer dedicated modes of mouthpiece ventilation. Presets facilitate the setting of the parameters and even provide unique touch trigger

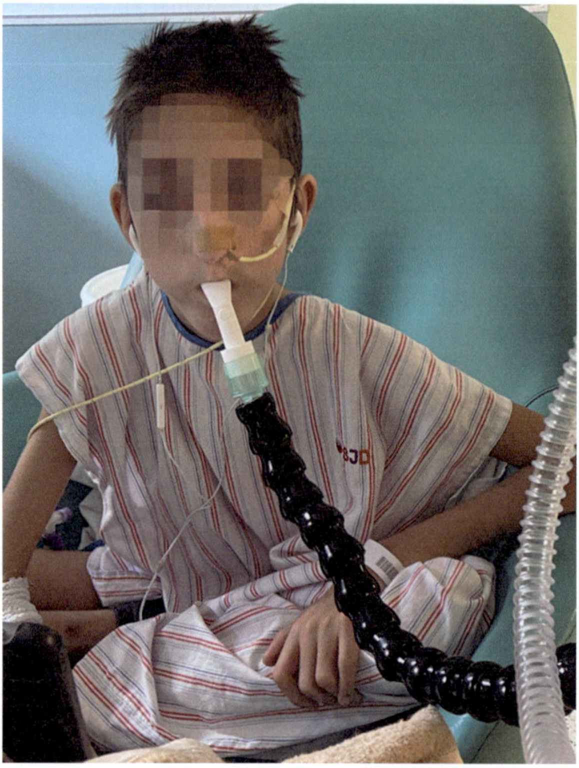

Fig. 2 Mouthpiece ventilation

sensitive to the tongue. Patients may combine daytime on mouthpiece ventilation and nighttime on nasal or oronasal NIV [19].

The most outstanding experience published is in neuromuscular patients who should have remarkable expertise managing secretions, currently with cough assistance devices.

2 Transferring Noninvasively Ventilated Patients to Home

General considerations focused on mechanical ventilation:

2.1 Transfer from NICU to Home

In this section, a crucial point is that most neonatal ventilators are not prepared to provide well-synchronized bilevel support. Additionally, leak compensation in neonatal modes is commonly insufficient to cope with considerable leaks in patients using nasal prongs who do not tolerate the pacifier. Suppose that the NICU takes care of the patient until their discharge. In that case, the team should be prepared to use hospital ventilators capable of covering the patient's needs and introduce ventilation settings not usual in preterm babies but sometimes required in PICU patients, like higher flows to compensate for the leaks. Growing evidence shows that modes with neural triggering (NAVA) may offer an advantage to keeping these patients on NIV and, therefore, prevent tracheostomy [5]. The commonest population are preterm babies with moderate-severe bronchopulmonary dysplasia (BPD), mild congenital neuromuscular diseases, and selected patients with mild congenital central hypoventilation disorder (CCHD). Last but not least, patients with moderate-severe sleep obstructive apnea due to craniofacial deformities or maxillary hypoplasia may require CPAP to stabilize the airway.

A progressive "weaning" process should be planned when using NAVA, switching from neural triggering to flow triggering in the same NICU/PICU ventilator. Later, the tolerance of a home ventilator with the most sensitive trigger available should be checked. Again, there are limitations in average home ventilators, especially regarding the appropriate monitoring of the tidal volumes in small infants weighing less than five kilograms. However, a few ventilators support patients weighing 3.5 to 5 kilograms.

When discussing noninvasive ventilation, the appropriate selection of interfaces is crucial [22]. In some places, RAM cannulas are used as alternatives to nasal masks to prevent pressure sores and improve patients' comfort (Fig. 3). For patients on CPAP, this is a good option; however, if the patient needs bilevel support, it will be challenging to avoid asynchrony.

Total face interfaces are frequently used in pediatric intensive care in some countries for infants with respiratory failure [23]. So, the smallest size, XXS, can be an

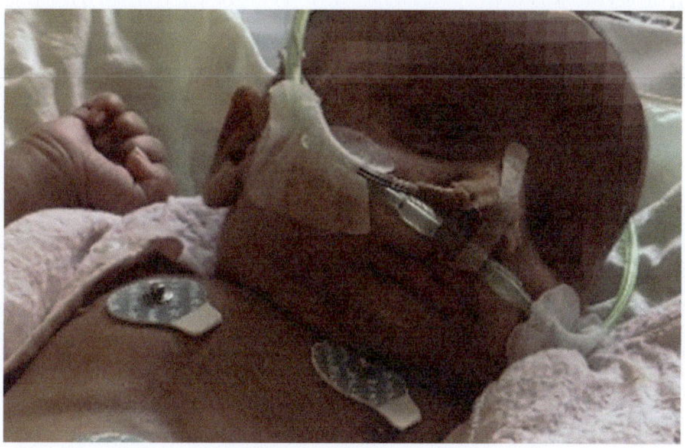

Fig. 3 RAM cannula

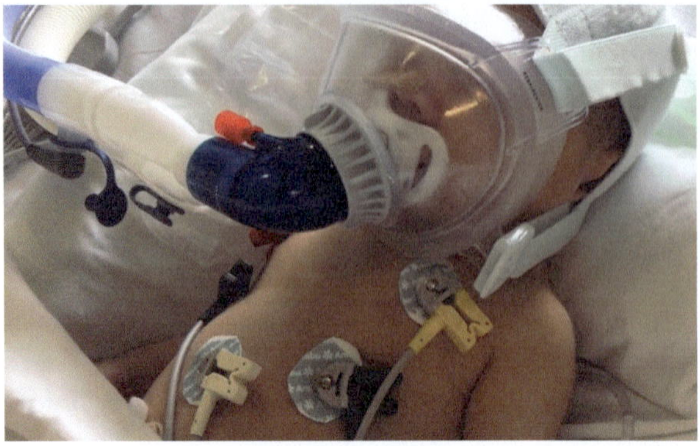

Fig. 4 Total face mask fitted under the chin

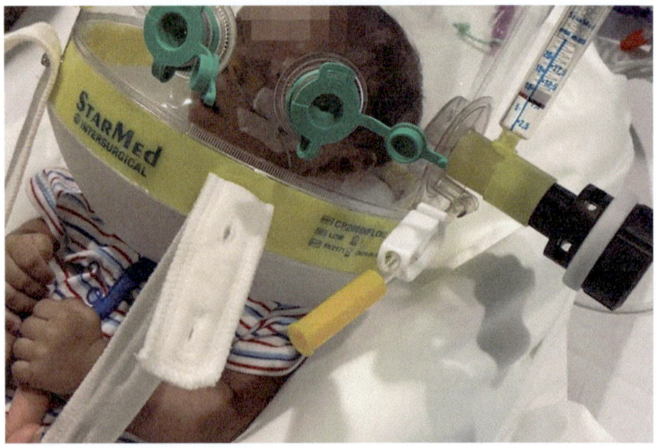

Fig. 5 Helmet interface

option for older ex-preterm patients weighing around three kilograms, knowing that they may sometimes be cautiously placed under the chin to fit appropriately (Fig. 4). The intended use is preferably during this transitioning period in the hospital when patients are at higher risk of NIV failure. Switching to a nasal mask is our favorite option before discharge. Commercial oronasal interfaces for small patients are not available in many countries, so they are not a realistic option.

Last but not least, helmet may also be an alternative in selected patients, especially those suffering from cranial-facial deformities requiring CPAP (Fig. 5).

2.2 *Transfer from PICU to Home*

Patients who currently may have prolonged mechanical ventilation in the PICU and end up needing home ventilation support suffer from a great variety of diseases, from neuromuscular patients after an acute decompensation or postoperative complications to postoperative cardiac patients dealing with unsolved problems (for example, mitral valve insufficiency) or sequelae like diaphragmatic palsy or vocal cord palsy, or neurological postoperative sequelae. Last but not least, ex-preterm babies stable on NIV may be transferred to the PICU before their discharge.

Strategies already proven effective in managing preterm babies, like NIV NAVA or kangaroo care, should be incorporated into the PICU [24]. Trained parents may be excellent caregivers for calming down BPD patients.

Each patient and condition will demand a different approach. Different interfaces may be selected based on age, weight, and severity. Some patients are at risk of needing tracheostomy, so they may need NIV support 24 hours per day for a prolonged period.

Recently, a new population of spinal muscular atrophy type I with a modified natural history is seen in our hospitals after the introduction of new treatments. These children require early and intensive NIV support, and families should be trained in the use of cough assistance techniques.

As a general rule, those patients who do not tolerate short breaks (bilateral diaphragmatic palsy), develop airway collapse with rapid deterioration (associated tracheomalacia), or have "blue spells" (Ondine's curse) should not be kept on NIV support. They should go straightforward to tracheostomy to guarantee their safety.

A progressive weaning from NIV support, at least four to six hours/day, should be achieved in two to three weeks. Otherwise, the stay may be prolonged excessively, and discomfort and a lack of environmental interaction could have side effects. Nowadays, patients diagnosed with BPD are intermittently placed in HFNC to facilitate the process.

2.3 Transfer from General Ward to Home

Generally speaking, this is the most uncomplicated patient transfer. Electively ventilated patients can benefit from an adaptation in a general ward or a step-down unit.

Most of them are stable patients diagnosed with sleep obstructive apnea or nocturnal hypoventilation. So, they may be quickly discharged after finding the best interface, titrating the appropriate settings, and training the parents.

These patients are definitively less risky than the invasively ventilated population; however, parents or caregivers should receive appropriate training to prevent the commonest complications, like pressure sores, and identify the clinical signs and symptoms of patient deterioration for an early consultation.

Interface selection is vital to success, so sometimes, it requires finding new options available in the market and appropriate training on how to fit them properly. Nowadays, it is becoming more common to offer an alternative interface (oronasal or total face mask) to families just in case of sudden deterioration at home causing severe hypoxemia. Usually, two to three nights at the hospital are required to sort out discomfort and asynchronies. Built-in software should be analyzed to identify asynchronies and fine-tune the parameters [25], especially in small infants and patients who cannot express the reasons that generate discomfort.

Nowadays, families are used to traveling despite the limitations imposed by ventilator dependency, so the selection of the ventilator may be influenced not only by technical issues but also by practical aspects like the ventilator's weight and the battery's length [12].

Mode selection will depend on the patient's needs, most commonly CPAP in patients diagnosed with obstructive sleep apneas and S/T mode or PS mode in patients diagnosed with nocturnal hypoventilation [18].

Close monitoring during the first month may help prevent loss of treatment adherence or complications like pressure sores. Telemedicine potentially facilitates it through the data clouds offered by ventilator companies [25].

Having said that, adaptation at home has also been published in selected groups of patients, but it seems limited to wealthy countries with plenty of resources [26].

References

1. Jardine E, Wallis C. Core guidelines for the discharge home of the child on long-term assisted ventilation in the United Kingdom. UK Working Party on Paediatric Long Term Ventilation. Thorax. 1998;53(9):762–7.
2. Sterni LM, Collaco JM, Baker CD, et al. An official American Thoracic Society clinical practice guideline: pediatric chronic home invasive ventilation. Am J Respir Crit Care Med. 2016;193(8):e16–35.
3. Nixon GM, Edwards EA, Cooper DM, et al. Ventilatory support at home for children: a consensus statement from the Australasian paediatric respiratory group. 2008 [accessed 2 July 2022]. Available from: http://www.thoracic.org.au/journalpublishing/command/download_file/id/10/filename/Ventilatory_Support_at_Home_for_Children._A_Consensus_Statement_from_the_Australasian_Paediatric_Respiratory_Group.pdf.
4. Park S, Suh E-S. Home mechanical ventilation: back to the basics. Acute Crit Care. 2020;35(3):131–41.
5. Shetty S, Evans K, Cornuaud P, et al. Neurally adjusted ventilatory assist in very prematurely born infants with evolving/established bronchopulmonary dysplasia. AJP Rep. 2021;11(4):e127–31.
6. Olguin Ciancio M, Cambra FJ, Pons-Odena M. Tracheal opening manoeuvre (PEEP-20) in a patient with bronchopulmonary dysplasia and severe tracheobronchomalacia with neurally adjusted ventilatory assist (NAVA). BMJ Case Rep. 2020;13(1):e229471.
7. McKinney RL, Agarwal A. Transition from intensive care unit to a portable ventilator in children with severe bronchopulmonary dysplasia. Pediatr Pulmonol. 2023;58(3):712–9.
8. Tobin M. Chapter 9: Pressure support ventilation. In: Principles of mechanical ventilation. 3rd ed. McGraw-Hill. p. 231.
9. Lemyre B, Deguise MO, Benson P, et al. Nasal intermittent positive pressure ventilation (NIPPV) versus nasal continuous positive airway pressure (NCPAP) for preterm neonates after extubation. Cochrane Database Syst Rev. 2023;7(7):CD003212.
10. Lujan M, Sogo A, Pomares X, et al. Effect of leak and breathing pattern on the accuracy of tidal volume estimation by commercial home ventilators: a bench study. Resp Care. 2013;58(5):770.
11. Gregoretti C, Navalesi P, Ghannadian S, Carlucci A, Pelosi P. Choosing a ventilator for home mechanical ventilation. Breathe. 2013;9(5):394–409.
12. Henningfeld JK, Maletta K, Ren B, Richards KL, Wegner C, D'Andrea LA. Liberation from home mechanical ventilation and decannulation in children. Pediatr Pulmonol. 2016;51(8):838–49.

13. López-Jardón P, Martínez-Fernández MC, García-Fernández R, et al. Utility of intermediate care units: a systematic review study. Healthcare (Basel). 2024;12(3):296.
14. Caggiano S, Pavone M, Cherchi C, et al. Children with medical complexity and pediatric palliative care: data by a respiratory intermediate care unit. Pediatr Pulmonol. 2023;58(3):918–26.
15. Bishara J, Keens TG, Perez IA. The genetics of congenital central hypoventilation syndrome: clinical implications. Appl Clin Genet. 2018;11:135–44.
16. Khayat A, Medin D, Syed F, et al. Intelligent volume-assured pressured support (iVAPS) for the treatment of congenital central hypoventilation syndrome. Sleep Breath. 2017;21(2):513–9.
17. Pluym M, Kabir AW, Gohar A. The use of volume-assured pressure support noninvasive ventilation in acute and chronic respiratory failure: a practical guide and literature review. Hosp Pract (1995). 2015;43:299–307.
18. Fauroux B, Abel F, Amaddeo A, Bignamini E, et al. ERS statement on paediatric long-term noninvasive respiratory support. Eur Respir J. 2022;59(6):2101404.
19. Bach JR. Noninvasive respiratory management of patients with neuromuscular disease. Ann Rehabil Med. 2017;41(4):519–38.
20. Gonçalves MR, Bach JR, Ishikawa Y, et al. International Study Group on Continuous Noninvasive Ventilatory Support in Neuromuscular Disease (CNVSND). Continuous noninvasive ventilatory support outcomes for patients with neuromuscular disease: a multicenter data collaboration. Pulmonology. 2021;27(6):509–17. https://doi.org/10.1016/j.pulmoe.2021.06.007. Epub 2021 Oct 14. PMID: 34656524.
21. Pinto T, Chatwin M, Banfi P, Winck JC, Nicolini A. Mouthpiece ventilation and complementary techniques in patients with neuromuscular disease: a brief clinical review and update. Chron Respir Dis. 2017;14(2):187–93.
22. Castro-Codesal ML, Olmstead DL, MacLean JE. Mask interfaces for home non-invasive ventilation in infants and children. Paediatr Respir Rev. 2019;32:66–72. https://doi.org/10.1016/j.prrv.2019.03.004. Epub 2019 Mar 23. PMID: 31130424.
23. Toni F, Lasaosa FJC, Conti G, et al. Comparison in the management of respiratory failure due to bronchiolitis in a pediatric ICU between 2010 and 2016. Respir Care. 2019;64(10):1270–8.
24. Xie X, Chen X, Sun P, et al. Kangaroo mother care reduces noninvasive ventilation and total oxygen support duration in extremely low birth weight infants. Am J Perinatol. 2021;38(8):791–5.
25. Janssens J-P, Cantero C, Pasquina P, Georges M, Rabec C. Monitoring long term noninvasive ventilation: benefits, caveats and perspectives. Front Med. 2022;9:874523. https://doi.org/10.3389/fmed.2022.87452.
26. Duiverman ML, Vonk JM, Bladder G, et al. Home initiation of chronic non-invasive ventilation in COPD patients with chronic hypercapnic respiratory failure: a randomised controlled trial. Thorax. 2020;75(3):244–52.

Evaluation of the Child with Home Ventilation

Jia Liu and Robert J. Graham

The goals of prolonged mechanical ventilation for children with chronic respiratory failure are to prolong survival, relieve dyspnea, normalize gas exchange, optimize cardiopulmonary interactions, treat sleep-disordered breathing, improve daytime function, mitigate acute on chronic respiratory processes, and promote or sustain growth and development. For many patients with progressive disorders, the implementation of chronic mechanical ventilation, whether noninvasive or transtracheal, has altered the natural history of their diseases [1]. Even for those with static, chronic conditions, the use of home ventilation may mitigate cumulative morbidities or allow for support during intercurrent illnesses. In addition, the use of chronic respiratory support has been shown to reduce the number of days spent in the hospital as well as overall healthcare costs.

Following the decision to pursue technology supports, the reality of home care can be daunting for families and challenging for all members of the care team, community and hospital based. This chapter outlines the considerations for home provision of the range of respiratory technology supports for children with pediatric neuromuscular diseases and their families. "Evaluation" is broad in scope and begins prior to the initial discharge. "Re-evaluation" is essential, thereafter. This should occur at regular intervals, coinciding with routine visits, intercurrent illnesses, circumstance marking progression or resolution of the underlying conditions, or other medical, surgical, and social/family events that may be consequential.

J. Liu
Division of Critical Care Medicine, Boston Children's Hospital, Boston, MA, USA

Department of Anesthesia, Pain and Perioperative Medicine, Critical Care Medicine, Children's National Medical Center, Washington, DC, USA
e-mail: jliu@childrensnational.org

R. J. Graham (✉)
Division of Critical Care Medicine, Boston Children's Hospital, Boston, MA, USA
e-mail: robert.graham@childrens.harvard.edu

A. Kawaguchi et al. (eds.), *Prolonged and Long-Term Mechanical Ventilation in Children*, https://doi.org/10.1007/978-981-97-8903-0_18

Anticipating issues and optimizing supports are important for all stakeholders and essential to improving outcomes.

1 Preparation

There are both emotional and practical challenges associated with the integration of technology supports into routine home care. Adequate preparation is essential for a safe transition and should include considerations for safe discharge planning, adaptations of the home care setting, availability of required equipment and supplies, appropriate training of families and home care personnel, and safe transportation to, and from, the home. Family and provider expectations should align with infrastructure (e.g., transitional care facilities, telehealth capacity, equipment options, housing) and systems (e.g., home nursing, primary care and specialist relationships, home and community therapies, insurance coverage, school accommodations), which vary dramatically throughout the world and within different healthcare systems.

1.1 Discharge Planning

Discharge planning for the child going home with respiratory supports should begin as soon as possible during the sentinel admission to allow for multidisciplinary coordination of the child's transition to the home. Successful transition to the home may be aided by establishing a medical home that is co-managed by a generalist/primary care and a respiratory subspecialist [2]. Integration of the medical home with other subspecialties may be necessary, depending upon the child's underlying conditions (e.g., stem cell transplants with pulmonary complications, complex congenital heart disease, or solid organ transplants). Early identification and communication with the child's medical home can allow for discussions on timing and requirements for discharge and whether bridging to home via a subacute inpatient facility or rehabilitation center will be necessary. Coordination of community-based services and outpatient follow-up should be initiated as an inpatient and then transitioned to the designated outpatient provider with care to ensure detailed handoff of ongoing needs [2].

Prior to transitioning to home care with chronic ventilation, the medical team must ensure that the patient has demonstrated medical stability for a period of time on home equipment and unchanged ventilator settings prior to discharge. Readiness determination should include indirect respiratory outcomes, such as adequate weight gain for infants and progression of physical therapy and mobility. Tolerance of transition to the portable home ventilator should be ensured, as this may require some time and multiple attempts for success [3]. Capacity to wean fiO2 for safety and feasibility of home provision is essential; factors to consider include altitude, bias flow and dilution of the specific ventilator, capacity of home oxygen sources (portable and stationary), and maximal provision and duration of increased fiO2 during acute stressors. Establishing a period of stability prior to transition home allows time to ensure that the appropriate medications and equipment will be available in the home, and it may minimize unplanned readmissions [4]. Subsequent hospitalizations, whether elective or unplanned admissions, should serve as an opportunity to revisit home care provision to ensure ongoing safe care in the home and to address any issues prior to discharge [5]. Contingency plans, as outlined below, are essential.

1.2 Adaptations of the Home Care Setting

An on-site, or virtual, evaluation of the home and surroundings can be very informative and should be pursued well in advance of discharge. Modifications to the home may be required to ease care and optimize safety. Ramps for wheelchair access will permit safe ingress and egress. Lift systems can minimize physical burden and risk of injury to home care providers. Doorways can be expanded to permit access to multiple rooms. Alternative bath and toileting accommodations may be needed. Most importantly, electrical system upgrades with grounding and increased amperage are often required for equipment demand and safety. Emergency power options should also be reviewed, recognizing the need for ongoing supports in the context of power outages. Families should also receive counseling in preparation for how the implementation of respiratory supports in the home will affect their daily lives, family dynamic, and outside relationships [6].

1.3 Equipment and Supplies

Ideally, the equipment intended for use at home will be tested prior to discharge home. Individual hospital policy regarding the use of home equipment varies, but evaluation for a period of time, minimum of 24 hours, ensures proper function and family understanding (see below) as well as patient tolerance and efficacy. The American Thoracic Society guidelines for pediatric chronic home invasive ventilation provide some guidance regarding necessary home supplies (Table 1) [7]. Delivery of monitoring (pulse oximetry) and backup devices (e.g., tracheostomy tubes, backup ventilators, batteries, suctioning supplies, portable oxygen and/or electric oxygen concentrators) as well as emergency supplies (self-inflating resuscitation bag) should be confirmed. If the child is being discharged on noninvasive positive-pressure ventilation (NIPPV), a variety of available NIPPV interfaces and headgear should be trialed prior to discharge to assess for optimal fit. If possible, alternating masks can mitigate pressure points and risk of skin ulceration or midface hypoplasia [8]. It may also allow for modification during illness as compared to routine support. Medication supplies and refills should be sufficient to allow for the scheduling of follow-up visits. Providers responsible for recertification or reordering should be identified prior to discharge.

Table 1 ATS-suggested home equipment for pediatric patients requiring chronic invasive Home ventilation

ATS-suggested home equipment
Ventilator
Backup ventilator
Batteries
Heated humidifier
Self-inflating resuscitation bag and mask
Portable suction machine
Oxygen supply
Pulse oximeter and probes
Medical air compression and nebulizer (if prescribed)
Backup tracheostomies (if invasive airway in place)

1.4 Training for Family Caregivers

Standards for training and evaluation of competency for family caregivers vary between institutions and across providers. Families and their medical teams should come to an agreement on minimum safety preparation and number of responsible parties available to assist in the home. For patients requiring invasive mechanical ventilation, it is recommended a minimum of two family caregivers be fully trained in all aspects of the child's care prior to discharge. This may not be possible for single-parent households, but alternatives should be explored for safety and sustainability; friends, extended family, and neighbors may be willing and could be essential during an emergency with the child or periods when the parent needs to leave the home or if incapacitated by an illness or other circumstances. Competency evaluation and training should focus on routine management of the ventilator and tracheostomy tube, as well as less common but often more urgent scenarios such as tube obstruction, decannulation, and bleeding from the airway [7]. In addition to hands-on training at the bedside, family caregivers may often require additional educational experiences, especially to address emergent scenarios that may not occur during the child's hospitalization. In these situations, simulation sessions with nursing and/or respiratory therapists may be beneficial [9]. CPR training should be completed by all family caregivers, and any additional home care personnel should be certified as well. Assumption of full care by families while in the hospital can be informative for all stakeholders and reassuring to families; supported replication of the demands of home care prior to discharge is ideal.

1.5 Transportation

Discharge planning for a child or young adult with technology dependence should include safe transportation to, and from, the child's home. For infants, or those with severe hypotonia, car seat tests or modification to a car bed may be needed. Personal vehicles may require modifications, including lifts and power inverters, and adaptive car seats or car beds may need to be purchased. It may also be necessary for an additional caregiver to tend to the child during transportation while the other is driving, and any emergency response required en route should involve pulling off the road to allow for safe care provision and call for emergency medical assistance if needed. For the initial transition from hospital to home, ambulance transport may be appropriate, taking into consideration the proximity and location of the home (rural vs. urban), child's mobility, weather, and need for monitoring *en route*. Long-term transportation considerations should factor in school, routine family excursions, and extended travel, including vacations.

2 Ongoing Home Monitoring and Assessment

Conceptually, monitoring is used to detect early physiologic changes, determine adequacy of ventilation, and minimize cumulative morbidities or risk of mortality. Continuous direct observation, however, is often not practical, nor desirable, in the community setting. Recommendations for monitoring children and young adults requiring home respiratory support vary based on underlying pathophysiology and lability, care setting (e.g., home, long-term care facility, school, work, or in transport via car), and adjuvant supports (e.g., home nursing or personal care assistant). The child's individual risks as well as the environmental circumstances determine the balance of extrinsic monitoring (e.g., pulse oximetry and heart rate) and intrinsic device alarms. Provider and family evaluation and calibration of the alignment of a child's underlying vulnerability and mechanical supports are necessary; that is, transtracheal supports, while seemingly more challenging, may provide a modicum of safety that may not be present without an artificial airway and only NIPPV options in the same clinical circumstances. There are also pragmatic considerations when determining monitoring parameters, as recurrent false alarms will lead to alarm fatigue and desensitize providers and may also disturb the child's sleep.

2.1 Ventilator Alarms

Internal ventilator alarm settings, for both NIPPV and transtracheal ventilators, are utilized to monitor for high- and low-pressure parameters, high and low respiratory rates, and minute ventilation. Stakeholders must acknowledge, however, that internal alarms may be insufficient in the setting of a large mask or peritracheal leak or in the event of a device malfunction. Certain low-pressure alarms may not alarm when there has been accidental decannulation in patients with smaller tracheostomies, as the resistance within the tube is enough to generate a pressure in the ventilator that exceeds the low-pressure alarm threshold [10]. Setting a low minute ventilation alarm to approximately half of the measured minute ventilation may provide an alternative method for detection. Disabling of alarms is common in devices without leak compensation or those with modifications to allow for mouthpiece interface. Home care providers and prescribing staff must understand the risk versus benefit when implementing modifications to minimize “signal-to-noise” and optimize lived experience and outcomes in the community.

2.2 Extrinsic Monitoring

Pulse oximetry can be used intermittently or on a continuous basis with oxygen and heart rate parameters determined on a case-by-case basis. Hypoxemia is likely to be an early indicator of inadequate ventilation in infants and small children, making it a helpful monitor for early detection of airway obstruction or equipment malfunction [2]. This benefit must be balanced against the frequency of false alarms contributing to alarm fatigue, which may negate the benefit of early detection using pulse oximetry. There is often need to adjust default oximetry settings, which may be intended for adults or those with intrinsic lung disease; thresholds for those with limited reserve and neuromuscular conditions may be set at 94% saturation rather than 92% or 88%. Similarly, heart rate parameters in the context of neuromuscular conditions, with and without associated cardiomyopathy, as effective nocturnal respiratory supports often result in lower sleeping heart rates; parents should be calibrated to signs of adequate perfusion and normal heart rate variability. Typically, capnography is not available, except in cases of central hypoventilation syndromes, but can complement oximetry. Simple audio and video monitors can be used to augment surveillance and may help families in their activities of daily living. Trials for telemonitoring with home ventilation have been conducted and shown to be feasible; however, there are currently no standards in place, and it is not widely available to patients and families [11, 12].

2.3 Home Care Personnel

In addition to family caregivers, additional home care personnel may be in the form of home care nursing, hospice, personal care assistants, extended family, or friends. Allowances for home care nursing from insurance companies vary based upon the child’s age, independence, medical condition, technology dependence, goals of care, and other factors. These individuals may require additional training, but augmenting numbers of proficient home care providers is crucial for safety and consistency of care. Of note, there are often no standards for evaluation of competency in non-licensed personnel; therefore, training should be tailored to the child’s needs and the prior experience of a given provider in addition to general safety considerations. When considering home care provision, families should be thoughtful about the type of personnel and how additional supports would impact the patient and family—this includes allowing the child to attend school, providing time for family members to work or maintain the household, and continuing care when a family caregiver is sick or incapacitated. Availability and the challenges of establishing, training, and maintaining a home care staff require time and tolerance, recognizing that safety is the priority [13].

2.4 Environmental Regulation

Extreme temperatures, heat or cold, variability in humidity, and other environmental variables can greatly impact the well-being of a child with underlying cardiorespiratory insufficiency. Home adaptations to permit climate monitoring and control for the child's room may be required. Families may consider prewarming, or cooling, vehicles for routine excursions, and limitations on day-to-day activities are warranted at times. Augmented hydration needs should be reviewed with medical providers, along with routine sunscreen and preventative measures. That said, accommodations for a variety of seasonal outdoor activities, including adaptive skiing, power soccer, hiking, sailing, and biking, are increasingly available and feasible via a growing number of national and regional nonprofit organizations such as Outdoors for All Foundation, Tetradapt, and AccessSportAmerica.

3 Community Resources

3.1 Durable Medical Equipment (DME) Companies and Pharmacies

A good working relationship with a DME company is essential to safely caring for children who require home respiratory support. In addition to ensuring that all the appropriate supplies are delivered to the home and functioning prior to initial discharge, DME companies must provide 24-hour availability as a resource to families and to service the equipment. This includes same-day replacement of malfunctioning equipment if needed [7]. Similarly, access to compounding pharmacies may be essential for individuals who rely upon enteral feeding tubes for medication administration.

3.2 Educational and Therapy Programs

Integration into community services requires evaluation of the child's developmental needs as well as adaptations to the school environment to allow for ongoing medical care. This may include additional staffing, equipment, and adaptations of the physical space to allow for safe ingress and egress. Advocacy to optimize access to school and workplace for individuals with chronic ventilator support may be required; families and providers can reference local and federal/national statutes (e.g., in the United States, the Americans with Disabilities Act, Education for All Handicapped Children Act P.L. 94-142, and the Affordable Care Act all have safety and accommodation mandates and guidelines).

A trained caregiver should accompany the child at school, and an emergency plan should be delineated. Personal care assistants may be required for feeding, toileting, transfers, or other activities of daily living in the educational or work setting. Bone health, or rather vulnerability to pathologic fractures, is always a concern in non-weight-bearing conditions and may be potentiated in those with hypotonia; care with transfers, positioning, and applications of braces should be emphasized. Backup devices and supplemental oxygen should be readily available in the school environment as well. Physical, occupational, speech-language/feeding, and other therapists benefit from hospital-based assessments as well as outlines of expectations, restrictions, and uncertainties. Clear communication between the medical teams, family, and therapy programs is important as the trajectory of any specific neuromuscular disease varies dramatically from one individual to another, especially with the progress of gene-targeted, gene-replacement, and other disease-specific treatments. Therapy advancements may affect both disease trajectory and goals for supportive therapy programs.

3.3 Utilities

Alerting local housing, power, and water authorities to a child's medical necessities can facilitate prioritization of service restoration during natural disasters or other interruptions, as well as identify programs to defray incurred costs with increased technology-driven electrical usage (e.g., home ventilators, oxygen concentrators, and climate control).

3.4 Financial

The majority of families have reported additional financial burdens related to home ventilation that are often not covered by insurance. Financial strains have included higher utility bills due to ventilator maintenance, additional supplies not covered by insurance, and gas for transportation to medical appointments. Inability to fill caregiver hours with home care nursing may lead to family members quitting jobs or school to become full-time caregivers [14–18]. Certain state-based funding may be available through "catastrophic illness" funds, many of which are specific to the pediatric population. Discussions can be had with landlords and property managers for those families who are renting their homes regarding funding for adaptations to the home to maintain compliance with the Americans with Disabilities Act. Families may find additional resources through faith-based institutions, nonprofit and advocacy groups (e.g., Kiwanis, Shriners, Boy Scouts), philanthropic organizations, and condition-specific entities, such as the Muscular Dystrophy Association. Additional considerations should also be paid to personal trusts, wills, and estate planning, as all of these have implications for long-term benefits and financial supports for the individual with special healthcare needs.

4 Routine Health Maintenance and Evaluation

Primary care, specialty collaboration, and proactive management are essential for optimal "routine" care in the community [19–21]. This may require alterations in standard care models. In addition to scheduled "well-child" clinic sessions, home visits, telehealth, use of remote adjuvants, portable and noninvasive measurement of gas exchange, use of downloadable data from home ventilators with a focus on child-derived variables (i.e., dependent and not controlled), weights, activity diaries, and open multidisciplinary input can be utilized to optimize the medical home.

4.1 Airway Evaluation

There is no standard for regular airway assessment for children requiring chronic home ventilation, specifically those with transtracheal support, but annual evaluation should represent the minimum [22]. Office-based transtracheal tube endoscopy can facilitate assessment of tube upsizing for linear growth, presence of granulation tissue, airway inflammation, and general mucosal integrity. Formal diagnostic laryngoscopy and bronchoscopy under general anesthesia are required to assess for suprastomal and laryngeal level pathology as well as the rare, acquired trachea-esophageal fistula. Determination of frequency of evaluation should also include considerations around anesthetic management and risk, such as difficult airway management (due to limited mouth opening, cervical spine instability or rigidity) or tolerance of general anesthesia (due to underlying cardiovascular disease or limited pulmonary reserve). Of note, independent of routine evaluation, recurrent or unexpected tracheal bleeding may warrant evaluation for a tracheo-vascular fistula via CT angiogram and/or bronchoscopy.

4.2 Bacterial Colonization

Chronic respiratory failure lends itself to airway bacterial colonization due to alterations in secretion clearance, aerodigestive interactions, presence of artificial airways with the development of biofilms, and other factors. Hydrophilic and Gram-negative bacteria (e.g., *Pseudomonas*, *Serratia*, and *Stenotrophomonas*) are not uncommon [23]. There is currently no standard of care for determining pathogenicity versus colonization for bacteria that are isolated from tracheal aspirates. Use of systemic or inhaled antibacterial agents to decrease colonization load, frequency of tracheostomy tube exchanges to reduce biofilm accumulation, utility of viral screening, and threshold for treatment of tracheitis or an acute lower airway process are often provider and case dependent. Providers should appreciate that recurrent empiric antibacterial treatment may select for resistant bacterial strains and have implications for enteric bacterial colonization.

4.3 Dental Care

Routine daily and office-based dental care should follow standard recommendations for all children. Extrapolation from the acute care setting and general population would suggest that oropharyngeal care and minimization of bacterial overgrowth can impact the risk of superimposed respiratory illness in children with chronic respiratory failure and long-term cardiovascular outcomes, respectively. Special consideration with respect to aspiration risk, developmental tolerance, and need for antibiotic prophylaxis or procedural sedation prior to intervention may require engagement of specialty providers.

4.4 Immunizations

There are no immunizations specifically indicated for individuals receiving chronic mechanical ventilation. Routine provision is recommended, including seasonal vaccinations for viral pathogens (e.g., *influenza* and *respiratory syncytial virus*). Expansion of exposure precautions, as we experienced during the COVID-19 pandemic, also remains essential. Strict hand hygiene is advised for all individuals caring for these children.

4.5 Medical Home

Coordination of routine health maintenance for these children can often be complex and requires thoughtful planning to avoid excessive burden on the family and home care providers. Establishment of a medical home allows for patient/family-centered care that ensures effective implementation of a comprehensive care plan that avoids duplication or redundancy in care by clearly delineating the roles and responsibilities of each provider within the child's care team [7]. Due to the unfamiliarity with technology dependence amongst community-based general practitioners, care coordination may fall upon a specialty ventilator or other service; this is feasible, but integration of care is essential to optimize outcomes [24, 25]. Maintaining a medical home as these children transition through adolescence into young adulthood will facilitate the eventual transition from pediatric to adult care providers [26].

The balance of in-person (office- or home-based) and remote evaluations depends upon the individual needs. The advent of telehealth options for both routine and acute issues has improved accessibility and holds the potential for more efficient resource utilization [12]. Clustering/coordination of in-person evaluations amongst specialists minimizes the travel burden on families and attenuates safety considerations for the child. Combined/multidisciplinary clinics also enhance communication and care coordination [27].

5 Contingency Planning

While the incidence of serious complications for pediatric patients requiring chronic home ventilation is relatively low [28], the consequences of those complications can be quite severe if appropriate action is not taken in a timely manner. Given this risk, careful contingency planning is required to address emergency situations safely and effectively.

5.1 Home Evaluation/Preparations

A formal safety plan should be posted in an easily accessible location in the home that includes emergency contact numbers and essential medical information that includes ventilator settings, medications, and allergies [7]. As children with chronic respiratory support transition into young adults, clarification of resuscitation status and life-sustaining therapies may be included as well. Children who require invasive mechanical ventilation should always have an emergency "go-bag" at hand that includes items such as a backup tracheostomy, self-inflating resuscitation bag, flashlight, and suction catheters [7, 29] (Fig. 1). A functioning phone, either a landline or a devoted mobile phone, should remain with the child at all times in case of emergency. An established working relationship with a primary provider, whether it is a community-based pediatrician or specialty provider, is essential to allow for timely communication and for management to remain in the home.

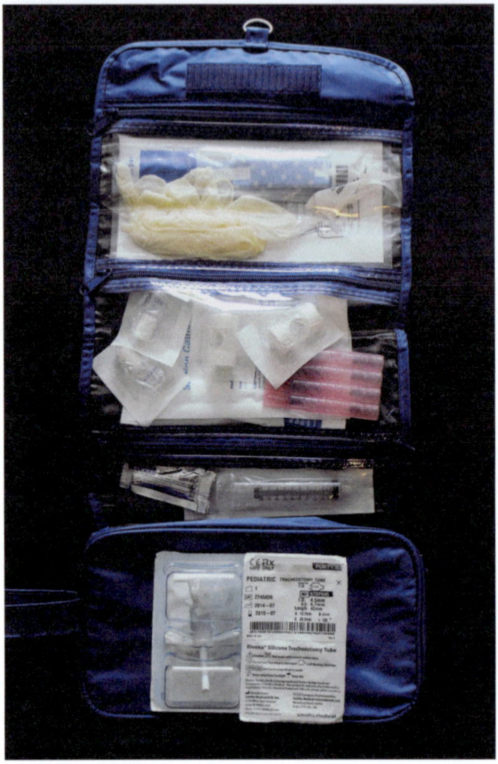

Fig. 1 Contents of go bag

5.2 *First Responders*

Outreach to local first responders can be made when a child transitions to chronic home respiratory support. Communication with local police, fire departments, and ambulance services may include the child's baseline needs, special condition-specific interventions or precautions, identification of equipment that may need to be taken with the child in the event of an emergency, determination of emergency destination (i.e., local hospital versus referral center), and clarification of resuscitation status and life-sustaining therapies.

5.3 *Subacute Care*

The child with technology dependence will experience intercurrent illnesses or unexpected accidents that will require evaluation, but may not always necessitate transport to tertiary care or referral centers. Therefore, local resources for medical services should be identified in advance. As noted above, this begins with the primary care and first responders but also extends to local and regional hospitals. It is important to determine the range of available services at these institutions, and if possible, specific providers should be identified who can familiarize themselves with a given case and establish channels of communication with the child's primary providers [30]. Again, telehealth with the medical home, or specialty services, can play a role in optimizing management of intercurrent illnesses and mitigate the need for hospital-based evalautions [12]. Individual care plans can be developed in conjunction with the family and local providers, including thresholds for transfer to a tertiary care center. Families should also consider bringing home equipment and supplies when presenting to local or unfamiliar hospital settings. Devices, such as pediatric NIPPV masks and cough assist machines, or compounded medications may not be available at every facility.

5.4 Acute and Emergency Care

Children who are technology dependent have a higher likelihood of requiring critical care services and are therefore more likely to present for acute and emergency care, due to the nature of their needs and associated vulnerabilities as well as hospital infrastructure/systems [31, 32]. Progression of underlying illnesses (e.g., heart failure, worsening neuromuscular weakness), planned surgical interventions (e.g., spinal instrumentation, bronchoscopy surveillance, cardiac catheterization, tendon releases), or superimposed acute illnesses (e.g., pneumonia, gastroenteritis, appendicitis, recurrent seizures) may necessitate readmission [4]. Once hospitalized, children with chronic ventilator dependence are at a higher risk for medical error and recurrent readmissions when compared with otherwise healthy children [33–35]. Patients and families should be encouraged to develop a medical passport and reference list of providers to facilitate communication and consistency of care. Referencing established care guidelines and, again, developing individualized care plans may be helpful.

5.5 Transportation

In addition to routine travel (i.e., school, medical appointments), children with chronic respiratory support may occasionally require long-distance travel, either by ground or by air. If traveling long distances, advanced planning might include identification of hospitals along the route and reciprocal equipment companies to assist with unexpected supply needs. A caregiver should be available for the duration of the trip and backup equipment, and supplies should be readily accessible. If travel by plane is anticipated, contingencies should be made for additional oxygen support at altitude, as most commercial airlines pressurize their cabins to the equivalent of 5000–8000 feet, which correlates to a decreased partial pressure of oxygen. Portable oxygen sources may have less liter flow capacity than stationary or home devices, and there is also a need to differentiate continuous versus on-demand flow options. Supplemental oxygen is provided by some airlines; however, the availability and flow rate vary by airline. Certain portable oxygen concentrators that are FAA approved may be used in flight as well; however, clear communication should take place with the airline ahead of planned travel to ensure that the device is approved. There are no standards for preflight testing in adults or pediatrics; however, for patients who are at high risk for developing hypoxia in-flight, a hypoxia altitude simulation test should be considered prior to travel [36, 37]. Space and limited supplies in-flight should also be considered. Power wheelchairs are prone to damage when placed in cargo holds, and ground crews likely require explicit instructions. Providers may need to write letters for airport security and airlines for excess baggage, electronic equipment, medication, and fluid allowance. Families can also consider sending additional supplies to the final destination in advance of the flight.

6 Quality of Life

Children and young adults of increasing complexity and technology dependence are thriving in the home care setting due to advances in medical care, shared decision-making, community services, and, most notably, vigilant and proactive care efforts by their families. Adaptations allow for participation in all aspects of family, school, and community activities [11]. Service dogs can be successfully incorporated into the lives of children and young adults with neuromuscular disease to assist with physical tasks and mobility as well as alerting other family members to medical emergencies such as low oxygen saturation. Use of service dogs in this population has been shown to improve independence and quality of life while simultaneously reducing stress and anxiety [38, 39]. While individual trajectory and subsequent needs may be difficult to predict, all stakeholders should acknowledge the impact of chronic care on the family unit and health-related quality of life [16, 17, 40]. The evolution of a medical home for this cohort of children will require provisions for family mental health, sibling supports, respite, and other measures to optimize outcomes.

"Evaluation" should encompass advanced care planning when optimizing quality of life for children and young adults in the home care setting. It has been shown that end-of-life discussions frequently occur for children on chronic respiratory support in the setting of an acute hospitalization or deterioration [41]. Value and goal-oriented discussions should be had with families and young adult patients, ideally during periods of medical stability, to help guide the medical team during periods of acute deterioration. Young adults should strongly consider appointing a healthcare proxy or durable power of attorney for healthcare to assist in medical decision-making if needed. If advance care directives, such as a living will or MOLST/POLST forms are created, copies should be provided to both primary and local medical institutions. In addition, copies should be easily identifiable in the home, especially if out-of-hospital do-not-resuscitate orders are included as part of the advance care directive.

Lastly, home care provision can be impacted by the unexpected. In the context of severe weather, natural disasters, and other unforeseen events, such as the COVID-19 pandemic, families experience reductions in home care nursing availability, inconsistency of equipment provision, changes in personal demands at work, and elimination of community-based/school-based service for therapies and routine education. Coupled with the fear of acquired infections, pragmatic challenges greatly impact parental fatigue, mental health, activities of daily living, and, ultimately, parent and child safety.

In summary, "evaluation" of the child, or young adult, with home ventilator needs requires a proactive approach to optimize outcomes and the lived experience of the child and family. System adaptations will be required as the complexities, capacity, and reach of home care technologies are ever increasing.

References

1. Panitch HB. Respiratory implications of pediatric neuromuscular disease. Respir Care. 2017;62(6):826–48.
2. Sobotka SA, Dholakia A, Agrawal RK, et al. Discharge practices for children with home mechanical ventilation across the United States. Key-informant perspectives. Ann Am Thorac Soc. 2020;17(11):1424–30.
3. Willis LD, Lowe G, Pearce P, et al. Transition from an ICU ventilator to a portable home ventilator in children. Respir Care. 2020;65(12):1791–9.
4. Kun SS, Edwards JD, Davidson Ward SL, Keens TG. Hospital readmissions for newly discharged pediatric home mechanical ventilation patients. Pediatr Pulmonol. 2012;47(4):409–14.
5. Sobotka SA, Lynch E, Peek ME, Graham RJ. Readmission drivers for children with medical complexity: home nursing shortages cause health crises. Pediatr Pulmonol. 2020;55(6):1474–80.
6. Nelson KE, Mahant S. Shared decision-making about assistive technology for the child with severe neurologic impairment. Pediatr Clin N Am. 2014;61(4):641–52.
7. Sterni LM, Collaco JM, Baker CD, et al. An official American thoracic society clinical practice guideline: pediatric chronic home invasive ventilation. Am J Respir Crit Care Med. 2016;193(8):e16–35.
8. Castro-Codesal ML, Olmstead DL, MacLean JE. Mask interfaces for home non-invasive ventilation in infants and children. Paediatr Respir Rev. 2019;32:66–72.
9. Graham RJ, Amar-Dolan LR, Roussin CJ, Weinstock PH. Bridging the stressful gap between ICU and home: medical simulation for pediatric patients and their families. Pediatr Crit Care Med. 2019;20(4):e221–4.
10. Kun SS, Nakamura CT, Ripka JF, Davidson Ward SL, Keens TG. Home ventilator low-pressure alarms fail to detect accidental decannulation with pediatric tracheostomy tubes. Chest. 2001;119(2):562–4.
11. Trucco F, Pedemonte M, Racca F, et al. Tele-monitoring in paediatric and young home-ventilated neuromuscular patients: a multicentre case-control trial. J Telemed Telecare. 2019;25(7):414–24.
12. Casavant DW, McManus ML, Parsons SK, Zurakowski D, Graham RJ. Trial of telemedicine for patients on home ventilator support: feasibility, confidence in clinical management and use in medical decision-making. J Telemed and Telecare. 2014;20(8):441–9.

13. Sobotka SA, Dholakia A, Berry JG, et al. Home nursing for children with home mechanical ventilation in the United States: key informant perspectives. Pediatr Pulmonol. 2020;55(12):3465–76.
14. Sobotka SA, Lynch E, Quinn MT, Awadalla SS, Agrawal RK, Peek ME. Unmet respite needs of children with medical technology dependence. Clin Pediatr (Phila). 2019;58(11–12):1175–86.
15. Sobotka SA, Foster C, Lynch E, Hird-McCorry L, Goodman DM. Attributable delay of discharge for children with long-term mechanical ventilation. J Pediatr. 2019;212:166–71.
16. Seear M, Kapur A, Wensley D, Morrison K, Behroozi A. The quality of life of home-ventilated children and their primary caregivers plus the associated social and economic burdens: a prospective study. Arch Dis Child. 2016;101(7):620–7.
17. Henderson CM, Raisanen JC, Shipman KJ, Jabre NA, Wilfond BS, Boss RD. Life with pediatric home ventilation: expectations versus experience. Pediatr Pulmonol. 2021;56(10):3366–73.
18. Edwards JD, Panitch HB, Constantinescu A, Miller RL, Stone PW. Survey of financial burden of families in the U.S. with children using home mechanical ventilation. Pediatr Pulmonol. 2018;53(1):108–16.
19. Graham RJ. Specialty services for children with special health care needs: supplement not supplant the medical home. Arch Dis Child. 2008;93(1):2–4.
20. Graham RJ. An opportunity: critical care beyond the intensive care unit. Pediatr Crit Care Med. 2005;6(3):327–8.
21. Sobotka SA, Gaur DS, Goodman DM, Agrawal RK, Berry JG, Graham RJ. Pediatric patients with home mechanical ventilation: the health services landscape. Pediatr Pulmonol. 2019;54(1):40–6.
22. Sherman JM, Davis S, Albamonte-Petrick S, et al. Care of the child with a chronic tracheostomy. This official statement of the American Thoracic Society was adopted by the ATS Board of Directors, July 1999. Am J Respir Crit Care Med. 2000;161(1):297–308.
23. Wasserman MG, Graham RJ, Mansbach JM. Airway bacterial colonization, biofilms and blooms, and acute respiratory infection. Pediatr Crit Care Med. 2022;23(10):e476–82.
24. Graham RJ, McManus ML, Rodday AM, Weidner RA, Parsons SK. Chronic respiratory failure: utilization of a pediatric specialty integrated care program. Healthc (Amst). 2017;5(1–2):23–8.
25. Graham RJ, McManus ML, Rodday AM, Weidner RA, Parsons SK. Pediatric specialty care model for management of chronic respiratory failure: cost and savings implications and misalignment with payment models. Pediatr Crit Care Med. 2018;19(5):412–20.
26. Willis LD. Transition from pediatric to adult care for young adults with chronic respiratory disease. Respir Care. 2020;65(12):1916–22.
27. Ali SO, Yeung T, McKeon M, et al. Patient and caregiver experiences at a Multidisciplinary Tracheostomy Clinic. Int J Pediatr Otorhinolaryngol. 2020;137:110250.
28. Edwards JD, Kun SS, Keens TG. Outcomes and causes of death in children on home mechanical ventilation via tracheostomy: an institutional and literature review. J Pediatr. 2010;157(6):955–959 e952.
29. Kohn J, McKeon M, Munhall D, Blanchette S, Wells S, Watters K. Standardization of pediatric tracheostomy care with "Go-bags". Int J Pediatr Otorhinolaryngol. 2019;121:154–6.
30. Conners GP, Kressly SJ, Perrin JM, et al. Nonemergency acute care: when it's not the medical home. Pediatrics. 2017;139(5):e20170629.
31. Dosa NP, Boeing NM, Ms N, Kanter RK. Excess risk of severe acute illness in children with chronic health conditions. Pediatrics. 2001;107(3):499–504.
32. Boss RD, Williams EP, Henderson CM, et al. Pediatric chronic critical illness: reducing excess hospitalizations. Hosp Pediatr. 2017; https://doi.org/10.1542/hpeds.2016-0185.
33. DeCourcey DD, Silverman M, Chang E, et al. Medication reconciliation failures in children and young adults with chronic disease during intensive and intermediate care. Pediatr Crit Care Med. 2017;18(4):370–7.
34. Berry JG, Hall DE, Kuo DZ, et al. Hospital utilization and characteristics of patients experiencing recurrent readmissions within children's hospitals. JAMA. 2011;305(7):682–90.

35. Berry JG, Graham DA, Graham RJ, et al. Predictors of clinical outcomes and hospital resource use of children after tracheotomy. Pediatrics. 2009;124(2):563–72.
36. Withers A, Wilson AC, Hall GL. Air travel and the risks of hypoxia in children. Paediatr Respir Rev. 2011;12(4):271–6.
37. Mohr LC. Hypoxia during air travel in adults with pulmonary disease. Am J Med Sci. 2008;335(1):71–9.
38. Allen K, Blascovich J. The value of service dogs for people with severe ambulatory disabilities. A randomized controlled trial. JAMA. 1996;275(13):1001–6.
39. Stace LB. Welcoming max: increasing pediatric provider knowledge of service dogs. Complement Ther Clin Pract. 2016;24:57–66.
40. Graham RJ, Rodday AM, Weidner RA, Parsons SK. The impact on family of pediatric chronic respiratory failure in the home. J Pediatr. 2016;175:40–6.
41. Edwards JD, Kun SS, Graham RJ, Keens TG. End-of-life discussions and advance care planning for children on long-term assisted ventilation with life-limiting conditions. J Palliat Care. 2012;28(1):21–7.

Care and Management of HMV Patients at Hospital

Karl Reiter

1 Introduction

Home mechanical ventilation (HMV) in children and adolescents is a multifaceted challenge not limited to proper respiratory care, although this is the central task. Most children on HMV have many more special needs depending on their underlying disease and developmental state, which should be addressed at home and after admission to the hospital.

HMV initiation may be viewed as a replication of intensive care into the home environment, where a dedicated and trained home care team successfully manages many of the inherent risks and problems in a ventilator-dependent child. Nevertheless, every child on HMV will—for acute or chronic reasons—be readmitted to and cared for in a PICU more than once and often multiple times during their life.

There is a scarcity of data regarding the type and acuity of emergency admissions to hospitals in HMV children. Our own published data spanning 295 patient-years of HMV in 54 patients showed a rate of 0.2 per patient-year of severe emergencies leading to acute PICU admission [20]. In a literature review including more than 12,000 pediatric patients, causes of death in decreasing order were progression of underlying disease, respiratory illness, and LTV accident with an overall mortality of 18% [10].

Healthcare systems varied widely within and between countries. Others have reported emergency treatment requirements in 1019 children and adolescents averaging 1.56 times per year per subject and hospitalizations averaging 160.8 days per year per subject [16]. In a cohort of infants with invasive HMV, rehospitalization was most commonly due to viral respiratory illness [2]. Educational level and

K. Reiter (✉)
University Children's Hospital at Dr. von Haunersches Kinderspital, Ludwig-Maximilians-University Munich, Muenchen, Germany
e-mail: karl.reiter@med.uni-muenchen.de

A. Kawaguchi et al. (eds.), *Prolonged and Long-Term Mechanical Ventilation in Children*, https://doi.org/10.1007/978-981-97-8903-0_19

availability of specialized home care among other factors certainly have a prominent influence on hospitalization rates.

Elective hospital admissions may vary from unit to unit and country to country depending on local resources (e.g., availability of PICU or IMC beds) and unit policy. Many stable patients may be regularly evaluated in day clinics although overnight studies should be done at least in unclear cases and patients with unacceptable symptoms. The opportunity to observe the patient (and caretaker's actions) over an extended period of time during a day and nighttime stay in the PICU often clarifies causes of symptoms otherwise unobtainable.

Very few data exist on specific problems, their handling, and outcomes in the hospitalized patient who is on chronic home mechanical ventilation. This text reflects in many respects our local experience spanning about 25 years of running a pediatric HMV program and will focus on respiratory and emergency issues.

2 Indications for Hospital Admission

Indications, albeit not an exhaustive list, for hospital admission are various and may be categorized into acute and elective.

- Acute:
  - Declining or low oxygen saturation by pulse oximetry
  - Infections: upper airway, lower airway, pneumonia
  - Aspiration
  - Atelectasis
  - Pneumothorax, cutaneous emphysema
  - Acute complications related to a tracheal cannula
  - Postischemic/hypoxic, post-resuscitation
  - Non-respiratory problems
  - Equipment malfunction
- Elective:
  - Control of efficiency and adequacy of HMV (e.g., polysomnography, tracheal cannula control by bronchoscopy), interface problems (e.g., leaks, pressure lesions, meteorism)
  - Echocardiography: pulmonary arterial hypertension, right-heart strain
  - Deteriorating neurology, failure to thrive, increasing frequency of hospital admissions
  - Tracheostomy-related surgery, adenotonsillectomy
  - Gastrointestinal surgery: gastrostomy/jejunostomy, fundoplication
  - PEG placement
  - Scoliosis surgery
  - Parent exhaustion

3 Setting and General Considerations

It is always a special challenge to the hospital care team when a pediatric HMV patient is admitted to the hospital. Patients and families usually adhere to daily routines taking care of many individual preferences, which involve all aspects of ventilatory care, care of the tracheostomy, positioning in neuromuscular patients, and timing of procedures among many others. It is paramount to take a history of all details of care including for example preferred positioning, anxieties regarding certain procedures, what a patient likes and dislikes, and what is calming a patient. Many patients are disabled in various respects, and, e.g., the application of hearing aids or glasses, if the patient is provided with these aids, should not be overlooked. It is always helpful to involve caretakers as much as possible in the hospital care of these patients.

In any case of hospital admission, it is advantageous for patients and the hospital care team to use their own equipment, especially the ventilator and the cough assist machine if equipped with this device with them. Patients are used to their ventilator and often are irritated by different flows and trigger sensitivities if an intensive care ventilator is used instead, although all parameters are selected identically in both machines. In addition, in NIV patients, intensive care ventilators often appear to be oversensitive regarding ventilation leaks leading to disturbingly frequent alarms in the absence of a threat to the patient. If the use of the patient's ventilator is not possible for any reason in this situation, usually a change in interface to reduce leaks is necessary. On the other hand, it can be very revealing for the hospital care team to directly observe the quality of ventilation provided by the patient's own ventilator and interface. Certainly, more sophisticated intensive care ventilators have to be used when more severe respiratory complications are apparent.

Patients are often supplied with a broad variety of ventilators and devices. Respiratory therapists, nurses, and physicians should feel safe in the handling of various home mechanical ventilators, cough assists, and suctioning and other auxiliary devices. The establishment of an experienced specialized team in an HMV program will be necessary to achieve this and be of invaluable help to the PICU or HDC team in caring for these complex patients.

Depending on local resources and the availability of a PICU bed, HMV patients are often cared for in a high-dependency unit (HDU). Ideally, this unit should be located near or within a PICU to have competent and trained personnel immediately available in the case of an acute emergency. Guidelines have been published on the requirements for physicians and nurses acutely caring for an HMV patient. They have to be knowledgeable and trained in tracheostomy care, cannula complications, and mechanical ventilators and other devices used in HMV. Guidelines have been published by the American and Australian/New Zealand societies [1, 5, 21].

4 Care of the Electively Admitted or Non-severe Acute HMV Patient

Various indications for hospital admission of the non-acute patient are detailed above, but most often embrace persistent suboptimal oxygenation or infectious complications. Suboptimal oxygenation, and airway infections accompanied by an increase in secretions, can often be handled at home by increasing ventilation pressures and inhalational therapy with physiotherapy. A physician-preset "infection mode" may be used at home in these circumstances. This, for example, can be characterized by an increase of 2–3 cmH_2O driving pressure and 1 or 2 cmH_2O PEEP. Admission to the hospital is often necessary when supplemental oxygen is needed despite these measures.

In the stable patient and if resources are available once yearly, control evaluations including a night at the hospital appear helpful. In our experience, during the years of COVID-related limitations leading to omissions of yearly controls at the hospital, several severe and unexpected HMV complications occurred. These were mostly related to tracheal cannula complications including tracheal perforations at the tip of the cannula and chronic underventilation.

Overnight stays at the hospital are useful in chronic HMV care for various reasons:

- In patients only ventilated at nighttime, an examination during a clinic visit during the day may include important data on the efficiency of HMV, but details of ventilation performance may be overlooked and HMV is therefore suboptimal.
- Respiratory physiology is different during supine positioning and sleep versus upright positioning during the day. This relates to reduced TLC caused in particular by upward pressure of the abdominal organs in the prone position and a decrease in ventilation of posterior parts of the lung among other factors.
- Triggering of the ventilator may be compromised during sleep, and ventilation leaks will be more prominent.
- In NIV patients, a decrease in muscle tone of the upper airways may lead to relevant obstruction.
- Ventilator adjustments can be probed within short time frames clinically and by controlling blood gases.
- Families without nursing coverage are at risk of getting exhausted either chronically or due to increased care requirements during infections or other complications of HMV and find some relief during hospital stays of their child.
- Guidance on how to deal with respective complications of HMV may be delivered more efficiently to parents during a hospital stay.

At admission, history is of paramount importance: thriving, rate of infections, quantity and quality of secretions, mental or activity deterioration, and headaches among many other often subtle symptoms hinting at inadequate ventilation. A detailed handover from the home care team is essential. A readout of monitoring devices and ventilator stored data will deliver objective data on the course of disease and ventilator use.

Clinical examination will clarify interface leaks and pressure injuries as well as excessive gastric air in NIV patients, adequacy of thoracic excursions and expiration time, gross ventilator synchrony with patient efforts, and abnormal auscultatory findings. Several blood gas checks in addition to pulse oximetry during awakeness and sleep and supine vs. upright position complement clinical findings. If available, transcutaneous or end-tidal CO2 measurements may be used, but values should be controlled by blood gas analysis.

In a patient with persistent suboptimal or unstable oxygenation, several possibilities have to be considered. Inadequacy of mechanical ventilation may be caused by inadequate ventilator mode or settings, especially too much reliance on spontaneous breathing efforts, patient-ventilator asynchrony/inconsistent triggering, or too low a PEEP. Increased quantity of bronchial secretions may be caused by chronic low-grade aspiration, persistent bacterial bronchitis, weak cough, or deteriorating muscular strength. Swallowing function, gastroesophageal reflux, and bacteriology of bronchial secretions or BAL should be investigated. Mechanical cough assistance should be initiated if weak cough is present. We have encountered massive bronchial secretion caused by too rapid weaning efforts from mechanical ventilation leading to microatelectases and noninfectious inflammation. Often, several etiological factors are in play.

5 Care of the HMV Patient with Acute Deterioration

In an emergency situation, general principles of intensive care are followed. In parallel to excluding non-respiratory acute diseases, in the HMV patient, special focus is on airway and pulmonary complications.

6 Acute Hypoxemia

Tracheal cannula dislocation or obstruction is easily identified and treated by reinsertion, handbag ventilation, and suctioning or cannula change. When insertion problems are encountered, a smaller cuffed cannula has to be used which always should be at hand in cannulated patients. If reinsertion is not successful or a smaller cannula is insufficient for ventilation, the tracheostomy has to be dilated in an emergency procedure using bougies under general anesthesia.

In noninvasively ventilated patients, an airway obstructed by secretions or vomitus has to be cleared by pharyngeal suctioning, handbag mask ventilation, and—in the case of tracheal or bronchial secretions—intensive physiotherapy. When the patient is used to a cough assist, this may be used. Rapid switching from mask ventilation to cough assist and back has to be performed because cough assist devices are not provided with supplemental oxygen flow. If less acute, ventilatory pressures and oxygen supplement may be increased to achieve sufficient chest excursions and oxygenation. Sometimes, only obstructed nasal passages caused by rhinitis need to be suctioned and decongestant nose drops applied to achieve major relief.

A chest X-ray is obligatory and may disclose pneumothorax, pneumonia, overinflation, pleural effusion, and atelectasis. A thoracic ultrasonography will show pleural effusions more quantitatively and may be equally sensitive for the diagnosis of pneumothorax in experienced hands.

In patients with secondary pulmonary arterial hypertension due to chronic respiratory disease in whom a shunt (e.g., ASD) is present, pulmonary hypertensive crises present with acute cyanosis and hemodynamic compromise. Echocardiography is essential in diagnosis and treatment monitoring.

7 Tracheal Cannula Complications

The most frequently encountered cannula complications are obstruction by thick tenacious secretions or dislocation. Both can easily be diagnosed clinically and corrected by suctioning and inhalational therapy or reinsertion, respectively. Sometimes, mucosal injury at the tip of the tracheal cannula may lead to obstructing granulomata. These should be diagnosed by flexible endoscopy through the cannula. Inserting a longer cannula bypassing the lesion will be the most important step in treatment. We use a salve containing steroids and an antibiotic applied on the cannula for local treatment of large granulomata, which accelerates healing significantly. If the lesion is close to the tracheal carina and bypassing by a longer cannula is not possible, a shorter cannula keeping distance to the lesion should be used and steroids applied by inhalation.

A rare tracheal cannula complication is perforation of the tip of the cannula through the posterior tracheal wall leading to mediastinal and cervical emphysema and inefficiency of ventilation. Here, bypassing the lesion using a longer cuffed cannula or tube will rescue the patient. In the majority, posterior tracheal perforations or traumatic dehiscence will eventually heal without surgery.

Bleeding in the tracheotomized patient is often concerning to the care team but in the majority of cases is caused by tracheobronchitis and does not interfere with oxygenation. Tracheoscopy through the tracheal cannula will reveal inflamed mucosa but is needed to exclude other causes of lower airway bleeding (e.g., overaggressive suctioning, cannula tip granuloma). In case of persistent local bleeding adrenaline, vasopressin or tranexamic acid can be applied locally through the bronchoscope.

Rarely, massive and life-threatening bleeding occurs when the tip of the cannula erodes the ventral tracheal wall and perforates into the truncus arteriosus. Here, a lifesaving measure is to bypass the erosion with a longer cannula or endotracheal tube introduced into the tracheostomy. Cuffed cannula or tubes have to be used to exert pressure on the bleeding site or at least to prevent blood aspiration to the lower airways. Emergency cardiothoracic surgery is needed to repair the arterial lesion.

Life-threatening lesions of the tracheal wall induced by a tracheal cannula tip should be preventable by regular bronchoscopic control investigations to direct the optimal cannula length and placement and identify lesions early. These controls will also show lesions induced by deep suctioning, which should lead to intensified teaching of the care team.

Intensive parent and caregiver education and the establishment of a dedicated team for tracheostomy care have been shown to reduce readmissions to hospital due to tracheal cannula complications [23]. Tracheostomata may narrow or develop scarring, which may hinder reinsertion of the cannula. There should always be a smaller sized cannula at hand, which should be routine during a hospital stay as well.

8 Pneumonia

Pneumonia with or without atelectasis is a major cause of hypoxemia or acutely deteriorating respiratory insufficiency in the HMV patient (Table 1).

Pneumonia is a clinical and radiological diagnosis confirmed by PCR and/or culture of bronchial secretions and in some cases positive blood culture. On the other hand, positive bacteriological findings in tracheobronchial secretions, especially *Pseudomonas* species, are often found in tracheotomized children and should be regarded as colonization unless clinical symptoms indicate infection [17, 25]. There are insufficient data to guide treatment in tracheostomy-related infections [14], and there is a risk of overuse of antibacterial agents with selection of resistant strains [18]. If infection is thought to be present, the choice of antibiotic treatment should take known colonization and local incidences into consideration but need not necessarily include *Pseudomonas* in the initial regimen as these bacteria seldom cause severe infection primarily. Fungal tracheobronchitis is rare with the exception of patients with disorders of granulocytes or severe immunodeficiency. Recently in adult, critically ill patients with influenza or COVID-19, severe tracheitis caused by *Aspergillus* species has been reported [9].

There are no data on the optimal length of antibiotic treatment in HMV patients. Especially in patients with reduced force of coughing secretion, clearance will be impeded significantly which may be favoring bacterial persistence in the peripheral airways or lung parenchyma. A prolonged antibiotic course therefore should be anticipated probably until all pertinent symptoms and signs have subsided. Equally unclear is when intravenous antibiotics may be switched to an orally/enterally applied antibiotic. Here, several factors usually have to be taken into account such as severity of disease, time since start of improvement, and reliability of the enteral route for sufficient absorption.

A recent cohort study in adult OSAS patients demonstrated an up to threefold increase in hospitalizations due to pneumonia compared to patients without OSAS [13]. Viral pneumonia may also be more frequent and severe in OSAS as has been

Table 1 Hypoxemia in the pediatric HMV patient

Symptom	Causes	Management principles
Hypoxemia		
Acute	Respiratory infection Aspiration Atelectasis Tracheostomy complications Pneumothorax Equipment malfunction	Pathogen identification, X-ray, antibiotics if indicated Bronchoscopy, X-ray, antibiotics X-ray, optimization of mechanical ventilation, positioning, physiotherapy, bronchoscopy Bronchoscopy, cannula change X-ray, drainage, optimization of mechanical ventilation Exchange for PICU devices
Subacute/ chronic	Excessive bronchial secretions: Recurrent aspiration Insufficient mechanical ventilation Inappropriate weaning Decreasing cough strength Infection (persistent bacterial bronchitis) Insufficient mechanical ventilation: Ventilatory leaks Inappropriate MV parameters Non-respiratory causes: Cardiovascular Abdominal: meteorism, hepatomegaly	Swallowing function, GERD Anticholinergics or Botox injections for excessive saliva Optimization of mechanical ventilation (increase PEEP) Stop or reduce weaning Physiotherapy, cough assist BAL in selected cases, antibiotics Optimize NIV interface Larger tracheal cannula or use of cuffed cannula Adjust according to blood gases and physiology Echocardiography

shown in adult individuals with influenza [22]. Recurrent microaspiration has been involved in pathogenesis as a predisposing factor. Although this has been studied in adult patients with OSAS, a proportion of pediatric NIV patients still may have upper airway obstruction in phases of suboptimal ventilation, and an analog mechanism may be at work.

9 Atelectasis

Atelectasis commonly underlies deterioration of oxygenation in HMV patients leading to or prolonging hospitalization (Fig. 1). Risk factors are severe neuromuscular disease, reduced force of cough, thickened or excess secretions, inflammation, and insufficient mechanical ventilation. Anatomical factors may be related to deformities of the thoracic cage with asymmetric restrictive physiology sometimes

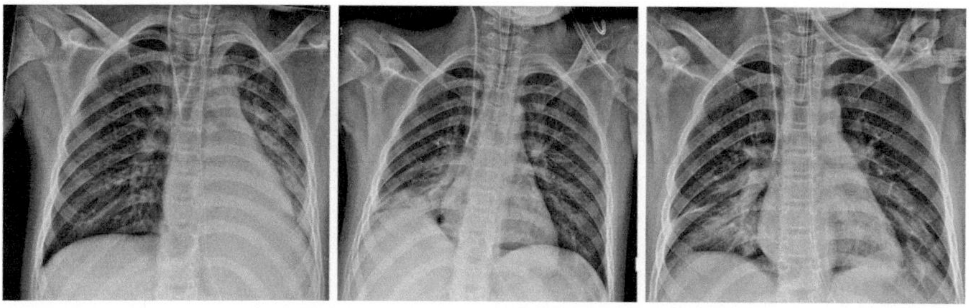

Fig. 1 Typical case of difficult weaning from invasive mechanical ventilation in a neuromuscular patient: 14-year-old patient, medullary tumor, tetraparesis. Recurrent atelectasis in varying localizations. No signs of infection. Patient and family declined tracheostomy. Successful extubation to noninvasive ventilation after 6 weeks using extensive physiotherapy, inhalational therapy with hypertonic saline, cough assist, and early mobilization. Bronchial stenosis was excluded by flexible endoscopy. Extubated at a PEEP of 8 cm H2O on pressure support of 17 cm H_2O. Sequence of chest X-rays within 14 days: atelectasis in left lower lung field, right lower lung field, both lower lung fields with improvement on the right, and deterioration on the left side

accompanied by distortion of bronchial anatomy and stenosis, e.g., in severe scoliosis. Bronchi may be compressed by enlarged lymph nodes. The diagnostic process should include tracheobronchial cultures. When bronchial stenosis is suspected (e.g., with refractory atelectasis or recurrence in the same location), bronchoscopy is indicated. This may be supplemented by chest CT to clarify anatomical relationships with adjacent vessels or lymph nodes.

Treatment of atelectasis includes intensive physiotherapy and positioning (keeping the affected side up, prone positioning with posteriorly located atelectasis). The use of a cough assist may be of great value. Inhalational treatment using normal or hypertonic saline to loosen thick secretions is essential. Concentrations up to 5.85% saline may be used if effective, but with higher concentrations, mucosal irritation and bronchoconstriction are a concern. Mucolytics per inhalation or systemically such as acetylcysteine may be worth a trial. Sometimes, an overwhelming effect is seen when acetylcysteine is started with loads of fluidic secretions, which may compromise respiration especially in NIV patients. Although evidence is lacking, many atelectatic regions will be colonized with bacteria, and antibiotic treatment should therefore be contemplated in every case.

Often, a prominent causal factor leading to atelectasis is suboptimal mechanical ventilation or overenthusiastic weaning efforts. Ventilation leaks through ill-fitting masks or small tracheal cannula should be sought and corrected. PEEP stability is essential, and an increase in PEEP is often helpful in atelectasis.

In refractory cases, many centers will use flexible bronchoscopy to check for mucus plugs or bronchial stenosis. Local application of mucolytics, DNase (if granulocyte-rich mucus is suspected), or surfactant may be discussed in individual cases. Rarely, plastic bronchitis may be encountered, and bronchial casts have to be removed by bronchoscopy. No recommendations exist on the timing of bronchoscopy in persistent atelectasis. Our local practice is to consider bronchoscopy when other measures are unsuccessful after 1 or 2 weeks.

10 Aspiration

Massive aspiration leading to hypoxemia usually is evident by history including vomiting and/or presence of food remnants in pharyngeal secretions. In tracheotomized patients, diagnosis is straightforward by finding food by tracheal suctioning. Further clinical signs and symptoms are acute dyspnea, rales by auscultation, and opacities in the chest X-ray.

If aspirated material contains solid parts, urgent bronchoscopy is indicated. With liquid food aspiration, aggressive physiotherapy and antibiotic treatment should be initiated. In many instances, bronchoconstriction is prominent, and inhalational therapy with beta-sympathomimetics is helpful. Placement of an enterostomy tube should strongly be considered in patients with compromised swallowing function, which additionally may help optimize nutritional status [24].

When the acute event has subsided, evaluation for the presence of gastroesophageal reflux should be considered. Fundoplication is often necessary, especially in patients with neuromuscular disease [7].

Gastroesophageal reflux may also lead to chronic low-grade aspiration going unnoticed by caretakers as most times no acute events are apparent and gastric contents may be of minimal volume. Recurrent aspiration causes chronic bronchial inflammation with ensuing increase in secretions, bronchial hyperreagibility, bronchiectasis, and chronic parenchymatous pulmonary injury. The diagnostic process includes gastroscopy, esophageal pH-metry or impedance probe, radiography, and bronchoscopy with bronchoalveolar lavage. Lipid-laden macrophages in the BAL fluid are regarded as a sign of aspiration but lack adequate sensitivity and specificity.

11 When to Intubate a Child on NIV?

The indication for tracheal intubation of a child on NIV will follow general intensive care rules although these are not well defined and not validated in larger numbers of patients.

Major points to be considered are the following:

- An NIV patient in severe dyspnea, with severe hypoxemia and/or a decrease in vigilance, should be endotracheally intubated immediately.
- The noninvasive interface should be optimized if possible, e.g., by the use of a full-face mask.
- Deteriorating oxygenation with requirement for stable high PEEP (e.g., >8 cm H_2O) and/or high peak pressures (>25 cm H_2O). SpO_2/FIO_2 <200 may be used as the clear limit below which invasive ventilation should be established. A value of SpO_2/FIO_2 below 264 is defined as ARDS [1001].
- Severe problems with secretions despite intensive physiotherapy, inhalations, mucolytics, and intensive use of a cough assist (e.g., +30 – 35 cm H_2O inspiratory pressures; −30 – 35 cmH_2O in expiratory phase).
- Shock and coma are clear indications for endotracheal intubation.

12 Mechanical Ventilation

Apart from following general rules of mechanical ventilation, specific considerations in the HMV patient include minimizing ventilatory leaks and optimizing upper airway patency. In noninvasively ventilated children, a nasal mask may need to be substituted by a full-face mask or a helmet. Rarely, negative-pressure devices are used for mechanical ventilation, although this mode is in principle more physiological than positive-pressure ventilation. Negative-pressure ventilators are not available as easy as other machines, nursing access to the patient is compromised, and most importantly collapse of the upper airways by the induced negative airway pressure is a major limitation.

Cautious suctioning of the nasal passages and applying adstringent nasal drops should not be overlooked in the NIV patient with upper airway infection.

In tracheotomized patients with difficult ventilation, a switch to a larger sized tracheal cannula can be considered or a cuffed one if this has not been used before. In neuromuscular patients, use of a cough assist may be of great help in both noninvasively and invasively ventilated patients.

13 Weaning from Invasive Mechanical Ventilation

If significantly higher ventilation pressures compared to their respective chronic ventilation parameters have to be applied during acute respiratory deterioration, a weaning strategy has to be considered. There are several studies on pediatric critically ill patients comparing different approaches and using various respiratory parameters to predict successful extubation [4, 6]. No single strategy has been shown to be superior, and physician experience may be as good as detailed algorithms. Additional complexity arises due to different targets in HMV patients as these persistently need mechanical ventilation and as a first goal will be extubated to continuous NIV.

Even the previously normal child will lose muscle volume and strength when undergoing prolonged mechanical ventilation. In adult critically ill and ventilated patients, it has been shown to take weeks for them to regain their muscle strength. In pediatric HMV patients who in the majority start with reduced muscle strength due to neuromuscular disease, recovery of respiratory muscle strength should be anticipated to last significantly longer.

For a successful weaning strategy, several aspects will have to be considered. These include timing and sequence of reductions in mechanical ventilation support, measures to support recovery of muscle strength, avoiding or treating contractures, avoiding or reducing delirium, adequate nutrition, and aggressive management of airway secretions among others.

In many patients with neuromuscular disease, recovery of muscle strength is not an issue due to their underlying disease. In children with less severe muscle hypotonia or other than neuromuscular disease having led to HMV, reconditioning of respiratory muscle strength may be achieved by intermittent training. There is no clear evidence of the efficiency of any strategy to do this [19], especially in the HMV population. Nevertheless, our suggested practice is to intersperse short periods of pressure-reduced assisted spontaneous ventilation modes (e.g., PSV). These will be kept until increasing respiratory frequency or even minimal signs of distress appear and will be cautiously extended daily. No training effect on respiratory muscles has been shown for increasing trigger thresholds.

A recently put forward concept of early mobilization in PICU patients embraces many of these issues including broad anti-delirium measures and physical mobilization of the mechanically ventilated child [12]. A dedicated multiprofessional team is essential. Unfortunately, resources may be too limited in many hospitals to achieve this.

14 When to Extubate?

When a child on chronic NIV HMV has been endotracheally intubated due to acute-on-chronic respiratory insufficiency and is improving, the optimal time point for extubation cannot be assessed by conventional ICU criteria. The aim is to achieve a level of ventilatory support to result in safe NIV after extubation, which should be in the order of previous ventilatory parameters.

If any mode of respiratory muscle function monitoring using, e.g., esophageal pressures will be of help as a further quantitative parameter of muscle strength in the decision to extubate has not been investigated [15].

Guidance may be derived from the work by Bach in SMA patients [3]. Criteria for extubation readiness have here been specified as follows:

- The child has to be afebrile
- No supplemental oxygen supply to achieve SaO2 >94%
- Chest X-ray cleared or clearing
- No respiratory depressants
- Airway suctioning only required 1 or 2 times during 8 h
- Clear nasal airway

International recommendations on weaning the pediatric patient from mechanical ventilation [1] are available but do not specifically give advice on the HMV patient. Two large RCTs comparing protocolized vs. non-protocolized liberation strategies in critically ill children did not reach consistent results [4, 6]. Therefore, an optimal weaning strategy has not been shown. A major confounding factor identified in these studies, namely residual sedation level, is most probably at play in HMV patients as well.

15 When to Bronchoscope?

A list of suggested indications for bronchoscopy and proposed management is provided in Table 2. In tracheotomized patients, tracheoscopy through the tracheal cannula should routinely be performed at least once a year to control for cannula position and any lesions at the tip of the cannula or at the position of the cannula cuff as well as inflammatory changes caused by, for instance, persistent bacterial infection or recurrent aspiration. This can be done in non-anesthetized pediatric

Table 2 Indications for bronchoscopy in the hospitalized pediatric HMV patient

	Symptoms and causes	Management
Massive or large-particle aspiration	Hypoxemia, atelectasis	Suctioning or foreign body extraction
Persistent atelectasis	Hypoxemia Mucus plug, plastic bronchitis Bronchial stenosis (e.g., lymphadenopathy, intrinsic, vascular compression) Foreign body Persistent infection	Suctioning or foreign body extraction Local DNase, surfactant (in selected cases) Often CT helpful BAL, antibiotics
Hemoptysis	Infection (most common cause) Tracheostomy related: Cannula tip granuloma Erosion of artery Tracheitis Overaggressive suctioning Mucosal desiccation Bronchial artery bleeding (in cystic fibrosis)	Antibiotics, if acute bacterial Change cannula length (bypass granuloma), less stiff cannula, local steroid Local epinephrine/vasopressin/tranexamic acid, bypass with cuffed cannula or endotracheal tube, position cuff to compress bleeding site/prevent aspiration, surgery when massive Antibiotics, if acute bacterial Instruct caregivers Increase humidification Local epinephrine/vasopressin/tranexamic acid, endobronchial blocker if massive Embolization by interventional radiology
Difficulty with cannula insertion	Constrictive stoma, narrow channel-like stoma	Interventional dilatation, surgery if unsuccessful
Persistent pulmonary infection	Pneumonia with resistant or atypical pathogen	BAL (in selected cases)
Obstruction of the upper airway in NIV patients	Inefficient ventilation	Depending on cause: nasal steroid, adenotomy may be options
Suspected perforation of the posterior tracheal wall	Mediastinal and cutaneous emphysema	Change cannula length (bypass defect), use cuffed cannula (surgery rarely needed)

patients. Any sign of new and persistent airway stenosis should lead to bronchoscopy. This may include stridor, need for increased ventilator pressures, or overinflation of one or both lungs or specific lobes.

In a child with acute respiratory distress, foreign body aspiration should also be taken into consideration. Urgent bronchoscopy will be lifesaving. In a child with neuromuscular disease, tenacious secretions may behave like a foreign body as patients may not have force enough to completely cough them out.

Further urgent indications for bronchoscopy are massive tracheobronchial bleeding referred to above and the inability to introduce the tracheal cannula. This may be caused by narrowing of the tracheostoma by a scar or a granuloma, which may occur in the trachea as well. As an emergency procedure, a smaller cannula should be introduced if possible and the stomal canal dilated with a metal dilator to a size accepting the usual cannula of the child. If scarring of the tracheostomy recurs, a surgical approach should be considered.

Many practitioners will refer to bronchoscopy when atelectasis is refractory to conservative measures within a time frame of 1 or 2 weeks. An exception is an atelectatic pneumonia where bronchoscopy will only be of value in cases refractory to standard antibiotic treatment, and atypical bacteria or fungi are suspected to identify microbial agents in bronchoalveolar lavage specimens.

In pediatric patients on NIV, bronchoscopy will require anesthesia or deep sedation in almost any case which obviously entails much more risk to the patient compared to a bronchoscopy through a tracheal cannula. Therefore, in nonurgent situations, it seems to be wise to be hesitant. If there are signs of increasing upper airway obstruction, endoscopic investigation may be limited to the nasopharyngeal airway and supraglottic and glottic structures which can be performed using local anesthesia with or without light sedation.

Adenotonsillar hypertrophy is a finding frequently encountered in children with obstructive sleep apnea and can significantly impede nasal ventilation. In this case, adenotomy or adenotonsillectomy depending on the size of the tonsils should be undertaken.

Posterior laryngitis identified by laryngoscopy hints at gastroesophageal reflux although specificity and sensitivity appear moderate.

16 Various Issues

In the adult critically ill population, prophylactic anticoagulation is standard in the absence of contraindications. This generally is extended to young adults. There is no evidence or guidelines regarding chronically ventilated and immobile pediatric patients if prophylactic anticoagulation should be considered in these patients. Incidence rates of thromboembolism in this patient group have not been reported but in our experience seem to be very low.

Prophylactic anticoagulation in the pediatric HMV patient may be considered when further risk factors such as genetically determined thrombophilia or local vascular factors are present.

17 Special Needs

Families caring for an HMV child carry a large burden in their daily life regarding constraints of own activity, disturbed sleep, and many worries and anxiety concerning the well-being of their child. These are aggravated with acute complications leading to hospital admission [11]. Decisions regarding the continuation of treatment or letting a child die for not prolonging suffering sometimes emerge with complications and are very hard to bear for many parents. Feelings of guilt and incompetence may occur and should be addressed. Special attention should be given to healthy siblings whose needs are often underestimated. In addition, hospital admission often creates problems with the parent's workplace as they want to stay with their child at hospital. If resources are available, these should be dealt with by a dedicated team of social workers and psychologists.

Patients with severe muscular hypotonia due to neuromuscular disease need meticulous positioning and frequent change of position for their comfort and to avoid pressure ulcers. Experienced and intensive physiotherapy and positioning sometimes including special mattresses are essential.

Optimal care of the pediatric HMV patient at hospital is accomplished best by establishment of an experienced and committed interprofessional team. In addition to medical care entailing many challenging issues, special needs of the patient and the family have to be addressed. The experience of home caregivers is often invaluable and rich in details to be considered in the care of an HMV patient. This information should actively be sought as it facilitates care and rehabilitation often enormously.

The need for social and psychological support for patients and their families or caregivers should not be underestimated, and if available expert advice by psychologists, child life specialists, and social workers is needed. Informational booklets have been developed (e.g., [8]) and are welcomed as supplementary information by many parents. In many cases, the involvement of palliative care specialists at an early time point will be of significant help to support patients, families, and caregivers. Helpful guidance in preparation for discharge from the hospital has been provided by the American and Australian societies [5, 21].

References

1. Abu-Sultaneh S, Iyer NP, Fernández A, Gaies M, González-Dambrauskas S, Hotz JC, Kneyber MCJ, López-Fernández YM, Rotta AT, Werho DK, Baranwal AK, Blackwood B, Craven HJ, Curley MAQ, Essouri S, Fioretto JR, Hartmann SM, Jouvet P, Korang SK, Rafferty GF, Ramnarayan P, Rose L, Tume LN, Whipple EC, Wong JJM, Emeriaud G, Mastropietro CW, Napolitano N, Newth CJL, Khemani RG. Executive Summary: International Clinical Practice Guidelines for Pediatric Ventilator Liberation, A PALISI Network Document. Am J Respir Crit Care Med. 2022; https://doi.org/10.1164/rccm.202204-0795OC. Online ahead of print.
2. Akangire G, Manimtim W, Nyp M, Townley N, Dai H, Norberg M, Taylor JB. Factors leading to rehospitalization for tracheostomized and ventilator-dependent infants through 2 years of age. J Perinatol. 2017;37(7):857–63.

3. Bach JR, Niranjan V, Weaver B. Spinal muscular atrophy type 1: a noninvasive respiratory management approach. Chest. 2000;117:1100–5.
4. Blackwood B, Tume LN, Morris KP, Clarke M, McDowell C, Hemming K, Peters MJ, McIlmurray L, Jordan J, Agus A, Murray M, Parslow R, Walsh TS, Macrae D, Easter C, Feltbower RG, McAuley DF, Collaborators S. Effect of a sedation and ventilator liberation protocol vs usual care on duration of invasive mechanical ventilation in pediatric intensive care units: a randomized clinical trial. JAMA. 2021;326:401–10.
5. Chawla J, Edwards EA, Griffiths AL, Nixon GM, Suresh S, Twiss J, Vandeleur M, Waters KA, Wilson AC, Wilson S, Tai A. Ventilatory support at home for children: a joint position paper from the Thoracic Society of Australia and New Zealand/Australasian Sleep Association. Respirology. 2021;26(10):920–37.
6. Curley MA, Wypij D, Watson RS, Grant MJ, Asaro LA, Cheifetz IM, Dodson BL, Franck LS, Gedeit RG, Angus DC, Matthay MA, Investigators RS, the Pediatric Acute Lung I, Sepsis Investigators N. Protocolized sedation vs usual care in pediatric patients mechanically ventilated for acute respiratory failure: a randomized clinical trial. JAMA. 2015;313:379–89.
7. Durkin ET, et al. Early laparoscopic fundoplication and gastrostomy in infants with spinal muscular atrophy type 1. J Paediatric Surgery. 2008;43(11):2031–7.
8. Edwards JD, Panitch HB, George M, Cirrilla A, Grunstein E, Wolfe J, Nelson JE, Miller RL. Development and validation of a novel informational booklet for pediatric long-term ventilation decision support. Pediatr Pulmonol. 2021;56(5):1198–204.
9. Feys S, Gonçalves SM, Khan M, Choi S, Boeckx B, Chatelain D, Cunha C, Debaveye Y, Hermans G, Hertoghs M, Humblet-Baron S, Jacobs C, Lagrou K, Marcelis L, Maizel J, Meersseman P, Nyga R, Seldeslachts L, Starick MR, Thevissen K, Vandenbriele C, Vanderbeke L, Vande Velde G, Van Regenmortel N, Vanstapel A, Vanmassenhove S, Wilmer A, Van De Veerdonk FL, De Hertogh G, Mombaerts P, Lambrechts D, Carvalho A, Van Weyenbergh J, Wauters J. Lung epithelial and myeloid innate immunity in influenza-associated or COVID-19-associated pulmonary aspergillosis: an observational study. Lancet. Respir Med. 2022;10(12):1147–59. https://doi.org/10.1016/S2213-2600(22)00259-4. Online ahead of print.
10. Foy CM, Koncicki ML, Edwards JD. Liberation and mortality outcomes in pediatric long-term ventilation: a qualitative systematic review. Pediatr Pulmonol. 2020;55(11):2853–62.
11. Graham RJ, Pemstein DM, Curley MA. Experiencing the pediatric intensive care unit: perspective from parents of children with severe antecedent disabilities. Crit Care Med. 2009;37(6):2064–70.
12. Ista E, Redivo J, Kananur P, Choong K, Colleti J Jr, Needham DM, Awojoodu R, Kudchadkar SR, International P-PI. ABCDEF bundle practices for critically ill children: an international survey of 161 PICUs in 18 countries. Crit Care Med. 2022;50:114–25.
13. Khemani RG, Smith LS, Zimmerman JJ, Erickson S; Pediatric acute lung injury consensus conference group. Pediatric acute respiratory distress syndrome: definition, incidence, and epidemiology: proceedings from the Pediatric Acute Lung Injury Consensus Conference. Pediatr Crit Care Med. 2015;16(5 Suppl 1):S23–40.
14. Lutsey PL, Zineldin I, Misialek JR, Full KM, Lakshminarayan K, Ishigami J, Cowan L, Matsushita K, Demmer RT. Obstructive sleep apnea and subsequent risk of hospitalization with pneumonia, respiratory infection, and total infection: the Atherosclerosis Risk in Communities Study. Chest. 2023;163:942–52.
15. Morrison JM, Hassan A, Kysh L, Dudas RA, Russell CJ. Diagnosis, management, and outcomes of pediatric tracheostomy-associated infections: a scoping review. Pediatr Pulmonol. 2022;57(5):1145–56.
16. Mortamet G, Crulli B, Fauroux B, Emeriaud G. Monitoring of respiratory muscle function in critically ill children. Pediatr Crit Care Med. 2020;21(5):e282–90.
17. Pai S, Kung P, Chou W, Kuo T, Tsai W. Survival and medical utilization of children and adolescents with prolonged ventilator-dependent and associated factors. PLoS One. 2017;12(6):e0179274.

18. Perez-Losada M, Graham RJ, Coquillette M, et al. The temporal dynamics of the tracheal microbiome in tracheostomised patients with and without lower respiratory infections. PLoS One. 2017;12(8):e0182520.
19. Perez-Losada M, Graham RJ, Coquillette M, et al. Tracheal microbiota in patients with a tracheostomy before, during and after an acute respiratory infection. Pediatr Infect Dis J. 2018;37(11):e269–71.
20. Ramnarayan P, Blackwood B, Khemani RG. What's new in paediatric ventilator liberation? Intensive Care Med. 2022;48:1635–7.
21. Reiter K, Pernath N, Pagel P, Hiedi S, Hoffmann F, Schoen C, Nicolai T. Risk factors for morbidity and mortality in pediatric home mechanical ventilation. Clin Pediatr (Phila). 2011;50:237–43.
22. Sterni LM, Collaco JM, Baker CD, Carroll JL, Sharma GD, Brozek JL, Finder JD, Ackerman VL, Arens R, Boroughs DS, Carter J, Daigle KL, Dougherty J, Gozal D, Kevill K, Kravitz RM, Kriseman T, MacLusky I, Rivera-Spoljaric K, Tori AJ, Ferkol T, Halbower AC, ATS Pediatric Chronic Home Ventilation Workgroup. An official American Thoracic Society clinical practice guideline: pediatric chronic home invasive ventilation. Am J Respir Crit Care Med. 2016;193(8):e16–35.
23. Tsai M, Chen H, Li H, Tsai Y, Yang Y, Liu C, Lee Y, Hsu C, Lee L. Sleep apnea and risk of influenza-associated severe acute respiratory infection: real-world evidence. Nat Sci Sleep. 2022;14:901–9.
24. Van Horn A, Kim HM, Helman J, Valora H, Epperson M, Fayson S, Brown D, Zopf D. Reduction in inpatient readmissions following implementation of a dedicated tracheostomy care team. Int J Pediatr Otorhinolaryngol. 2022;162:111282.
25. Wadman RI, De Amicis R, Brusa C, Battezzati A, Bertoli S, Davis T, Main M, Manzur A, Mastella C, Munot P, Imbrigiotta N, Schottlaender L, Sarkozy A, Trucco F, Baranello G, Scoto M, Muntoni F. Feeding difficulties in children and adolescents with spinal muscular atrophy type 2. Neuromuscul Disord. 2021;31(2):101–12.
26. Wasserman MG, Graham RJ, Mansbach JM. Airway bacterial colonization, biofilms and blooms, and acute respiratory infection. Pediatr Crit Care Med. 2022;23(10):e476–82.

Complications of Prolonged Mechanical Ventilation

Julio Parrilla

1 Introduction

Patients requiring prolonged mechanical ventilation (PMV) are rapidly increasing in number, as improved ICU care has resulted in many patients surviving acute respiratory failure only to then require prolonged mechanical ventilatory assistance during convalescence [1].

PMV has become a realistic alternative to death from progressive respiratory failure for many children with chronic respiratory illness. Estimated 2.5–3% of the population admitted to pediatric ICUs require prolonged ventilation [2].

The earliest reported experiences of PMV in children came from the polio epidemic that began in the 1930s and ended in the late 1950s. The polio epidemic was a powerful driver of the development of intensive care units and life support technologies. Practically, all of these patients were treated with negative-pressure devices [3].

Emphasize that a wide number of iatrogenic factors have been associated with PMV. First among these is the delay of weaning due to failure to appreciate ventilator liberation capabilities by not using appropriately frequent assessments or using inappropriately slow reductions in support strategies. Inappropriate ventilator settings can also slow the withdrawal process through imposed muscle loading or patient-ventilator asynchrony [4]. The result is unnecessary sedation, due to either asynchrony or poor monitoring of the actual need for sedation. As noted above, PICU-related stress, as well as sleep deprivation, can lead to altered mental status that can lead to overemployment of sedatives [5].

Nowadays, there is limited evidence to determine the definition of PMV in children. PMV has been defined by the National Association for Medical Direction on Respiratory Care as the need for at least 6 h of ventilatory support per day for 21

J. Parrilla (✉)
Virgen del Rocio Hospital, Seville, Spain

A. Kawaguchi et al. (eds.), *Prolonged and Long-Term Mechanical Ventilation in Children*, https://doi.org/10.1007/978-981-97-8903-0_20

consecutive days. In a recent paper, Colleti et al. reviewed 30 articles for qualitative analysis and found a wide variety of definitions, varying from 48 h to 6 months. The most frequently used definitions of prolonged mechanical ventilation were greater than 7 days, greater than 14 days, and greater than 21 days. The variety of definitions is a sign of the need for a consensus definition of pediatric PMV [6].

Increasing the duration of mechanical ventilation can lead to many challenging complications such as ventilator-associated pneumonia (VAP), neuromuscular disorders, diaphragmatic atrophy, laryngeal and tracheal lesions, lung complications, an increased length of ICU stay, and an unfavorable discharge destination [7].

PMV includes at least three differentiated groups of patients:

Patients successfully weaned from the ventilator after 14 days in the PICU
Patients weaned from the tube but switched to home noninvasive ventilation (VNI)
Patients requiring tracheostomy and long-term ventilation

Although they will share some complications in common, the kind and frequency of these complications will vary among the groups.

2 Complications of PMV in the PICU

2.1 Infectious Complications

Ventilator-associated tracheobronchitis (VAT) is a common infection during PMV. Several studies suggest that VAT results in longer ICU stay and hence an increase in healthcare costs. Uncertainties remain, however, regarding the cost/benefit balance of VAT treatment with antibiotics. The importance of VAT resides in its possible association with VAP. Frequent changes and manipulation of endotracheal tube (ETT) or tracheostomy tube (TT), the use of saline solution during secretion suctioning, and the presence of *Pseudomonas aeruginosa*, *Staphylococcus epidermidis*, and *Candida albicans* in the ETT correlate positively with VAP [8]. Infection of tracheostomy site is more frequent in the immediate postoperative period and could affect wound healing.

However, VAP is the most important infectious complication associated with mechanical ventilation (MV) due to possible consequences in terms of morbidity and mortality. The reported incidence of VAP varies widely between studies, ranging from 5% to 67%, with 1 to 63 episodes per 1000 ventilator days, and may account for approximately 20% of PICU nosocomial infections [9]. In summary, VAP occurs in approximately 10% of mechanically ventilated patients, of which 13% are fatal complications [10].

It is generally accepted that nosocomial bacteria or the patient's own flora colonizes the upper respiratory tract prior to lung infection, but only a small proportion of patients develop pneumonia. In the pediatric population, risk factors associated with nosocomial bacterial airway colonization include duration of MV, prolonged artificial airway (especially tracheostomy tubes), and humidification and suction systems. Ventilation for more than 48 h, underlying respiratory disease, genetic syndrome, immunodeficiency, discharge from pediatric intensive care unit to this unit, use of H2 antagonists, immunosuppressants, neuromuscular blocking agents, anesthetics, previous use of antibiotics, blood flow infection, gastroesophageal reflux, altered level of consciousness, and coma are risk factors for developing VAP [11].

The most commonly accepted clinical definition of VAP is pneumonia that occurs after a patient is intubated and supported by mechanical ventilation [12].

Although no minimum time has been established before an infection is defined as VAP, it is generally accepted that this should be greater than 48 h. The initial diagnosis is based on clinical suspicion and the presence of at least one of the following features on two or more serial chest radiographs: new or progressive radiologic infiltrates, consolidations, cavities, and pneumatoceles in infants younger than 1 year of age. In addition, standard diagnostic criteria include at least two or three of the following (under 12 years of age only): fever >38 °C or hypothermia <36.5 °C; changes in sputum volume or characteristics, or need for more suctioning; new-onset or worsening cough or dyspnea or tachypnoea or apnea; rales or bronchial breath sounds; or wheezing or rhonchi [10].

The concept of VAP is defined as a preventable injury leading to a worsening of the lung status and requiring increased ventilatory support. The diagnosis of VAP in pediatric patients requires an increase in mean airway pressure (MAP) greater than or equal to 4 cmH2O, or an increase in FiO2 of greater than or equal to 0.25 after two or more days of minimum daily MAP or FiO2 stabilization or decline. As a diagnostic criterion, we must consider an increase in PEEP levels greater than or equal to 2 cm H2O [13].

When abnormal temperature (<36 °C or >38 °C) or higher or lower white cell count (WBC ≤4000 or ≥15,000 cells/ml) is present and one or more antibiotics not prescribed before are given that are continued for at least 4 days, we can confirm the diagnosis of VAP. A positive diagnostic test for respiratory infection or the presence of purulence would meet the criteria for a possible pneumonia, while those with both purulence and positive quantitative or semiquantitative cultures have probable pneumonia. Probable pneumonia can also be triggered by suggestive histopathological features, positive pleural-fluid cultures, or diagnostic tests for legionella and selected viruses. Serum biomarkers such as C-reactive protein (CRP) or procalcitonin (PCT) can help in diagnosis [14].

2.2 *Neuromuscular Complications*

These effects depend largely on the drug used to optimize MV. The main drugs used are sedatives, analgesics, and neuromuscular blocking agents. Understanding the pharmacokinetics and pharmacodynamics of these drugs can help reduce their side effects so that when they do occur, they can be identified and treated appropriately. Muscle weakness associated with neuromuscular blocking agents has been reported in neonates and children, especially in patients with renal insufficiency or those receiving concomitant corticosteroids. In children, critical illness polyneuropathy can be difficult to diagnose, but it remains an important cause of morbidity. It is less common than in adult patients and is usually more benign and resolves more quickly [15].

Physical therapy started as soon as possible after the onset of MV can help shorten the time to return to function, although it does not appear to reduce the number of days in MV and length of PICU stay. We must not forget the effect of invasive MV on diaphragm function, whether atrophy from underuse or diaphragm damage from excessive use [16].

2.3 Laryngeal and Tracheal Lesions

Adequate and continuous humidification of inhaled gas and frequent suctioning of respiratory secretions are required during PMV to prevent obstruction of the artificial airway. During bronchial aspiration, the mucous membrane may be damaged due to negative pressure, resulting in granulomas in the airway. Although the most common lesion is located on the tracheal wall, with subglottic stenosis predominating, these complications are due to the fact that this area is the narrowest part of the airway in infants and children [17]. If the pressure of the tracheal cuff is above 20–25 mmHg, the blood flow of the mucosa may be reduced, resulting in ischemia, and the tracheal wall in the corresponding area may be easily damaged. Airway obstruction can also resolve spontaneously or with medical treatment, mainly due to granulomas. However, when fibrotic changes occur in the tracheal wall, they are usually irreversible and surgery may be required to restore adequate tracheal lumen [18].

Other lesions such as vocal cord dysfunction, fibrin pseudomembrane formation, tracheal dilation, and tracheomalacia are less common.

2.4 Pulmonary Complications

The application of excessive stretching force (strain), overpressure (stress), and periodic opening of the alveoli allow the penetration of most of the intracellular mediators into the extracellular space, either by rupturing the cell (trauma) or by activating signaling pathways, called mechanotransducers in epithelial, endothelial, or inflammatory cells. Some mediators directly damage the lungs, and others can initiate processes that lead to pulmonary fibrosis. The biological response to mechanical force is called biotrauma. Due to damage to the epithelium and alveolar capillary membrane, bacteria, inflammatory mediators, and degradation products can be transferred to the intravascular space. This translocation may be the cause of multiple organ dysfunction in mechanically ventilated critically ill patients. This theory explains the effects of ventilator-induced lung injury (VILI) but not its activation [19].

We have to consider the barotrauma theory or injury due to high transpulmonary pressure during MV. High alveolar distension pressures are associated with high mortality from alveolar rupture, which can accumulate air in the extra-alveolar space, leading to serious complications such as pneumothorax, mediastinal emphysema, subcutaneous emphysema, and, less commonly in pediatric patients, pneumoperitoneum, pneumopericardium, or air embolism. However, this theory may be questioned as it does not fully account for VILI, since the airway pressures of up to 150 cm H2O observed during musicians' performances only exceptionally cause extra-alveolar air leakage. Likewise, the volutrauma theory or overdistension injury may influence the pathogenesis of VILI, whereby lung volumes are able to produce diffuse alveolar damage characterized by lung hyperinflation and endothelial and epithelial cell damage, affecting capillary permeability changes, and nonhydrostatic lung function improves edema [20].

Similarly, the volutrauma theory or overstretching injury may influence the pathogenesis of VILI, whereby lung volumes are able to produce diffuse alveolar damage characterized by lung hyperinflation and endothelial and epithelial cell damage, affecting capillary permeability changes, and nonhydrostatic lung function improves edema. The periodic opening and closing of the alveoli produce an inflammatory process, from which the atelectatic trauma theory gets its name. Lung-protective ventilation strategies involving recruitment maneuvers and high positive end expiratory pressure can minimize VILI, but no studies have provided conclusive evidence of an overall reduction in mortality, even though the use of this ventilation strategy appears to be associated with the higher mortality relevant. However, the clinical impact of ergotrauma on VILI remains still scarce, but, according to experimental studies, this theory has possibly overcome the limitations of the hypotheses described before [21].

According to the most recent studies, VILI could be caused by the amount of energy that the ventilator applies to the lung, per unit of time, during MV. It has been shown that there is an energy threshold above which VILI is produced. Mechanical power increases mainly by increasing tidal volume, driving pressure (the difference between the alveolar pressure measured with an inspiratory pause and the alveolar pressure measured during an expiratory pause), flow, and respiratory rate, but it also increases, although to a lesser extent, with the increase of PEEP, resistance, and elastance [22].

Another important contributor to lung injury is oxidative stress, which is due to the formation of oxygen free radicals at high inspired oxygen concentrations. In this condition, cells within the lungs are exposed to factors that promote apoptosis due to damage to the lipids and surfactant molecules of the cell membranes and activation of the inflammatory cascade. This in turn promotes the release of inflammatory mediators, including interleukins and tumor necrosis factor, to keep the cycle going. Of particular note is that cell death can have a dramatic impact on lung development in very preterm infants, who are born with alveolarization while still in infancy. Again, this theory explains what VILI does rather than its genesis [23].

2.5 Other Complications

Patients receiving PMV may suffer from severe mental disturbance, especially when sedation and analgesia are inadequate. These patients endure repeated painful surgeries, limited voluntary movement, separation from family members, and difficulty communicating, all of which contribute to heightened anxiety. Insufficient sedation can lead to accidental device removal or increased anxiety, which may have lasting psychological and behavioral consequences after ICU discharge. Excessive sedation is associated with PMV, increased risk of unexpected failed extubation, confusion, prolonged PICU length of stay (LOS), and development of tolerance and iatrogenic withdrawal. The ideal depth of sedation exhibits significant intra- and inter-individual variability depending on the disease process being treated, stage of disease development, invasiveness of therapy required, and developmental abilities to cooperate with treatments and therapies [24]. The management and monitoring of sedoanalgesia are important measures in improving the efficacy of procedures and MV, as well as reducing adverse effects and preventing withdrawal syndrome, and delirium PICU [25].

During PMV, gastrointestinal and nutritional complications can be appeared. When the demand for oxygen exceeds the contributions, complications such as mucosal injury (stress ulcers) and abnormal motility (ileus) occur more easily. There is also a reperfusion injury that occurs when the splanchnic flow is restored after a long period of hypoperfusion. Repeated cycles of hypoperfusion-reperfusion are responsible for the mesenteric ischemia observed in critically ill patients. The phenomena may be amplified by the activation of the inflammation cascade, which, in turn, may activate the immune system so that it can implement a systemic inflammatory response syndrome [26].

We must not forget that patients with PMV often require drugs that reduce bowel motility, such as benzodiazepines. In these patients, it may be difficult to provide the correct energy input, so caloric supplementation may require adjustment of the diet provided. If tolerance is incorrect and this persists over time, a possible malnutrition could occur. In addition, patients with PMV may need additional tests or therapeutic procedures that indicate discontinuation of enteral nutrition for hours, or even overnight, which will significantly reduce caloric intake [27].

In adults, PMV is known to be associated with longer hospital stays and higher morbidity and mortality. Although these associations have also been observed in pediatric populations, it remains unclear whether children requiring PMV have the same characteristics and the same risk factors [7].

Last but not least, the impact in the mental health and quality of life of the parents and siblings is an aspect of vital consideration. Some papers have analyzed these aspects, comparing through standardized self-reported questionnaires carried out in cohorts with ventilated and non-ventilated children, evaluating the quality of life and mental health of families with these children with PMV. Among the results obtained, the PMV is one factor that impairs the quality of life of affected children and their families due to an increase in disease burden. These parents reported a reduced child's overall quality of life especially regarding the physical and psychological well-being and social integration and also in some aspects of their mental health compared to healthy children [28].

3 Complications of PMV Out of the PICU, Home Ventilation

PMV is an indispensable method for providing support in patients with serious diseases or injuries; occasionally, it will be necessary to send the patient home, continuing with this support. The main problems of pediatric home ventilation are its negative psychosocial impact on family life, limited home care resources, financial burden, and the fact that the equipment is usually designed for adults, although in recent years these technical aspects have improved significantly.

Safety incidents in patients with home ventilation are an issue that requires detailed analysis. A retrospective observational review of on-call logs was published a few years ago. Of the 188 on-call logs that were positive for a patient safety incident, where each call could yield more than one incident type, 227 different incident types were identified. Patient incident types included medical device issues (99 device failures, 41 user errors, 12 equipment availability), documentation (20 unavailable labels/prescriptions, 4 unclear information), clinical processes (16 inadequate treatment or general care), and clinical administration (10 inadequate handover or transfer of care). Patient incidents were associated with mild harm in 87 cases [29].

Home ventilation is a hot topic in pediatrics, leading to publications describing patient selection and special considerations in children, its modes and technical setup, follow-up, monitoring and weaning, and potential risks [30].

The main complications during PMV at home can be divided according to the need for invasive or noninvasive airway isolation.

3.1 Home Invasive Ventilation

Children who require medical technology, including tracheostomies, ventilators, feeding tubes, and other medical devices, require complex care not only during hospitalization and rehabilitation but also at home by family caregivers.

3.1.1 Tracheostomy-Related Complications

When a tracheostomy is necessary, complications appear with more frequency, and healthcare levels have to increase. Compared to adults who receive a tracheostomy, children have higher reported complication rates.

These complications occur as a consequence of the surgical procedure or as a result of long-term use. The most frequently reported complications include irritation or abrasion at the stoma site, infection, granuloma formation within the airway or at the stoma, obstruction of the cannula lumen, inadvertent decannulation, pneumothorax, subcutaneous emphysema, accidental reinsertion into a false track, and tracheocutaneous fistula following elective decannulation.

Recently, the American Association for Respiratory Care (AARC) has published a clinical practice guideline about the management of pediatric patients with tracheostomy in the acute care setting [31].

Feeding disorders and gastrostomy use are highly prevalent in children with invasive PMV. Feeding in these children is complicated by the presence of a tracheostomy, lung vulnerability, and medical complexity. The potential comorbidity of swallowing disorders and atypical early feeding experiences can result in complex feeding difficulties. To improve long-term feeding outcomes and maximize oral feeding in this vulnerable population, children would benefit from earlier feeding opportunities during critical developmental windows, standardized protocols for advancing oral feeding, and involvement of intensive, comprehensive therapies throughout hospitalizations and early childhood.

Long-term tracheostomy in itself represents a real risk for bacterial colonization, a risk factor for respiratory infections. *Pseudomonas aeruginosa*, *Serratia marcescens*, and *Staphylococcus aureus* are the species most frequently isolated. Colonization of respiratory tract with *Pseudomonas aeruginosa* is associated with living in a medical care home and the use of cuffed tracheostomy tube [32].

3.2 Home Non-invasive Ventilation

During home NIV, specific risks may have equivalent life-threatening implications to a tracheostomy. These include partial displacement of the mask obstructing the infant or child's airway, impaired clearance of airway secretions and/or vomit, imposition of additional dead space or rebreathing when the mask or ventilator is not operating properly, risk of skin pressure sores, and abnormal growth of the midface due to prolonged pressure of the mask. The influence of mask pressure can be reduced by changing different mask models, mouthpiece ventilation used during the day, etc. The application of adhesive pads and/or cushioning solutions may also be beneficial to minimize these complications in patients that need PMV [33].

The most important factor determining successful NIV application is the choice of an appropriate mask that minimizes leakage and maximizes patient's comfort.

3.2.1 Facial Deformities

In children, facial deformity can occur due to the pressure applied by the mask on growing facial structures. These complications are more frequent in case of a daily NIV use exceeding 10 h per day [34]. Facial flattening may be produced and concerned the forehead, malar area, and maxilla. A concave face may be observed in severe cases. Maxillary retrusion, midface hypoplasia, and dental malocclusion are complications observed in certain cases.

3.2.2 Facial Injuries

Skin injury is a frequent complication during the application of NIV; the contact zone of the interface with the patient's face will cause erythema that will be transient if the caregivers handle it properly. However, on certain occasions, if these lesions are prolonged, even skin necrosis may appear, and skin sores will be most common and severe on the forehead and the glabella. Mask exchange, ensuring adequate vascularization of the support area and the use of solutions that protect the skin, will be key to minimizing these frequent complications [34].

In patients with lagophthalmos, the use of interfaces with poorly controlled leaks can cause corneal ulcers. It is important to periodically review this type of complication, especially in patients with little participation in the environment.

4 Conclusions

Despite improvements in the understanding of respiratory muscle physiology and the pathophysiology of respiratory failure, no one mode or strategy of ventilation has been shown to be more effective than others in weaning children from mechanical ventilation. Data on the benefits of respiratory muscle rest in adults are conflicting, and the effects of respiratory muscle rest in children remain to be studied. However, to successfully wean from mechanical ventilation, the balance between the pumping capacity of the respiratory muscles and respiratory effort must be restored [35].

Advances in neonatal and pediatric intensive care over the past few decades have significantly improved the chances of survival for critically ill infants and children. Many children fully recover from serious illness and live long and healthy lives. Others develop chronic disease or disability because vital organ functions have not fully recovered. A subset of the latter group developed chronic respiratory failure and remained dependent on MV for varying periods of time. Finally, the stressful, costly, labor-intensive nature of the ventilator-assisted child's care creates many important psychosocial, ethical, and economic issues for children and families [36].

References

1. MacIntyre NR, Epstein SK, Carson S, Scheinhorn D, Christopher K, Muldoon S, National Association for Medical Direction of Respiratory Care. Management of patients requiring prolonged mechanical ventilation: report of a NAMDRC consensus conference. Chest. 2005;128(6):3937–54.
2. Sarkar M, Roychowdhoury SR, Bhakta S, Raut S, Nandi M. Tracheostomy before 14 days: is it associated with better outcomes in pediatric patients on prolonged mechanical ventilation? Indian J Crit Care Med. 2021;25(4):435–40.
3. Kelly FE, Fong K, Hirsch N, Nolan JP. Intensive care medicine is 60 years old: the history and future of the intensive care unit. Clin Med (Lond). 2014;14(4):376–9.
4. MacIntyre NR. The ventilator discontinuation process: an expanding evidence base. Respir Care. 2013;58(6):1074–82.
5. Kamdar BB, Needham DM, Collop NA. Sleep deprivation in critical illness: its role in physical and psychological recovery. J Intensive Care Med. 2012;27(2):97–111.
6. Colleti J, Azevedo RT, de Oliveira Caino FR, de Araujo OR. Prolonged mechanical ventilation in children: review of the definition. Pediatr Crit Care Med. 2021;22(11):e588–93.
7. Liu Y, Wang Q, Hu J, Zhou F, Liu C, Li J, et al. Characteristics and risk factors of children requiring prolonged mechanical ventilation vs. non-prolonged mechanical ventilation in the PICU: a prospective single-center study. Front Pediatr. 2022;10:830075.
8. Telias I, Brochard LJ, Gattarello S, Wunsch H, Junhasavasdikul D, Bosma KJ, Camporota L, Brodie D, Marini JJ, Slutsky AS, Gattinoni L. The physiological underpinnings of life-saving respiratory support. Intensive Care Med. 2022;48(10):1274–86.
9. Hotterbeekx A, Xavier BB, Bielen K, Lammens C, Moons P, Schepens T, Ieven M, Jorens PG, Goossens H, Kumar-Singh S, Malhotra-Kumar S. The endotracheal tube microbiome associated with Pseudomonas aeruginosa or Staphylococcus epidermidis. Sci Rep. 2016;6:36507.
10. Amanati A, Karimi A, Fahimzad A, Shamshiri AR, Fallah F, Mahdavi A, Talebian M. Incidence of ventilator-associated pneumonia in critically ill children undergoing mechanical ventilation in pediatric intensive care unit. Children (Basel). 2017;4(7):56.
11. Antalová N, Klučka J, Říhová M, Poláčková S, Pokorná A, Štourač P. Ventilator-associated pneumonia prevention in pediatric patients: narrative review. Children (Basel). 2022;9(10):1540.
12. Wu D, Wu C, Zhang S, Zhong Y. Risk factors of ventilator-associated pneumonia in critically ill patients. Front Pharmacol. 2019;10:482.
13. Klompas M. Complications of mechanical ventilation--the CDC's new surveillance paradigm. N Engl J Med. 2013;368(16):1472–5.
14. Spalding MC, Cripps MW, Minshall CT. Ventilator-associated pneumonia: new definitions. Crit Care Clin. 2017;33(2):277–92.
15. CDC. Paediatric Ventilator-Associated Event (PedVAE) For use in neonatal and paediatric locations only device associated module PedVAE January 2021. 11-1 to 11-19. Available in: https://www.cdc.gov/nhsn/acute-care-hospital/pedvae/. Accessed 21 Nov 2022.
16. Hermans G, Van den Berghe G. Clinical review: intensive care unit acquired weakness. Crit Care. 2015;19(1):274.
17. Goligher EC, Brochard LJ, Reid WD, Fan E, Saarela O, Slutsky AS, et al. Diaphragmatic myotrauma: a mediator of prolonged ventilation and poor patient outcomes in acute respiratory failure. Lancet Respir Med. 2019;7(1):90–8.
18. Gal JS, Yudkowitz FS, Rothschild MA. Pediatric otolaryngology. In: Anesthesiology and otolaryngology. New York: Springer; 2013. p. 333–64.
19. Aravena C, Almeida FA, Mukhopadhyay S, Ghosh S, Lorenz RR, Murthy SC, Mehta AC. Idiopathic subglottic stenosis: a review. J Thorac Dis. 2020;12(3):1100–11.
20. Relja B, Land WG. Damage-associated molecular patterns in trauma. Eur J Trauma Emerg Surg. 2020;46(4):751–75.
21. Amato MB, Barbas CS, Medeiros DM, Magaldi RB, Schettino GP, Lorenzi-Filho G, Kairalla RA, Deheinzelin D, Munoz C, Oliveira R, Takagaki TY, Carvalho CR. Effect of a

protective-ventilation strategy on mortality in the acute respiratory distress syndrome. N Engl J Med. 1998;338(6):347–54.
22. Albaiceta GM, Blanch L. Beyond volutrauma in ARDS: the critical role of lung tissue deformation. Crit Care. 2011;15(2):304.
23. Haudebourg AF, Tuffet S, Perier F, Razazi K, de Prost N, Mekontso Dessap A, Carteaux G. Driving pressure-guided ventilation decreases the mechanical power compared to predicted body weight-guided ventilation in the Acute Respiratory Distress Syndrome. Crit Care. 2022;26(1):185.
24. Cannavò L, Perrone S, Viola V, Marseglia L, Di Rosa G, Gitto E. Oxidative stress and respiratory diseases in preterm newborns. Int J Mol Sci. 2021;22(22):12504.
25. Smith HAB, Besunder JB, Betters KA, Johnson PN, Srinivasan V, Stormorken A, Farrington E, Golianu B, Godshall AJ, Acinelli L, Almgren C, Bailey CH, Boyd JM, Cisco MJ, Damian M, deAlmeida ML, Fehr J, Fenton KE, Gilliland F, Grant MJC, Howell J, Ruggles CA, Simone S, Su F, Sullivan JE, Tegtmeyer K, Traube C, Williams S, Berkenbosch JW. 2022 Society of Critical Care Medicine Clinical Practice Guidelines on Prevention and Management of Pain, Agitation, Neuromuscular Blockade, and Delirium in Critically Ill Pediatric Patients with Consideration of the ICU Environment and Early Mobility. Pediatr Crit Care Med. 2022;23(2):e74–e110.
26. Ekinci F, Yildizdas D, Horoz OO, Aslan N, Society of Pediatric Emergency Intensive Care Medicine of Turkey-Sedoanalgesia Study Group. Sedation and analgesia practices in pediatric intensive care units: a survey of 27 centers from Turkey. J Pediatr Intensive Care. 2020;10(4):289–97.
27. Grootjans J, Lenaerts K, Derikx JP, Matthijsen RA, de Bruïne AP, van Bijnen AA, van Dam RM, Dejong CH, Buurman WA. Human intestinal ischemia-reperfusion-induced inflammation characterized: experiences from a new translational model. Am J Pathol. 2010;176(5):2283–91.
28. Johannsen J, Fuhrmann L, Grolle B, Morgenstern L, Wiegand-Grefe S, Denecke J. The impact of long-term ventilator-use on health-related quality of life and the mental health of children with neuromuscular diseases and their families: need for a revised perspective? Health Qual Life Outcomes. 2020;18(1):219.
29. Yang L, Nonoyama M, Pizzuti R, Bwititi P, John G. Home mechanical ventilation: a retrospective review of safety incidents using the World Health Organization International Patient Safety Event classification. Can J Respir Ther. 2016;52(3):85–91.
30. Kwak S. Home mechanical ventilation in children with chronic respiratory failure: a narrative review. J Yeungnam Med Sci. 2023;40(2):123–35.
31. Volsko TA, Parker SW, Deakins K, Walsh BK, Fedor KL, Valika T, Ginier E, Strickland SL. AARC Clinical Practice Guideline: Management of Pediatric Patients with Tracheostomy in the Acute Care Setting. Respir Care. 2021;66(1):144–55.
32. Lepainteur M, Ogna A, Clair B, Dinh A, Tarragon C, Prigent H, Davido B, Barbot F, Vaugier I, Afif M, Roux AL, Rottman M, Orlikowski D, Herrmann JL, Annane D, Lawrence C. Risk factors for respiratory tract bacterial colonization in adults with neuromuscular or neurological disorders and chronic tracheostomy. Respir Med. 2019;152:32–6.
33. Chawla J, Edwards EA, Griffiths AL, Nixon GM, Suresh S, Twiss J, Vandeleur M, Waters KA, Wilson AC, Wilson S, Tai A. Ventilatory support at home for children: a joint position paper from the Thoracic Society of Australia and New Zealand/Australasian Sleep Association. Respirology. 2021;26(10):920–37.
34. Fauroux B, Lavis JF, Nicot F, Picard A, Boelle PY, Clément A, Vazquez MP. Facial side effects during noninvasive positive pressure ventilation in children. Intensive Care Med. 2005;31(7):965–9.
35. Hsieh MJ, Yang TM, Tsai YH. Nutritional supplementation in patients with chronic obstructive pulmonary disease. J Formos Med Assoc. 2016;115(8):595–601.
36. Long DA, Fink EL. Transitions from short to long-term outcomes in pediatric critical care: considerations for clinical practice. Transl Pediatr. 2021;10(10):2858–74.

Long-Term Mechanical Ventilation: Respiratory Therapist's Point of View

Nisha Cithiravel, Sarah Kuyntjes, Faiza Syed, and Tuyen Tran

1 What Is a Respiratory Therapist

Respiratory therapists (RTs) are regulated healthcare providers who are part of an interdisciplinary team to monitor, assess, and treat patients. In Canada, RTs complete either a 3-year advanced diploma or a 4-year joint diploma/degree program [1]. RTs specialize in cardiorespiratory care, treating patients from acute exacerbations to chronic respiratory care needs. The role is as diverse as the practice locations, ranging from supporting critical patients to providing education and to acting as a transitional care coordinator arranging oxygen and respiratory equipment for discharge home. The profession is challenging, complex, and varied day to day.

Many RTs work in the hospital setting, but they can also be found working in research, education, home care, diagnostics, and medical sales [1, 2]. In addition to holding their registered respiratory therapist (RRT) credentials, an RT can choose to obtain additional qualifications including Smoking Cessation Counsellor, Certified Tobacco Educator (CTE), Extracorporeal Membrane Oxygenation (ECMO) Specialist, or Certified Respiratory Educator (CRE) [2]. The Respiratory Therapy Society of Ontario has undertaken extensive research to outline in detail the role of the RT throughout multiple practice settings [2].

N. Cithiravel · S. Kuyntjes (✉) · F. Syed · T. Tran
Long-Term Ventilation Clinic, SickKids Hospital, Toronto, ON, Canada
e-mail: nisha.cithiravel@sickkids.ca; sarah.kuyntjes@sickkids.ca; faiza.syed@sickkids.ca; tuyen.tran@sickkids.ca

A. Kawaguchi et al. (eds.), *Prolonged and Long-Term Mechanical Ventilation in Children*, https://doi.org/10.1007/978-981-97-8903-0_21

2 The Long-Term Ventilation (LTV) Clinic at the Hospital for Sick Children (SickKids)

The SickKids LTV clinic runs weekly, providing an opportunity for the team to see patients in-person or virtually. The success of the LTV team for managing patients with various respiratory disorders is dependent on several factors including physical patient exam, assessment of ventilation effectiveness, checking equipment functionality, carrying out a personalized assessment and workup, and providing patient and family caregiver (FC) education.

The SickKids LTV RTs have diverse roles and responsibilities during in-person appointments. These include performing respiratory and diagnostic assessments such as capnography, auscultation, oxygen saturation, peak cough flows (PCFs), thoracic/spine casting and brace assessment, tracheal aspirate, and capillary blood gas (CBG) sampling and analysis. For patients who are invasively ventilated (IV), the RTs will assess ventilator downloads, check equipment and tracheostomy kit, and perform airway assessment such as minimal occlusive volume (MOV) for patients with cuffed tracheostomy tubes and/or transtracheal pressure to assess readiness for a speaking valve. In addition, noninvasive ventilation (NIV) initiations, mask fittings, and mechanical in-exsufflation teaching and device downloads are also performed.

The content that is described in this chapter will be based on the experiences, practices, and policies from this clinic and program.

3 Initiation of Long-Term Mechanical Ventilation (LTMV) and the Transition Home

3.1 Introducing the Need for LTMV

LTMV has decreased length of stay in the pediatric intensive care unit (PICU) after tracheostomy placement allowing earlier transition to home [3]. The hospital environment is not optimal for a child's emotional, mental, and intellectual health [4]. In addition, LTMV minimizes disruptions to the child's development and family life, increases life expectancy, improves quality of life (QOL), and prevents a dependence on institutions. It also helps avoid nosocomial infections, frees beds in hospitals, and reduces healthcare costs [4–7].

3.2 Initial Steps to Discharge Home

Prior to transition to home, the child should be medically stable including presence of a stable airway and ventilation settings. The amount of oxygen used should be ideally less than 40% to maintain SpO_2 above 95%. Lower SpO_2 targets are accepted if the patient has an underlying single ventricle physiology. An enteral feeding tube may be considered to optimize feeding and weight gain. This should involve an interprofessional team that decides on IV or NIV with continued follow-up to ensure a smooth and safe transition home [4, 8, 9]. The focus of RTs involved in the care of LTMV patients and discharge planning includes optimizing ventilator settings, appropriate equipment acquisition, educating family and community caregivers on the patient's respiratory care/equipment, and liaising with the interdisciplinary team [4]. The level of complexity, amount of equipment, and length of time to prepare the patient and family for discharge will be influenced by the mode of ventilation (NIV vs. IV) [10]. Typically, the length of training for IV can take approximately 6–8 weeks and less than 1 week for NIV [4]. However, barriers such as housing concerns, funding/availability of equipment, intercurrent illnesses, family social issues, and availability of trained home healthcare caregivers in the community can cause delays in discharge [3]. Having a protocol and clearly outlined pathway can help identify barriers to discharge and decrease delays to discharge. The Canadian Thoracic Society clinical practice guideline for LTMV for pediatrics recommends designating a case coordinator for these patients to facilitate discharge planning, decrease length of stay, and enhance safe transition home [3]. A review of this practice model completed by Tearl et al. highlighted the improvements noted in their discharge planning when an RT discharge coordinator was assigned for children going home with respiratory technology [11]. There was early identification and initiation of family education, an increase in the quality and consistency of the training provided, increased satisfaction in the discharge process from the medical team, and a decrease in patient's length of the stay [11].

3.3 Initiating Noninvasive Ventilation

Unlike IV which is always initiated through a PICU stay due to the need for surgical placement of the tracheostomy tube, NIV can be initiated either through an inpatient process similar to the IV process or electively through an outpatient process. Polysomnography (PSG) testing can be used to follow patients with underlying neuromuscular conditions who are at risk for respiratory deterioration. The LTV program follows the recommendations for the management of Duchenne muscular dystrophy (DMD) outlined by The Lancet in 2010 as a guide for initiating NIV electively for outpatients with underlying neuromuscular conditions.

In patients with DMD, it is typical that forced vital capacity (FVC) continues to increase as they grow until they become nonambulatory, and then FVC tends to plateau before beginning to deteriorate [12]. Earlier loss of ambulation in these patients is also associated with a more rapid decline in respiratory function [12]. As such, the point at which loss of ambulation occurs indicates a reasonable time to begin to monitor for sleep-disordered breathing (SDB) through annual baseline PSG testing [12]. The Lancet provides the following recommendations for initiating nocturnal NIV based on PSG findings [12]:

- End-tidal ($EtCO_2$) or transcutaneous carbon dioxide ($TcCO_2$) values of 50 millimeters of mercury (mmHg) or greater for 2% of the total sleep time
- Increase in carbon dioxide (CO_2) of 10 mmHg greater than the patient's awake baseline while asleep for 2% of the total sleep time
- Oxygen saturation (SpO_2) 88% or less for 2% of total sleep time
- SpO_2 88% or less for 5 min continuously
- Apnea-hypopnea index (AHI) of 5 or more

Initiating nocturnal NIV can also be done empirically based on signs and symptoms of SDB (Table 1). In some cases, patients may be asymptomatic despite the presence of hypoventilation. In these cases, The Lancet recommends NIV be initiated when FVC is less than 50% predicted or maximum inspiratory pressure (MIP) is less than 60 cm of water (cmH_2O) [12]. NIV is recommended for daytime use in the presence of daytime hypercapnia (CO_2 >45 mmHg) or SpO_2 <95% on room air [12].

Based on the recommendations above, NIV recommendations should be discussed with the patient and their family. The patient should then undergo a mask fit and air trial with the healthcare team. Typically, patients are placed on a continuous positive airway pressure (CPAP) of 5 cmH_2O to let them feel what it will be like to wear the mask on their face with some airflow and then progress to gentle NIV pressures such as inspiratory positive airway pressure (IPAP) 10 cmH_2O and expiratory positive airway pressure (EPAP) 5 cmH_2O. This provides an opportunity to assess mask leak to determine if a different interface should be selected. If the patient is being seen virtually, a virtual mask fitting process developed by the LTV RTs during the COVID-19 pandemic which will be outlined later in this chapter is completed. The patient will then be given their interface to utilize during the day while awake for up to 30 min as an opportunity to acclimate to the mask on their face prior to

Table 1 Signs and symptoms of sleep-disordered breathing [12]

Signs and symptoms of sleep-disordered breathing
Fatigue
Dyspnea
Headaches (upon awakening or continuous)
Frequent nocturnal awakenings
Difficult arousal
Hypersomnolence
Difficulty concentrating
Awakenings with dyspnea and tachycardia
Frequent nightmares

their NIV initiation PSG in the sleep lab. In some circumstances where the patient is known to tolerate the sleep lab poorly or is anticipated that they will have a difficult time acclimating to therapy, the LTV clinic will pursue an elective admission to the children's rehabilitation hospital for a slower and gentler start to NIV therapy.

Once initial settings have been determined by either PSG or overnight oximetry and capnography performed at the children's rehabilitation hospital, the patient and their family will receive education and training on use and maintenance of the NIV device and their interface. The RTs then follow to establish compliance with NIV ventilation in the home with recommendations tailored to their unique needs and experience with NIV.

3.4 Initiating Invasive Ventilation

Families with children requiring invasive ventilation have made an informed decision to pursue LTMV via a tracheostomy for their child in the PICU with the medical team including the LTV team that will follow the patient once discharged home. LTV RTs are involved in the initial conversations with family on life at home with a tracheostomy and mechanical ventilation. A cuffed tracheostomy tube is normally preferred to minimize air leak and maximize ventilation efficiency. Patients who receive a tracheostomy are sometimes unable to protect the lower airways due to bulbar impairment or weakened muscles of the upper aerodigestive tract. In addition, they may have a weak cough impairing secretion management, have uncontrolled gastroesophageal reflux, and/or have anatomic facial abnormalities [6]. After the tracheostomy is in place and the patient is stable, the RT transitions the patient to the home ventilator in the PICU using the PICU ventilation parameters as a reference. Typically, the first tracheostomy change is done in the PICU by the ears, nose, and throat (ENT) surgeon, with the RT changing them thereafter. The PICU team can start training the FCs if home healthcare provider resources are limited. This facilitates a smooth transition to home and prevents delay in discharge [3].

The selection of the home ventilator may be limited by the country, the healthcare system, and the family's budget. Long-term mechanical ventilators need to be user friendly, be portable, have internal batteries, have optional external batteries, have adjustable alarm settings, be safe to use with oxygen therapy, and have the ability to add humidification [4, 9, 13]. Early introduction of the home ventilator will facilitate compliance and allow the team to identify issues [4]. It also stresses the need for a home assessment and helps family and caregivers to arrange the home environment appropriately. The RT will provide the equipment list to the community healthcare agency during the home assessment to ensure that adequate space and safety measures are in place. The home assessment needs to consider accessibility in/out of the home, storage space for equipment and supplies, adequate electrical outlets, heating/cooling system, and telephone access for emergencies [4, 9, 13].

3.5 Equipment Acquisition

The RT leads the respiratory equipment acquisition, a process which varies based on the geographical area and financial support available. For invasively ventilated patients, an awake, alert, and trained caregiver is required for constant monitoring [4]. This can result in a significant loss of income for the family, as one of the parents often must stop working outside the home and become the primary caregiver [4]. Families can receive funding support through government grants, charitable programs, and private insurance (if available); however, these sources of funding do not cover all the costs incurred by the family. For this reason, assessing a family's financial situation and arranging for additional support are an important part of discharge planning. The RT is well versed in the funding and community support available for families related to respiratory technology; they work closely with social workers and community respiratory vendors to ensure that all required supplies are arranged and delivered in a timely manner. RTs support the family when there are problems with obtaining respiratory supplies due to limited inventory or discontinuation and have the expertise to recommend alternative options. A study on healthcare utilization and home mechanical ventilation (HMV) costs indicated high caregiver burden as 39% of monthly healthcare costs were of FC time [14]. In addition, increased ventilator dependence increased the monthly healthcare costs [14]. The LTV RTs collaborated with the hospital's outpatient pharmacy and created an initiative to help families with the rising costs and limited availability of tracheostomy and suction supplies through community vendors during the novel coronavirus disease 2019 (COVID-19) pandemic. Through this initiative, tracheostomy and suctioning supplies were provided at more cost-friendly price points for families by utilizing the hospital's purchasing power, and supplies were available to purchase during their visit to the hospital or could be shipped to the home.

It is important to ensure that there is a backup ventilator system available in case of equipment malfunction or electrical power failure. This includes a backup ventilator, external battery source, and a self-inflating resuscitator with tracheostomy adapter for invasively ventilated patients [9, 13]. The pulse oximeter device with audible alarms is used as an additional external monitor and is a part of the standard of care for the pediatric population [4, 13]. Other respiratory equipment may include portable suction device and supplies, oxygen therapy equipment, medication compressor, ventilator circuit replacements, tracheostomy tubes and tracheostomy care supplies, humidification adjuncts, communication adjuncts, sterile distilled water, disinfection supplies, and an emergency tracheostomy kit. The RT will ensure that the emergency tracheostomy kit has the following equipment: same-size tracheostomy tube with tracheostomy ties and obturator attached, one size smaller tracheostomy tube, scissors, water-soluble lubricant, saline nebules, and pre-cut tracheostomy dressing. Families are recommended to maintain 3 months' worth of supplies for all soft and replaceable goods to facilitate emergency uses and stock shortages.

3.6 Optimizing Ventilation

Establishing ventilation settings with adequate volumes, support, comfort, and synchrony is important. This includes considering the underlying medical condition. The modes commonly used include synchronized intermittent mandatory ventilation (SIMV), assisted pressure control (PC), pressure support (PS), or spontaneous timed (ST) and volume-assured modes [5]. Depending on the ventilator used, there can be limitations including minimum weight requirements to be considered. Normally, inspiratory pressures between 12 and 22 cmH_2O are used [15] aiming to deliver tidal volumes (Vt) of approximately 8–10 milliliters per kilogram (ml/kg) to adequately ventilate the patient and account for the circuit's compressible volume [16, 17]. With neuromuscular patients, their chest wall compliance decreases as the disease progresses necessitating an increase in their ventilation pressures to achieve the target Vt [17]. For spinal muscular atrophy (SMA), 10 cmH_20 above positive end expiratory pressure (PEEP) can reduce pectus excavatum deformity, improve chest wall deformity, and normalize inspiratory muscle synchrony [4]. A low inspiratory pressure can be achieved in young infants due to their more compliant lungs and chest wall, but as the child gets older and develops scoliosis and obesity, higher inspiratory pressures may be necessary to overcome the restriction [16]. Some patients may need a backup rate to provide enough support to rest the respiratory muscles, such as in patients with underlying neuromuscular disease [17]. Due to a reduced chest wall and pulmonary compliance, the mechanical load on the weakened respiratory muscles is increased, leading to fatigue [16]. In addition, their intrinsic breathing pattern is fast and shallow resulting in a shorter inspiratory time (It), leading to smaller Vt and CO_2 retention. Therefore, setting a longer It helps increase Vt and achieve a normal CO_2 [15], ideally less than 50 mmHg. PEEP of 5–6 cm H_2O is typical, but higher settings may be required if airway obstruction or compression occurs. Adjusting trigger, rise time, and flow cycle sensitivity can improve patient comfort and synchrony on the ventilator. Setting appropriate alarms on the home ventilator and oximeter including low minute ventilation, circuit disconnect, high respiratory rate, and low SpO_2 is essential to notify caregivers of incidents such as accidental decannulation, ventilator disconnection, inadequate ventilation, and increased work of breathing. Once the initial settings are established on the home ventilator, the RT can use overnight oximetry, $EtCO_2$, $TcCO_2$, CBG, and bedside assessments to titrate the ventilator settings. The goal of customizing the ventilation settings for each patient is to achieve optimal oxygenation and CO_2 clearance, thereby improving neurocognitive development and maximizing the patient's QOL [5, 6].

Families must have an emergency plan in case of fire, prolonged power failure, or severe weather conditions requiring evacuation. The families will also be provided with a letter by the healthcare team to submit to their local electrical company for priority reinstation of service [4].

The patient may need an enteral feeding tube prior to discharge. If the child has bulbar impairment due to their neuromuscular disease, swallowing becomes difficult causing inadequate ingestion of nutrition and increasing the risk of aspiration [15]. The enteral feeding tube will allow for optimal nutrition, allow medication to be administered, and relieve any excess gas and bloating due to mechanical ventilation.

3.7 Caregiver Education

The home environment is preferable to the hospital environment for children who require LTMV support [18]. In addition, there is lower morbidity, minimal hospitalizations, and improvement in QOL [5].

Successfully transitioning children home requires an established home care program that provides ongoing educational support and establishes a clearly outlined education plan with objectives and a proposed timeline [3–7, 9, 18]. Children ventilated via a tracheostomy should be discharged home with at least two identified FCs due to their fragility and complexity. These FCs will require training in tracheostomy and ventilator care in order to care for their child at home [4]. Identifying and training as many caregivers (including both family and community healthcare providers) is essential to provide family with enough support to work, care for additional children, sleep, and relax [9].

FC training can be initiated in the PICU by the bedside RTs, registered nurses (RNs), and home and community support transition program team members (RTs, RNs). This team offers educational support through simulation-based workshops, webinars, and 24/7 live nursing support. Home and community caregivers (HCCPs) are offered just-in-time transition (JITT) through this program to help support transition home [4]. The aim of the program is to improve transition from hospital to home and to support community care for children with medical complexity and technology dependence [19]. The training program includes basic respiratory anatomy, hand hygiene and infection control practices, stoma and tracheostomy care, tracheostomy changes, ventilator care, suctioning and portable suction device, medication delivery, humidification delivery, cardiopulmonary resuscitation (CPR) and emergency management, and manual resuscitator [9, 13]. The PICU provides a safe and supportive environment to allow FCs to gain knowledge and confidence. Close to the time of discharge, knowledge and skills are reassessed through arrangements such as "care by parent" where FCs provide full care for their child in the hospital environment to practice learned skill independently. Other considerations for education and training include activities for daily life such as bathing, oral hygiene, physical activities, and going to school/work. For children who require daytime ventilation attending school, the preparation is similar to discharge home. It is important to always have a trained caregiver present with the child, appropriate nursing orders, a clear outlined plan for mobility/transportation to and from school, and an emergency plan [4].

As part of the healthcare team, the RTs can work on school nursing orders for safe care. For invasively ventilated children, the RT will consider appropriate suctioning and humidification adjuncts. If the child can be off ventilation during transportation, a heat and moisture exchanger (HME) can be added directly to the tracheostomy. However, if ventilation is required, an in-line HME will need to be added to the circuit for humidification. For suctioning, an in-line suction catheter can be added during transportation and at school to reduce the number of disconnections from the ventilator and reduce the risks from aerosol-generating procedures [20].

4 Outpatient Management: Long-Term Ventilation (LTV) Program

4.1 LTV Clinic

Ventilation data from invasive or NIV is important to determine if the patient's ventilation is effective and adequate. Computer programs are used to download data from the different types of home ventilators and the mechanical in-exsufflation device (M-IE). Different types of ventilators will provide slightly different data. Typically, Vt, leak value, apnea-hypopnea index (AHI), adherence data measured in hours, and percent triggered and cycled breaths are reviewed.

Leak values are displayed differently depending on the ventilator device. For example, some devices only report unintentional leaks, while others will report the total leak (intentional and unintentional leaks combined). Intentional leak is the leak from the ventilator that is intended to occur (e.g., from the presence of an exhalation valve in the circuit). For patients who are invasively ventilated via tracheostomy with a single-limb passive circuit, it will have an exhalation port to prevent rebreathing of CO_2 [17]. It will have a certain amount of intentional leak that changes depending on the pressure settings. By occluding the circuit to check the intentional leak, the RT can calculate the unintentional leak by subtracting the intentional leak from the total leak, which will help the RT determine if the patient is being optimally ventilated. Unintentional leaks can cause ineffective ventilation because it lowers the Vt that the patient may receive. These leaks may also be position dependent, particularly if the patient has low tone or scoliosis or if the patient has grown. If the leak is significant and making ventilation ineffective, the LTV team may recommend an upsize of the tracheostomy tube and/or inserting a cuffed tube to improve ventilation. If the patient already has an appropriately sized cuffed tracheostomy tube in situ, the RT can perform another minimal occlusive volume (MOV) to ensure a proper seal. The method includes fully deflating the tracheostomy tube with a syringe and then reinflating it with air or sterile water depending on the type of cuffed tracheostomy tube until no leak is heard on auscultation with a stethoscope. This ensures that the airway is sealed without overinflating the cuff and preventing tracheal injuries [21]. For patients who use NIV with high leak values on the download, the interface needs to be assessed. The RTs can try several strategies to minimize leak such as teaching how to adjust the mask, resizing the mask, or changing the interface from nasal to a full-face mask (FFM). Different adjuncts can be trialed including a chin strap if they use a nasal mask to prevent mouth leak or a nasal gel pad to seal the leak at the bridge of the nose.

Adherence data should be reviewed when the download data is obtained. Adequate usage helps prevent nocturnal hypoventilation and daytime hypercapnia. The data alerts the RT to discuss issues that limit the patient's tolerance to therapy and help address them. For example, if the patient is experiencing discomfort with the ventilation pressures, the pressures can be adjusted to accommodate acclimation. If the patient is experiencing asynchrony with the ventilator, the RT may adjust inspiratory time, rise time, trigger, and cycle [17]. If poor adherence is due to lack of support at nighttime, the healthcare team can advocate for the family to receive nursing support in the community.

The RT can also look at the percentage of breaths that are triggered and cycled by the patient (acceptable range dependent on the patient's underlying condition and the clinical settings) [17]. For neuromuscular patients, the aim is for a low percentage of triggered breaths (10–20%) to allow the respiratory muscles to rest overnight [17].

The LTV clinic uses PCFs to assess cough strength. Having an impaired cough can cause frequent atelectasis, ventilation-perfusion mismatch, pneumonia, and respiratory failure. PCFs above 250–270 liters per minute (LPM) have been shown to be sufficient to prevent pneumonia in adults [22]. The patient will use a PCF meter with either a full-face mask or a mouthpiece with nose clip. This test requires a good seal around the mouth and nose to capture the entire expiratory cough. A mask interface allows for coverage of the mouth and nose, which is better tolerated with improved measurements, especially in weaker children. The PCF maneuver requires the patient to cough into the interface with good effort. The best of three coughs is recorded. Pediatric patients may not be able to reliably complete the testing for reasons such as immaturity, cognition issues, general weakness, or an artificial airway in situ. In this case, the patient is assessed based on the observation of weak cough and secretion retention [4, 23]. To help with secretion management, a patient may be initiated on LVR or M-IE, which will be described in greater detail later in this chapter.

Facilitating speech in patients with a tracheostomy tube is important to improve QOL by enhancing their psychological well-being, communication, and swallowing/eating [24]. A speaking valve is a one-way valve that closes during exhalation. It redirects exhaled air into the pharynx, mouth, and nasal cavity enabling the patient to speak [25]. If the patient has a cuffed tracheostomy tube, they need to tolerate having the cuff deflated and the ability to manage their secretions to decrease risks of aspiration to initiate speaking valve use [24]. To assess if the patient can use a speaking valve who is either ventilator dependent or breathing spontaneously, the RT in clinic will perform a transtracheal pressure to ensure that there is adequate airflow through the upper airway with minimal resistance. The tracheal pressure in a healthy person during speech is 5–10 cmH_2O [24]. The RT will use a pressure manometer attached to a speaking valve and connected to the patient's proximal opening of the tracheostomy tube (Fig. 1). The patient is eligible for a speaking valve if their transtracheal pressure gradient on exhalation is less than 10 cmH_2O. For patients who will use the speaking valve with mechanical ventilation, some setting adjustments may be required. During the inspiratory phase, gas flows from the ventilator into the lungs and the larynx and exits through the upper airway during exhalation. Increasing ventilation pressures or volumes depending on the ventilation mode used may be necessary to compensate for the volume loss through the upper airway during the inspiratory phase. In addition, this volume loss can also cause alarms such as low minute ventilation and low exhaled Vt. Other strategies to improve speech while on the ventilator include the use of longer It and higher PEEP because it increases the impedance of the ventilator circuit causing more airflow through the larynx [24]. Some patients may complain of discomfort from the airflow through the upper airway due to drying of the pharyngeal membranes and/or inability to ventilate adequately. If the patient's status deteriorates from increased work of breathing and desaturations, remove the speaking valve immediately. If the patient tolerates the speaking valve in clinic, the patient is encouraged to increase the length of use at home.

Outside of clinic, monitoring and patient education are vital for providing consistent care. When a patient is newly initiated on ventilation, ventilation changes are made in clinic, or adherence needs improvement, the RTs will do a follow-up download to assess compliance and discuss barriers. The RTs also provide education on oximetry, M-IE, NIV, and tracheostomy management for families, home care

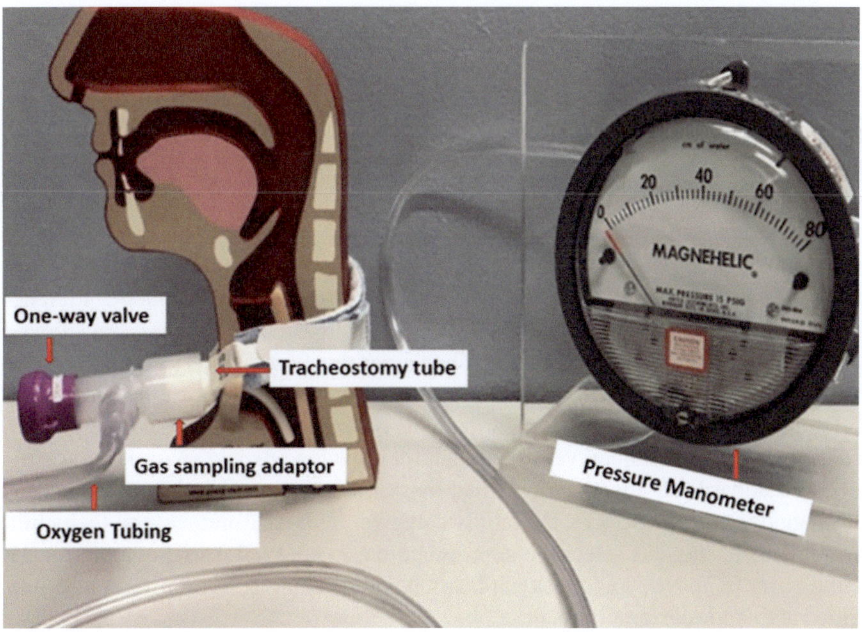

Fig. 1 Technique of transtracheal pressure measurements in a tracheostomy patient

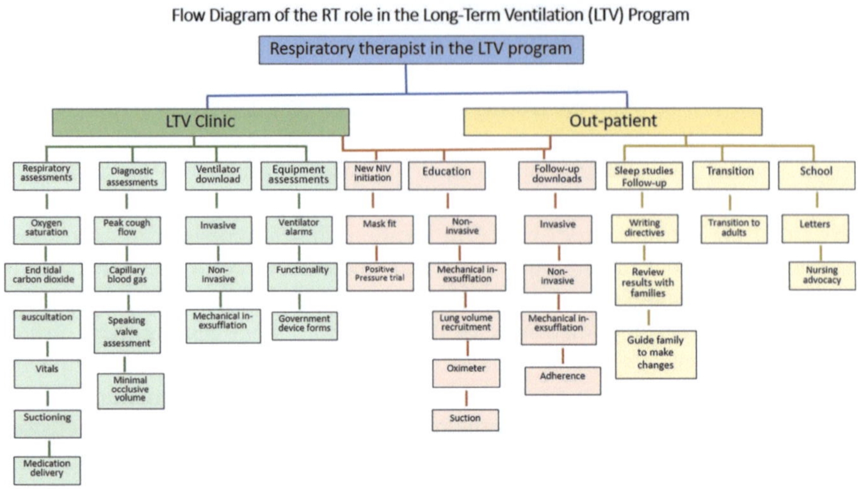

Fig. 2 Flow diagram of the RT role in the long-term ventilation (LTV) program

nurses, and staff. The RTs also partner with nurse practitioners and physicians for equipment troubleshooting and sick calls. Meeting the needs of our pediatric patients and helping fill the gaps that they may experience in the community are very important. Figure 2 provides a flow diagram of the roles of the RTs in the LTV program.

5 Remote and Virtual Care

The global pandemic from COVID-19 has significantly impacted services across the health system [6, 26]. In response to these challenges, rigorous public health strategies and policies were implemented; notably, physical distancing measures were enforced in public spaces, which included limiting in-person visits to hospitals. Teleconsultations and telemonitoring including telephone or video conferencing were utilized to mitigate these challenges [6]. Initially, the LTV clinic transitioned all in-person appointments to virtual. Challenges that faced the RTs during this time were obtaining downloads remotely, mask fitting new patients to be initiated on NIV, and assessing mask barriers for patients on existing NIV. In response, the RTs asked FCs to mail or email ventilator data for downloading and analysis and developed a standardized approach to virtual mask fitting for nasal and full-face masks. With guidance from the RTs, the family caregiver took measurements on their child which guided the RTs select the appropriate mask and mail it to the home for the child to try [27]. NIV and mask application and cleaning education were also provided at this virtual appointment.

The LTV team continued to deliver the same quality of care to patients remotely, without significantly compromising patient outcomes and satisfaction. Many families continue to choose virtual appointments over in-person. Although telemedicine technology shows excellent promise, it is not without its limitations. These include the absence of respiratory and diagnostic assessments and a potential loss of social interactions, which help create rapport and enrich the patient and family experience. Currently, evidence on the fact that telemonitoring benefits day-to-day care, mean- to long-term outcomes, and cost-effectiveness is very limited in children [6].

6 Pulmonary Clearance

Respiratory therapists have been providing pulmonary clearance therapies for infants, young children, and adolescents for many years with favorable outcomes. Treatments provided may include a combination of LVR, M-IE, and manual chest physiotherapy (CPT). Suctioning, humidity, and inhalation medications are also considered as adjunctive therapies.

In the critical care environment, pulmonary clearance therapies can be selected for acutely unwell patients where their normal mucociliary clearance mechanisms are altered. RTs will also encounter patients who are already established on pulmonary clearance therapies at home and have had a readmission to hospital. Patients may continue to be prescribed these therapies as they transition from PICU to a ward setting and on discharge home if required long term.

Pulmonary clearance is indicated in pediatrics where cough mechanics or ability to clear secretions is compromised, as suctioning alone is ineffective in clearing secretions in the lower airways [4, 28]. Indications include patients with underlying neuromuscular condition, deconditioning from long-term illness, respiratory infection, or presence of an artificial airway in situ impairing cough [4, 29]. Recommendations from the Canadian Thoracic Society (CTS) Home Mechanical Ventilation Guidelines define impaired cough by clinical assessment and/or maximum expiratory pressure (MEP) <60 cmH_2O and/or PCF in children ≥12 years <270 LPM and/or FVC <40% predicted [4]. Pulmonary clearance strategies are effective in preventing mucus plugging, improving gas exchange and pulmonary function, improving ventilatory support, decreasing length of hospital stay, and improving QOL [30, 31].

LVR is a manual pulmonary clearance and cough augmentation technique more commonly provided during the recovery phase of illness or introduced to patients seen in outpatient clinic for assessment. This requires full patient participation and is not ideal for a young child or a patient who is unable to follow instructions. The Lancet DMD guidelines recommend LVR for patients with an FVC <60% predicted to help preserve lung compliance [12]. LVR involves the use of a manual resuscitation bag with a one-way valve built in-line. With a good seal by mask, mouthpiece, or tracheostomy, breaths can be stacked to inflate the lungs to 60–80% total lung capacity [4, 32]. The interface is then removed to allow the patient to cough passively. Although the tracheostomy interface is an option, it is recommended to keep the cuff deflated to prevent air trapping. While stacking breaths, it is recommended to have patients hold their breath after each inflation.

M-IE outpatient initiation and management are established in the LTV clinic, and use in the PICU setting has gained momentum in the last 5–8 years. M-IE is recommended when PCF is less than 270 lpm, maximum expiratory pressure (MEP) less than 60 cmH2O, or FVC less than 50% predicted [12]. M-IE therapy involves delivery of positive pressure for a set time followed by a quick shift to negative pressure, simulating and/or supporting a weak cough. A brief pause time occurs before the next cough cycle is delivered. Pressures typically begin at +/−30 cmH_20 with a goal of prescribing therapeutic pressures of +/−40 cmH_20 [4, 31]. Three to five cough cycles and three to five sets are recommended per treatment session. The Canadian Thoracic Society guidelines suggest starting at two to four treatments per day (1 h after feeding) [4, 31]. For patients initiating therapy for the first time, it is recommended to suggest starting at two treatments per day, morning and night. This allows the patient to build tolerance to the device. Generally, for pediatrics, starting at the lower number of cough sets and cycles proves successful. An additional strategy that has proven effective is to end therapy on an insufflation (post-suctioning) to allow for lung recruitment. Some mechanical pulmonary clearance devices may have additional features to enhance therapy such as the oscillation feature to help mobilize secretions. Oscillation can be used in the auto or manual mode during either inhale, exhale, or both phases.

Commonly observed issues with M-IE are fear of high pressures required for effective cough, anxiety, and parent skill if therapy is not routinely performed. Once barriers are managed, treatments can be increased as the child tolerates it. To increase sessions, considerations around feeding schedules, medication administration, and other active therapies should be noted. In outpatient management, FCs are instructed to provide additional treatments as needed (e.g., when a child is sick) [31]. Often, with mechanical pulmonary clearance devices, manual and automatic modes are available. Automatic mode is preferred in pediatrics since the device can be set while the care provider focuses on delivering therapy. Good techniques include ensuring that the child's head is positioned and secured well, holding the interface firmly on the face and watching the screen to know what phase of cough is being delivered so that the caregiver can coach the patient accordingly. When these elements are not in place, leaking and asynchrony occur, which builds anxiety and leads to a negative experience for the child. Therapy can be provided via a tracheostomy using a simple attachment and is usually tolerated better. CPT can include a combination of manual techniques to loosen and remove secretions. CPT techniques include postural drainage, percussion, vibrations, deep breathing, and coughing. Physiotherapists work closely with RTs to suggest a combination of manual and mechanical techniques that are best suited for patients. Therapy sessions may also include inhalation medications or other aerosol treatments before and/or after prescribed pulmonary clearance techniques. Assisted cough techniques (ACTs) can also be applied to CPT, MI-E, or LVR techniques to further improve peak cough flow. Examples of ACTs are abdominal breathing and lateral costal breathing [23, 33, 34].

The cost of pulmonary therapy equipment and supplies can be high, especially MI-E devices. Funding for MI-E and other pulmonary clearance equipment and supplies varies. Although most centers acknowledge this as a required therapy for certain groups of patients, support for funding has been slow to implement in some jurisdictions.

7 Conclusion

Respiratory therapists are one of the many integral care providers for patients with prolonged mechanical ventilation needs. From hospital to community care, RTs collaborate with an interprofessional team and offer specialized knowledge of respiratory physiology, ventilation, and secretion management strategies. RTs provide tailored recommendations for respiratory equipment and supplies for transition home, and patient and family education and support. As there are continued technological advancements in respiratory equipment, RTs will play a role in adapting, incorporating, and educating their patients, families, and colleagues on the new therapies.

References

1. College of Respiratory Therapists of Ontario [Internet]. What is a respiratory therapist? [Cited 2022 Jul 2]. Available from https://www.crto.on.ca/public/what-is-respiratory-therapy/.
2. Respiratory Therapy Society of Ontario. Registered respiratory therapist role profile across multiple practice settings in Ontario. 2020 [cited 2022 Jul 2]. Available from: https://www.rtso.ca/wp-content/uploads/2020/10/RTSO-Role-Profile-2020-10-21.pdf.
3. Amirnovin R, Aghamohammadi S, Riley S, Woo M, Del Castillo S. Analysis of a pediatric home mechanical ventilator population. Respir Care. 2018;63(5):558–64.
4. Amin R, MacLusky I, Zielinski D, Adderley R, Carnevale F, Chiang J, et al. Pediatric home mechanical ventilation: a Canadian Thoracic Society clinical practice guideline executive summary. Can Jour Resp Crit Care Sleep Med. 2017;1(1):7–36. https://doi.org/10.1080/24745332.2017.1300463.
5. Cancelinha C, Madureira N, Mação P, Pleno P, Silva T, Estêvão MH, Félix M. Long-term ventilation in children: ten years later. Revista Portuguesa De Pneumologia (English Edition). 2015;21(1):16–21. https://doi.org/10.1016/j.rppnen.2014.03.017.
6. Praud JP. Long-term non-invasive ventilation in children: current use, indications, and contraindications. Front Pediatr. 2020;8:584334. https://doi.org/10.3389/fped.2020.584334.
7. Paulides F, Plötz F, Verweij-van den Oudenrijn L, van Gestel PJ, Kampelmacher M. Thirty years of home mechanical ventilation in children: escalating need for pediatric intensive care beds. Intensive Care Med. 2012;38:847–52. https://doi.org/10.1007/s00134-012-2545-9.
8. Sahetya S, Allgood S, Gay PC, Lechtzin N. Long term mechanical ventilation. Clin Chest Med. 2020;37(4):753–63. https://doi.org/10.1016/j.ccm.2016.07.014.
9. Cairo JM, Pilbeam SP, Gramlich T. Chapter 21: long term ventilation. In: Pilbeam's mechanical ventilation physiological and clinical applications. 5th ed. St. Louis, MO: Elsevier; 2012. p. 428–58.

10. McKim DA, Road J, Avendano M, Abdool S, Cote F, Duguid N, et al. Home mechanical ventilation: a Canadian Thoracic Society clinical practice guideline. Can Respir J. 2011;18(4):197–215. https://doi.org/10.1155/2011/139769.
11. Tearl DK, Cox TJ, Hertzog JH. Hospital discharge of respiratory-technology-dependent children: role of a dedicated respiratory care discharge coordinator. Respir Care. 2006;51(7):744–9.
12. Birnkrant DJ, Bushby K, Bann CM, Alman BA, Apkon SD, Blackwell A. Diagnosis and management of Duchenne muscular dystrophy, part 2: respiratory, cardiac, hone health, and orthopaedic management. Lancet Neurol. 2018;17(4):347–61. https://doi.org/10.1016/S1474-4422(18)30025-5.
13. AARC & Respiratory Home Care Focus Group. AARC clinical practice guideline. Long-term invasive mechanical ventilation in the home—2007 revision & update. Respir Care. 2007;52(8):1056–62.
14. Nonoyama M, McKim D, Road J, Guerriere D, Coyte P, Wasilewski M, et al. Healthcare utilisation and costs of home mechanical ventilation. Thorax. 2018;26(73):644–51. https://doi.org/10.1136/thoraxjnl-2017-211138.
15. Perrin C, Unterborn J, Ambrosio C, Hill N, MD. Pulmonary complications of chronic neuromuscular diseases and their management. Muscle Nerve. 2004;29:5–27.
16. Fauroux B, Khirani S, Griffon L, Teng T, Lanzeray A, Amaddeo A. Non-invasive ventilation in children with neuromuscular disease. Front Pediatr. 2020;8:482. https://doi.org/10.3389/fped.2020.00482.
17. Choi P, Adam V, Zielinski D. Noninvasive ventilation downloads and monitoring. Sleep Med Clin. 2020;15(4):569–79. https://doi.org/10.1016/j.jsmc.2020.08.012.
18. McDougall CM, Adderley R, Wensley D, Seear M. Long-term ventilation in children: longitudinal trends and outcomes. Arch Dis Child. 2013;98:660–5.
19. Connected Care [Internet]. Connected Care @ SickKids. [Cited 2022 Aug 13]. Available from https://www.connectedcare.sickkids.ca.
20. Amin R, Keilty K, Science M, Orkin J. COVID-19: Guidelines for the Delivery of Home and Community Care Services for Children with Medical Complexity at School [Internet]. Sickkids News 2020 [cited 2022Aug13]. Available from: https://www.sickkids.ca/siteassets/news/news-archive/2020/covid19-school-guidelines-medical-complexity.pdf.
21. Park H, Kim M, In J. Does the minimal occlusive volume technique provide adequate endotracheal tube cuff pressure to prevent air leakage?: a prospective, randomized, crossover clinical study. Anesth Pain Med (Soeul). 2020;15(3):365–70. https://doi.org/10.17085/apm.20020.
22. Mellies U, Goebel C. Optimum insufflation capacity and peak cough flow in neuromuscular disorders. Ann Am Thorac Soc. 2014;11(10):1560–8. https://doi.org/10.1513/AnnalsATS.201406-264OC.
23. Abdullahi A. Safety and efficacy of chest physiotherapy in patients with COVID-19: a critical review. Front Med. 2020;7:454. https://doi.org/10.3389/fmed.2020.00454/full.
24. Hess D. Facilitating speech in the patient with a tracheostomy. Respir Care. 2005;50(4):519–25.
25. Utrarachkij J, Pongsasnongkul J, Preutthipan A, Chantarojanasri T. Measurement of end-expiratory pressure as an indicator of airway patency above tracheostomy in children. J Med Assoc Thail. 2005;88(7):928–33.
26. Moynihan R, Johansson M, Maybee A, Lang E, Légaré F. Covid-19: an opportunity to reduce unnecessary healthcare. BMJ [Internet]. 2020;370:m2752. https://doi.org/10.1136/bmj.m2752.
27. Tran T, Nonoyama M, Cithiravel N, Syed F, Janevski J, Chiang J, Amin R. Virtual mask fitting in pediatric patients during COVID-19: a case series. Can J Respir Ther. 2021;57:93–8. https://doi.org/10.29390/cjrt-2021-023.
28. Morrrow B. Airway clearance therapy in acute paediatric illness: a state-of-the-art review. S Afr J Physiother. 2019;75(1):1295. https://doi.org/10.4102/sajp.v75i1.1295.
29. Guimarães F, Rocha Â. Weak cough strength and secretion retention in mechanically ventilated patients: is there a role for cough-assist devices. Respir Care. 2018;63(12):1583–4. https://doi.org/10.4187/respcare.06527.

30. Prevost S, Brooks D, Bwititi PT. Mechanical insufflation-exsufflation: practice patterns among respiratory therapists in Ontario. Can J Respir Ther. 2015;51:33–8.
31. Fauroux B, Guillemot N, Aubertin G, Nathan N, Labit A, Clement A, Lofaso F. Physiologic benefits of mechanical insufflation-exsufflation in children with neuromuscular diseases. Chest. 2008;133(1):161–8. https://doi.org/10.1378/chest.07-1615.
32. Bianchi C, Baiardi P, Bianchi C, Baiardi P. Cough peak flows: standard values for children and adolescents. Am J Phys Med Rehabil. 2008;87(6):461–7.
33. Spinou A. A review on cough augmentation techniques: assisted inspiration, assisted expiration and their combination. Physiol Res. 2020;69(Suppl 1):S93–S103. https://doi.org/10.33549/physiolres.934407.
34. Rose L, Adhikari NK, Leasa D, Ferguson D, McKim DA. Cough augmentation techniques for extubation or weaning critically ill patients from mechanical ventilation. Cochrane Database Syst Rev. 2017;1(1):CD011833. https://doi.org/10.1002/14651858.CD011833.pub2.

The Ethical Point of View in Prolonged Mechanical Ventilation and Home Ventilation

Samiran Ray and Joe Brierley

1 Introduction

Prolonged mechanical ventilation (PMV) evolved alongside the birth of mechanical ventilation and the development of intensive care, mainly during the polio pandemic of the early-mid-twentieth century.

Children would be quarantined in wards with multiple ventilated patients in negative-pressure ventilators, the so-called iron lungs. Children could remain dependent on these for long periods, even years. Although a technological advance, this was not universally viewed as desirable. Painting a grim picture of the times, a polio survivor in the USA documented:

> ... polio left kids crippled, and that was an image that this big strong post-war country simply couldn't abide. We had children lining up in wheelchairs, in iron lungs, whose very vitality was drained and everyone's hope for their future was shaken right at the most critical time in their childhoods ... There were many other diseases that were bad for America, but polio broke its heart. (Mark Sauer in the documentary *A Paralyzing Fear: The Story of Polio in America* [1])

Mechanical ventilation has become an acceptable and established part of in-hospital treatment in most developed healthcare systems. The need for mechanical ventilation is usually short-lived, with a triage of candidacy at admission, even in resource-rich healthcare systems. In a small proportion of patients, ongoing organ failure for weeks or months can make liberation from a ventilator difficult. Once in this prolonged phase of mechanical ventilation, decisions need to be made about whether the child's prognosis is so poor that mechanical ventilation should be withdrawn. When withdrawal of ventilation is not acceptable—either because of the

S. Ray (✉) · J. Brierley
Paediatric Intensive Care Medicine, Great Ormond Street Hospital NHS Foundation Trust, London, UK
e-mail: samiran.ray@gosh.nhs.uk; joe.brierley@gosh.nhs.uk

A. Kawaguchi et al. (eds.), *Prolonged and Long-Term Mechanical Ventilation in Children*, https://doi.org/10.1007/978-981-97-8903-0_22

prospect of eventual recovery or with acceptance that life-long ventilation can be maintained alongside a good quality of life—then PMV is continued.

For some children, technological advancements have moved ventilators outside the closely monitored confines of the intensive care unit, making a move to long-term ventilation units or home ventilation (HV) an option for many. This change may have resolved some of the problems recognised by Mark Sauer about PMV for children in the 1950s, but ethical deliberations surrounding PMV and HV use continue in many healthcare settings worldwide. Key to this is the moving boundaries of what is possible through advancing technology and the question 'just because we can do it, should we?'

In this chapter, we will explore the ethical issues involved in the use of PMV and HV. The adoption of PMV and HV varies globally—governed mainly by the resources available within the national health and social care setting, even within the economically developed world. Ethical viewpoints of what is appropriate similarly vary based on national moral norms. We will not focus on the issues surrounding PMV in the intensive care unit (ICU) setting where recovery and eventual discharge are likely but a recognised slow process (for example, recovery from critical illness myopathy). Instead, we will limit our discussion to those looking to progress to PMV outside the ICU, including HV. Firstly, we discuss critical ethical arguments that may shape practice. We then discuss the importance of ethical decision-making and the process that may help to achieve this, including steps taken to try and ensure shared decision-making between all parties involved and the processes needed if this is not achievable.

2 Key Ethical Determinants

Whilst many practices around the establishment and continuation of PMV and HV will be determined by resources and broader societal values, we identify questions that may arise in this context. However, the priority must be maintaining the 'best interests' of the child in decision-making, as outlined by Article 3 of the UN Convention on the Rights of a Child [2].

2.1 Clinical Feasibility

Whilst this may not be seen as an ethical principle, a question that needs to be addressed early on is whether PMV or HV is clinically feasible. Positive-pressure ventilation has long been recognised to cause lung injury, related to the amount of mechanical power being delivered to the lung by the ventilator, which is ultimately dependent on the disease process necessitating ventilation [3]. High-pressure ventilation for weeks or months can lead to ongoing lung damage, with associated multi-organ failure and death. Even if technologically feasible, PMV at high pressures is unlikely to be successful, which is crucial in discussions with families about PMV or HV.

PMV/HV can be provided either non-invasively via a mask, usually intermittently, or invasively usually continuously, via a tracheostomy tube. These interfaces are considered preferable to endotracheal tubes as they facilitate mobility, discharge from both ICU and hospital and child development (as lacking in the children with polio remarked upon by Mark Sauer above).

Whilst ventilators may be able to generate high pressures, delivering this to the patient non-invasively may be limited by the leak around the mask. Tight-fitting face masks worn continuously can lead to pressure ulceration, adding to patient morbidity [4]. Non-invasive PMV typically will rely on the ability to tolerate time off the ventilator to preserve skin integrity. Therefore, for high-pressure PMV, a tracheostomy will be necessary. Leak around a tracheostomy tube may still be problematic, and measures to counteract this (say, with a cuffed tube) run the risk of complete loss of airway patency if the tracheostomy tube gets blocked—a greater risk in smaller children with tracheostomies. Pragmatically, therefore, high-pressure ventilation may only be deliverable in an intensive care setting.

2.2 *Expected Benefits of PMV or HV*

PMV/HV is used to treat chronic respiratory failure, which may arise from disorders of respiratory drive, lung pathology, neuromuscular weakness, and, rarely, cardiac pathology. Broadly, PMV/HV is started with one of the two aims: (i) to act as a bridge to recovery or definitive treatment, whereby the eventual outcome is that the child no longer requires ventilation, or (ii) as a destination therapy, when there are no disease-modifying options, recovery is unlikely and the child is expected to need lifelong ventilation [5].

The benefit is rarely questioned in the first situation. Observational studies provide guidance where this is likely (Box 1). However, an overall view of the child's health needs to be considered carefully—children may have a limited lifespan due to conditions unrelated to the reason for which they need PMV/HV. For example, PMV/HV may not be of benefit for chronic lung disease of prematurity, which may recover, if the child also has metastatic cancer, which will not recover.

Box 1 Indications for Using LTV as a Bridge to Recovery/Definitive Therapy (Not Destination Therapy)

Airway

- Airway malacia
- Upper airway obstruction
- Subglottic stenosis

Chest wall and lung parenchymal disease

Chronic lung disease for which treatment exists or spontaneous recovery is possible

Lung hypoplasia

Chest wall deformities amenable to surgery

Cystic fibrosis with lung transplant as definitive therapy (may be dictated by national transplant programme criteria)

Cardiovascular

Congenital heart disease where surgical repair is more amenable later in childhood, e.g. valve disorders

Neurological

Reversible phrenic nerve injury

Reversible neuropathy/myopathy, e.g. Guillain-Barre syndrome and critical illness neuropathy

For destination therapy, the underlying disease will inform whether PMV/HV is appropriate. For example, some conditions may be non-progressive, such as congenital central hypoventilation syndrome, and children will live good-quality lives into adulthood with the support of PMV/HV. However, others, such as neuromuscular or metabolic diseases, may progress to a point where life cannot be sustained even with PMV/HV. In such cases, the trajectory of disease progression must be considered to contextualise the benefit gained.

One area where the benefit of PMV/HV can be questioned is when it is considered a bridge to emerging or experimental therapies. The recent explosion in the advancement of neuromuscular disease therapies, particularly in spinal muscular atrophy (SMA), brings this into focus. An international expert conference in the early 2000s advised against tracheostomy and home ventilation in children with SMA type 1, the most lethal form of the disease, with rapid progression of weakness in infancy [6]. However, a series of novel therapies have transformed the condition to a point where PMV/HV is considered ethically acceptable for many, if not all, children. Therefore, an ethical argument could be extended to other diseases for the use of PMV/HV whilst awaiting research or trial results for similar diseases and treatments. Information that may be relevant to consider includes the disease trajectory, the likelihood of treatment being effective and effect size and the timeliness of translation from research to clinical use. For scenarios of first-in-man use of therapies, the use of PMV/HV should be taken into account in the broader ethical review of the treatment to be given. A framework for the ethical evaluation of such speculative treatment has been published [7].

2.3 The Demands of PMV and HV

The objective of PMV/HV is to sustain life, improve its quality or hopefully both. However, PMV/HV is associated with potential increases in the demands of healthcare; many have been expressed by those adults able to communicate the effect of

PMV/HV on their quality of life [8–10]. Although some children may find it difficult to synchronise with the ventilator, which can be uncomfortable [11], newer ventilation technology has reduced this risk. However, this remains a challenge in children with small tidal volumes or lower inspiratory flow rates, those with poor voluntary muscle control or those with high leak volumes. Non-invasive ventilation can be associated with bloating [12]. Full-face masks, particularly in those with neuromuscular weakness, may increase the risk of aspiration. Pressure area sores from tight-fitting masks can be problematic, which means continuous PMV/HV with masks is undesirable.

Whilst PMV/HV via tracheostomy may overcome some of these problems, tracheostomy tubes can become obstructed, which leads to a potential (and catastrophic) loss of airway. Tracheostomy tube suctioning is needed to prevent this. Whilst suctioning of the tube is not painful, in reality, in children with an ineffective cough, the airway may be suctioned beyond the tracheostomy tube length—repetitive suctioning can cause discomfort and distress as expressed by intensive care unit survivors [13, 14]. A review of hospital use in children post-tracheostomy also identified a large number of hospital days spent by children with lower respiratory tract infections in the first year post-tracheostomy. However, it is unknown whether this is better or worse than for children with a mask interface or those before a tracheostomy [15].

The demands of PMV/HV have to be outweighed by the benefits when making an ethical argument for or against the use of PMV/HV. Most children with PMV/HV quantify the additional demands of healthcare as mild or moderate [16]. Adults similarly have found PMV/HV acceptable when it is provided for symptomatic relief or to prolong survival, even if the demands are high [9]. However, this may depend on the disease; patients with progressive neuromuscular disease expressed hopelessness due to their prognosis rather than the demands of PMV/HV itself [10]. One of the cautions against such qualitative evidence is that they are biased in favour of those patients who can express their opinion—PMV/HV can be most contentious in children unable to communicate—through either developmental age or disability. Facial expressions of pain or distress, alongside physiological indicators of pain such as changes in heart rate or blood pressure, may help but can be challenging to interpret.

A difficulty sometimes faced is when there may be no demonstrable benefits from providing PMV/HV but equally no demonstrable demands on the child—for example, if the child is considered so neurologically impaired that they cannot experience any pain or suffering. In most societies, it would not be ethical to provide treatment with no benefit; therefore, the argument would still persist not to provide PMV/HV. However, other factors, such as the sanctity of life and the status afforded to brain death, may determine the course of action [17].

2.4 *Locus of Choice and Autonomy*

Who decides whether a child should receive PMV/HV may be determined by societal values and healthcare systems. Ideally, this should be a shared decision between the clinical team, the child and their parents. The clinical team will usually determine whether there are clinical indications for PMV/HV whilst discussing the benefits and anticipated demands of PMV/HV with the patient and family. Where possible, the child's view must be sought and respected to uphold patient autonomy, and in accordance with Article 12 of the UN Convention on the Rights of the Child—respect for the views of the child [2].

In most settings where the child's voice cannot be heard, including when the child may not have the developmental competence for decision-making, those with parental responsibility share the decision-making on PMV/HV with the clinical team. However, parents may have overlapping interests [18]. The burden on parents and families in looking after children with HV is high and may inform their decision-making. The parent will know their child the best, even when they may have spent long periods of their life in hospital. A child is likely to share their parents' moral and religious values, so the parents' decision may be most representative of the child's. A caveat to this is that the child will have a unique experience of the condition they need PMV/HV for, which may affect the development of their personal values. Whilst a child may depend on their parents, the parents may still have some dependence on their child—this may be through emotional attachment, although in some societies, this can be financed through social support.

A shared decision, however, does not ensure ethical or moral validity. The clinical team and family may be complicit, often inadvertently, in not preserving the child's best interests [19]. More often, difficulties can arise when there is a difference in opinion between clinical teams and families. Societal values vary between countries and may dictate whose views are accorded primacy in such situations. As a result, an independent body may have to adjudicate based on the balance of best interests of the child, such as clinical ethics committees or the courts.

2.5 Cultural and Religious Values

Cultural and religious values often inform decisions around withholding and withdrawing life-sustaining treatment, which can influence decision-making around PMV/HV, both for individuals and in broader healthcare policy.

Withholding life-sustaining treatment in the case of a child with an irreversible disease may not be considered morally equivalent to the withdrawal of life-sustaining treatment. In some cultures, the latter may be seen as a more active process of ending life, whilst the former may be considered a more passive way of allowing 'nature to take its course'. Furthermore, cultural and religious views on the sanctity of life can vary; for some, it may be paramount to maintain life, regardless of the demands of PMV/HV incurred by the individual, family or society.

Where personal views are not reflective of wider society, there may be a risk of discrimination in not taking these into account. Mutual respect between the family and the clinicians should be maintained to allow understanding of opposing views without necessarily generating disputes. Where possible, cultural or religious representatives should be involved to help find common ground, provided that the best interest of the child is given primacy [20].

The societal differences between different countries and regions which influence decisions about PMV/HV were highlighted between the North and South of Europe in the Eurydice studies in paediatric intensive care units [21]. Such international variability in practice has also been demonstrated in adults [22]. The overarching principles around decision-making that affects survival, as PMV/HV can do, should reflect these societal values and be enshrined in professional body regulations (such as the General Medical Council in the UK) and national law.

The weight of cultural and religious values in decision-making is well exemplified in the case of Tafida Raqeeb in the UK [23]. Tafida was a 4-year-old girl when she sadly suffered a spontaneous intracranial bleed, leaving her with irreversible, extensive brain injury and minimally conscious. She was ventilator dependent in the intensive care unit. The clinical team treating her did not think that it was in her best interests to continue being ventilated and proposed to withdraw mechanical ventilation. Her parents, based on their religious beliefs, disagreed with this. A hospital in Genoa, Italy, was willing to continue prolonged mechanical ventilation. Tafida's parents requested a transfer to Italy, which the treating team refused based on their opinion that it was not in her best interests to continue to be ventilated, regardless of the location. The case was subject to judicial review, where it was argued that the clinical team had mainly focussed on the narrow area of medical best interests. As a 4-year-old, Tafida had demonstrated evidence of religious belief compatible with her parents. Based on this, it was deemed in her wider best interests to be allowed free movement under European Union law to do so. In doing so, the courts also concluded that whilst each region had an obligation to protect against unethical action in its territory, it did not have a monopoly over global ethical or legal matters. However, the judgement, particularly the faith aspects of a 4-year-old, has since been criticised [24] and not supported in subsequent rulings. Tafida was transferred to Genoa and remains mechanically ventilated at the time of writing.

2.6 Legal Frameworks

As the decision to initiate or withdraw PMV/HV in most instances will affect the survival of the child, legal frameworks will play an important role in safeguarding the quality of the decision-making process. This norm forms part of societal (and, by extension, the State's) responsibility towards protecting the welfare of children [25]. In the UK, the courts are asked to decide for the child if a mutual agreement cannot be reached between the clinical teams and the child and family, or rarely, if the best interests of the child are unclear or even at risk, even if clinicians and the family do agree. This process, whilst well established, may be seen as too adversarial and non-compassionate. It may also not necessarily ensure consistency in decision-making. Several examples of high-profile cases, in the UK and the USA, regarding the continuation of life-sustaining treatment in children (and often, by inference, providing PMV/HV) have highlighted how seemingly similar cases can lead to different judgements, even within the same country. An argument can be that each situation should be judged on its own merits and individual nuances; this can then be considered in each subsequent case as part of case law in common law jurisdictions. The importance, therefore, is in the due process of a legal judgement. Alternatively, others claim that judges should not hold moral authority over others, arguing that moral dilemmas should not translate to legal problems [26].

Another legal factor that may influence decision-making in this area is the definition of death, particularly the acceptance of neurological determination of death, whether whole-brain or brainstem death. The World Health Organization proposes the operational definition of death as *'the permanent loss of capacity for consciousness and all brainstem functions, as a consequence of permanent cessation of circulation or catastrophic brain injury'* [27]. Despite this, brain death in the absence of circulatory death is not recognised in all jurisdictions, notably with an East-West split [28]. Furthermore, even in countries that recognise brain death, there are differences in the legal interpretation of what this is, focussing on whether the brainstem or the entire brain needs to show irreversible loss of activity [29]. This area has been the focus of legal challenges in the USA, including in children. The consequence of this is the provision of PMV/HV to a child who could be declared dead in many other jurisdictions. The most well-known of these individual cases is that of Jahi McMath. Jahi McMath was a 13-year-old girl who suffered hypoxic brain damage following elective surgery. She was declared dead following a determination by neurological criteria in the US state of California. However, her parents contested this on the grounds of their religious beliefs that did not recognise brain death, holding that as Jahi's heart was beating, she was still alive. Despite the declaration of death being recognised by the courts, her family was allowed to take her body to New Jersey. In this state, patient or family religious objections to neurological verification of death prevent its use. Subsequently, Jahi, or her body depending on belief, was maintained on home ventilation for a further 5 years until asystole (incidentally following the complications of another surgical procedure) [30].

2.7 Justice

Although justice, the last of the four bioethical principles, is rarely explicitly stated as a factor in decision-making for PMV/HV, the resources needed to provide PMV/HV have a role to play in decision-making in any healthcare setting.

Most overtly, resource use determines whether PMV/HV is provided or not if the family has to bear the cost of PMV/HV due to a lack of public health support. Given the family's resources, the cost of providing PMV/HV may be exorbitant. Sadly, they will not receive ventilation, even though a similar child elsewhere in the world would. Decision-making in this instance is hardly ethical for this child but may be morally understandable if providing PMV/HV would mean others would die from a lack of basic healthcare. Unfortunately, this situation is the case for many of the world's population, where PMV/HV for a child is simply not an option.

Public healthcare systems are unlikely to support PMV/HV in every possible case, as all public healthcare systems have limits to resource availability. Therefore, rationing must occur, even though this is not overtly stated. Part of this happens through the determination of benefit—cost-effectiveness has to be considered for any treatment to be beneficial. In the UK National Health Service, the National Institute of Health and Clinical Excellence (NICE) sets a threshold for funding a treatment based on incremental cost per quality of life-adjusted years gained, i.e. the cost of the treatment divided by the number of years of life in perfect health the therapy can achieve. Typically, this has been between £20,000 and £30,000, although more recently, modifiers for treatments that prolong life or reduce the severity of illness allow higher cost treatments to be used [31]. For example, gene therapy for children with SMA type 1 was recently approved at a much higher treatment cost per individual, making it the most expensive therapy approved by the NICE. However, although no formal health economic evaluation has been undertaken for PMV/HV in the NHS, the cost has previously been estimated in the region of £200,000–£300,000 per year for a child with a tracheostomy on PMV/HV, i.e. ten times the cost of what NICE would typically consider cost-effective [32].

Beyond financial costs, workforce considerations also play a significant part. HV requires home nurses and carers to be trained and employed to help look after the child at home. These professionals are often sourced from the same workforce pool as hospital workers putting strain on the overall system. When new members of staff need to be recruited, the time taken to train can lead to prolonged stays for the child in the hospital, at an opportunity cost to other children who may need the intensive care unit or high-dependency unit bed. Although overtly considered within the welfare or best interest balance sheet for an individual child, these consequences are difficult to ignore.

Finally, by keeping alive children with PMV/HV who otherwise would have died in a public healthcare system, the overall size of the population is increased with an overall reduction in the quality of health of the population (for example, through the diversion of finite resources and opportunity cost). Whilst inherently this may be ethically justifiable, because of the inherent value of life, keeping many children alive with a poor quality of life diminishes overall population health. This could logically lead to what has been termed by the philosopher Derek Parfit as the Repugnant Conclusion or the mere addition paradox: whereby a large population exists whose average life quality is so poor that their lives collectively may not be worth living. Whilst unlikely to happen within a resource-constrained system, it cautions against keeping people alive when the cost to the population is greater than the quality of life gained.

3 Ethical Decision-Making Rather Than Ethical Decisions

Given the various complex, interrelated factors that determine the ethical quality of a decision, which may be challenging to balance fully, importance is placed instead on the decision-making process. This is based on the argument that following a robust process in which the child's best interests are held to be paramount will lead to reproducible results where ethical consistency is maintained.

The main decision points around PMV/HV involve a) the initiation of PMV/HV and b) the continuation of PMV/HV. Both are important. We propose practices that we have found to aid the process in achieving consistency and satisfaction between the parties involved.

Decision-making should involve the clinical team, the child where possible, and the family. The clinical team will bring together their knowledge of the experience of the disease, the likely prognosis based on the best evidence and observed trajectory in the individual patient of PMV/HV and what it entails based on feedback they receive from similar children needing PMV/HV. The clinical team should be representative of all those who are, and will be, looking after the child. This should ideally include those across healthcare settings (for example, the family doctor or community paediatricians), nurses, physiotherapists or respiratory therapists, and the relevant members of the HV team who will take over ongoing care. The child must be supported to express their thoughts and feelings on the matter, about their experience of the disease and their hopes and fears for the future. The parents and family will explore their unique knowledge about their child, their own values and beliefs, and hopes for their child, together with their insight on their capacity to look after a child on PMV/HV.

Decision-making is a process and cannot be achieved in a single meeting. Therefore, initial discussions have to centre around the diagnoses, prognosis and goals of care—Is PMV/HV planned to continue for the rest of the child's life, or is there an expectation of successful treatment or spontaneous recovery from the disease necessitating ventilation?

An honest account of what life entails for a child needing PMV or HV should be painted. This will depend on the services available locally—for example, home carers or home nursing packages, whether care responsibilities need to be shared with the family for parts of the week, equipment ordering and supply responsibilities and other costs that must be borne [33]. An idea should be given on how HV would affect family life—this includes housing, mobility, safety and ability to take holidays. Siblings and other members of the family are often affected by a child needing HV. This must be reflected in the conversation. If possible, families should be introduced to those looking after a child on PMV/HV to give a first-hand account of what this entails. However, each family unit will be different, and not all share the same experiences, even though common themes emerge from the literature [34].

The child and family's understanding should be checked intermittently. This is important to avoid frustration and disappointment later in treatment. In addition, a lot of information will be transferred in the course of the decision-making process, some of which clinical teams may think trivial. It is, therefore, essential to make sure that families understand the information given in line with the principles of providing informed consent.

Communication should be open, empathetic and non-judgmental. It is impossible to remain fully unbiased—all clinical team members will have their views on what they think is suitable for the child and family. It may help to acknowledge this, but to explicitly acknowledge that the decision is not based on a single person's opinion and that determining a child's best interest can be complex and difficult.

Alternatives, where available, should be discussed. In most cases, PMV/HV is needed to preserve and maintain life—without this, a child would die or remain in intensive care indefinitely. However, the time course may vary—a child with a neuromuscular disease may need PMV/HV to reduce carbon dioxide retention or improve sleep quality in the short term and prevent a decline in functional status. Not providing PMV/HV may hasten decline but may not lead to immediate death—this may be an acceptable alternative. Palliative care should be introduced where life is likely to be limited. Even though palliative therapies may not be immediately needed, the balance between active and palliative treatments may shift if the child deteriorates or finds PMV/HV less tolerable. This is often referred to as parallel planning.

The decision to continue with PMV/HV must be reviewed regularly once PMV/HV is established. This is important as the disease either progresses or improves or the child's experience of PMV/HV changes. The ethical basis of decision-making may not be the same as at initiation—what comprises the best interests of the child may have changed. Time should be dedicated to re-exploring this openly and transparently without the child or family feeling harassed or questioned.

Sadly, despite the best intentions, sometimes a shared decision cannot be agreed. When there is a difference in opinion between the clinical team or families, processes must exist to achieve resolution. One approach may be to give primacy to those with parental responsibility as they are the usual decision-maker for their child and carry the burden of whatever the decision made more than anyone else. However, as highlighted in the previous section, the parents' interests may not entirely overlap with those of the child, and both clinical teams and broader society are responsible for protecting children from harm. Some have looked to resolve such differences through independent mediation. This process allows an independent mediator, often with legal or clinical training, to get both parties to identify their goals and differences and try to reconcile some of these to find a mutually agreed solution. Most importantly, this process can facilitate resumed communication if this has broken down, allowing all parties to tell their side of the story and be heard [35].

Ethics support services can also prove helpful in considering moral questions about treatment, in this context, about PMV/HV decisions when the best interests of a child are either unclear or disputed. Hospitals usually put together clinical ethics committees with representation from clinical teams not involved in the child's care, lay members and philosophical/ethics, law and faith experts. Typically, the clinical team presents the case, outlining the ethical difficulties in determining the best course of action. Parents and children in our centre can also attend the meeting. After hearing the facts, the committee deliberates the values involved, determines the relevant ethical issues and then articulates the moral arguments for and against possible treatment options, including PMV/HV. They may make recommendations about whether the proposed treatment has an ethical basis but do not make any decision, which remains for the child if competent, and parents/those with parental responsibility to make, together with the clinical team. Whilst in many cases, the clinical ethics committee can provide sufficient guidance for both the clinical teams and families to accept, critics point out that they are affiliated with hospitals, with only a few members genuinely independent. Although there is guidance for the composition and operation of clinical ethics committees, shared learning within networks, governance and decision review may not be uniformly available [36].

As discussed above, where shared decisions cannot be reached, the courts are best placed to resolve disagreements. Although the process can be lengthy, expensive and adversarial, legal processes are independent and binding; they ensure consistency and robustness of process. This is warranted as decisions around PMV/HV may inevitably lead to a decision about life or death. Following high-profile cases, particularly in the UK, a statutory requirement to avoid court processes is being pursued to give processes such as mediation and clinical ethics committee review greater importance. Regardless of this, the judicial process will remain the ultimate arbiter of best interest disagreements.

4 Conclusion

PMV and HV have come a long way since the 1950s. Ventilators are more portable, smarter and more user-friendly. Pathways to home ventilation in children are better defined. The number of children on home ventilation has increased worldwide—with a spectrum from nocturnal non-invasive ventilation to continuous tracheostomy ventilation. As we can medically and technologically do more, we still need to ask whether we should, with ethical issues continuing to be identified. At all points, the best interests of the child should be maintained—but the determination of best interests may be difficult. A rigorous and consistent decision-making process is best placed to safeguard ethical practice. Ideally, this should be reached through open communication between the child, their family and clinicians. If this is unsuccessful, well-defined steps should be in place to resolve differences and ultimately adjudicate.

References

1. Wellner KL. Polio and historical inquiry. OAH Mag Hist. 2005;19(5):54–8.
2. UNICEF. The UN Convention on the Rights of the Child. 1989. https://www.unicef.org.uk/what-we-do/un-convention-child-rights. Accessed 13 Aug 2022.
3. Gattinoni L, Tonetti T, Cressoni M, Cadringher P, Herrmann P, Moerer O, Protti A, Gotti M, Chiurazzi C, Carlesso E, Chiumello D, Quintel M. Ventilator-related causes of lung injury: the mechanical power. Intensive Care Med. 2016;42(10):1567–75.

4. Lauderbaugh DL, Billman G, Popien TL, Hauseur S, Lee E, O'Haver J. A Comparison of the Braden Q and the Braden QD Scale to Assess Pediatric Risk for Pressure Injuries during Noninvasive Ventilation. Respir Care. 2021;66(8):1234–9.
5. Ray S, Brierley J, Bush A, Fraser J, Halley G, Harrop EJ, Casanueva L. Towards developing an ethical framework for decision making in long-term ventilation in children. Arch Dis Child. 2018;103(11):1080–4.
6. Benson RC, Hardy KA, Gildengorin G, Hsia D. International survey of physician recommendation for tracheostomy for Spinal Muscular Atrophy Type I. Pediatr Pulmonol. 2012;47(6):606–11.
7. Brierley J, Larcher V. Compassionate and innovative treatments in children: a proposal for an ethical framework. Arch Dis Child. 2009;94(9):651–4.
8. Huttmann SE, Magnet FS, Karagiannidis C, Storre JH, Windisch W. Quality of life and life satisfaction are severely impaired in patients with long-term invasive ventilation following ICU treatment and unsuccessful weaning. Ann Intensive Care. 2018;8(1):38.
9. Gale NK, Jawad M, Dave C, Turner AM. Adapting to domiciliary non-invasive ventilation in chronic obstructive pulmonary disease: a qualitative interview study. Palliat Med. 2015;29(3):268–77.
10. Ando H, Chakrabarti B, Angus RM, Cousins R, Thornton EW, Young CA. Experience of long-term use of non-invasive ventilation in motor neuron disease: an interpretative phenomenological analysis. BMJ Support Palliat Care. 2014;4(1):50–6.
11. Blokpoel RGT, Burgerhof JG, Markhorst DG, Kneyber MCJ. Patient-ventilator asynchrony during assisted ventilation in children. Pediatr Crit Care Med. 2016;17(5):e204–11.
12. Grychtol R, Chan EY. Use of non-invasive ventilation in cerebral palsy. Arch Dis Child. 2018;103(12):1170–7.
13. Van de Leur JP, Zwaveling JH, Loef BG, Van der Schans CP. Patient recollection of airway suctioning in the ICU: routine versus a minimally invasive procedure. Intensive Care Med. 2003 Mar;29(3):433–6.
14. Turner JS, Briggs SJ, Springhorn HE, Potgieter PD. Patients' recollection of intensive care unit experience. Crit Care Med. 1990 Sep;18(9):966–8.
15. Powell J, Keltie K, Sims A, Richardson H, Brodlie M, Powell S. National cohort study of health care resource use after pediatric tracheostomy. JAMA Pediatr. 2022;176(8):817–9.
16. Seear M, Kapur A, Wensley D, Morrison K, Behroozi A. The quality of life of home-ventilated children and their primary caregivers plus the associated social and economic burdens: a prospective study. Arch Dis Child. 2016;101(7):620–7.
17. Wilkinson D. Is it in the best interests of an intellectually disabled infant to die? J Med Ethics. 2006;32(8):454–9.
18. Wilkinson D. How much weight should we give to parental interests in decisions about life support for newborn infants? Monash Bioeth Rev. 2010;20(2):13.1–25.
19. Birchley G. Deciding together? Best interests and shared decision-making in paediatric intensive care. Health Care Anal. 2014;22(3):203–22.
20. Truog RD. Tackling medical futility in Texas. N Engl J Med. 2007;357(1):1–3.
21. Devictor DJ, Nguyen DT. Forgoing life-sustaining treatments in children: a comparison between Northern and Southern European pediatric intensive care units. Pediatr Crit Care Med. 2004;5(3):211–5.
22. Avidan A, Sprung CL, Schefold JC, Ricou B, Hartog CS, Nates JL, Jaschinski U, Lobo SM, Joynt GM, Lesieur O, Weiss M, Antonelli M, Bülow HH, Bocci MG, Robertsen A, Anstey MH, Estébanez-Montiel B, Lautrette A, Gruber A, Estella A, Mullick S, Sreedharan R, Michalsen A, Feldman C, Tisljar K, Posch M, Ovu S, Tamowicz B, Demoule A, DeKeyser GF, Pargger H, Noto A, Metnitz P, Zubek L, de la Guardia V, Danbury CM, Szűcs O, Protti A, Filipe M, Simpson SQ, Green C, Giannini AM, Soliman IW, Piras C, Caser EB, Hache-Marliere M, Mentzelopoulos SD. ETHICUS-2 Study Group. Variations in end-of-life practices in intensive care units worldwide (Ethicus-2): a prospective observational study. Lancet Respir Med. 2021;9(10):1101–10.

23. Van Leeuwen B. Free movement of life? The interaction between the best interest and the right to freely receive services in Tafida Raqeeb. Public Law. 2020;(3):398–408.
24. Cave E, Brierley J, Archard D. Making Decisions for Children-Accommodating Parental Choice in Best Interests Determinations: Barts Health NHS Trust v Raqeeb [2019] EWHC 2530 (Fam); Raqeeb and Barts Health NHS Trust [2019] EWHC 2531 (Admin). Med Law Rev. 2020;28(1):183–96.
25. Bridgeman J. 'Our legal responsibility… to intervene on behalf of the child'. Recognising public responsibilities for the medical treatment of children. Med Law Inter. 2021;21(1):19–41.
26. Paris JJ, Ahluwalia J, Cummings BM, Moreland MP, Wilkinson DJ. The Charlie Gard case: British and American approaches to court resolution of disputes over medical decisions. J Perinatol. 2017;37(12):1268–71.
27. Shemie SD, Hornby L, Baker A, Teitelbaum J, Torrance S, Young K, Capron AM, Bernat JL, Noel L, The International Guidelines for Determination of Death phase 1 participants, in collaboration with the World Health Organization. International guideline development for the determination of death. Intensive Care Med. 2014;40(6):788–97.
28. Yang Q, Miller G. East-West differences in perception of brain death. Review of history, current understandings, and directions for future research. J Bioeth Inq. 2015;12(2):211–25.
29. McGee A, Gardiner D. Differences in the definition of brain death and their legal impact on intensive care practice. Anaesthesia. 2019;74(5):569–72.
30. Biel S, Durrant J. Controversies in brain death declaration: legal and ethical implications in the ICU. Curr Treat Options Neurol. 2020;22:12.
31. National Institute of Health and Clinical Excellence (NICE). NICE changes to provide faster, fairer access to new drugs and devices. 2021. https://indepth.nice.org.uk/methods-review/index.html#group-section-Additional-resources-BVYgdxP8JQ. Accessed 12 Aug 2022.
32. Noyes J, Godfrey C, Beecham J. Resource use and service costs for ventilator-dependent children and young people in the UK. Health Soc Care Community. 2006;14(6):508–22.
33. Dybwik K, Tollåli T, Nielsen EW, Brinchmann BS. "Fighting the system": families caring for ventilator-dependent children and adults with complex health care needs at home. BMC Health Serv Res. 2011;11:156.
34. Carnevale FA, Alexander E, Davis M, Rennick J, Troini R. Daily living with distress and enrichment: the moral experience of families with ventilator-assisted children at home. Pediatrics. 2006;117(1):e48–60.
35. Meller S, Barclay S. Mediation: an approach to intractable disputes between parents and paediatricians. Arch Dis Child. 2011;96(7):619–21.
36. Brierley J, Archard D, Cave E. Challenging misconceptions about clinical ethics support during COVID-19 and beyond: a legal update and future considerations. J Med Ethics. 2021;47(8):549–52.

Prolonged Home Mechanical Ventilation: A Nursing Perspective

Sheila S. Kun, Josephine Ellashek, Sally L. Davidson Ward, and Thomas G. Keens

1 Introduction

Children's Hospital of Los Angeles (CHLA) discharged their first patient on HMV on November 29, 1977. At that time, it seemed bold, and perhaps reckless, to attempt to care for a ventilator-dependent child in the home. Such patients were only cared for in an ICU at that time. But it was successful, and this young man with the diagnosis of congenital central hypoventilation syndrome has done very well.

Having a child in the ICU has been shown to be a very stressful experience for mothers and fathers. The research work by leading nursing researchers since the 1980s [1–3] reported that the grief, depression, and role attainment of being a mother were stressors in the ICU setting. Interventions were needed before parents were ready for home care training. Carnevale et al. described the moral experience of families with ventilator-assisted children at home as "daily living with distress and enrichment." Parents were living with daily threat of death and feeling that there was "no free choice" in the matter [4].

The Resiliency Model of Family Stress, Adjustment, and Adaptation suggested by McCubbin and McCubbin offered sharp focus on family adjustment and adaptation when families are faced with stressful experiences. The goal was for the family to manage stress without major changes in their daily functioning [5].

S. S. Kun (✉) · J. Ellashek
Division of Pediatric Pulmonology and Sleep Medicine, Children's Hospital Los Angeles, Los Angeles, CA, USA
e-mail: jellashek@chla.usc.edu

S. L. D. Ward · T. G. Keens
Division of Pediatric Pulmonology and Sleep Medicine, Children's Hospital Los Angeles, Los Angeles, CA, USA

Keck School of Medicine, University of Southern California, Los Angeles, CA, USA
e-mail: sward@chla.usc.edu; tkeens@chla.usc.edu

A. Kawaguchi et al. (eds.), *Prolonged and Long-Term Mechanical Ventilation in Children*, https://doi.org/10.1007/978-981-97-8903-0_23

When clinicians were confronted with the questions of "What do you do with these HMV patients? And how do we respond to the needs of ICU parents?" nursing became the obvious discipline to **take on the task of the day-to-day care**. With the rich research work on family stress and adaptation strategies, nursing learned very quickly that all of the families devoted significant efforts toward normalizing their experience [4]. Families had to work with their new normal. This striving for normalcy and stability, however, was sometimes undermined by limitations in family finances, family cohesion, and unpredictability of the child's condition [4].

Nurses recognized that parent participation in care has been shown to decrease parental stress by giving parents control over particular areas of their child's care in the ICU setting [3]. With the HMV parents, they needed to be totally trained in all home care procedures, including the medical technology of the ventilator use. New technology for parents may be more challenged in their caregiver role [6]. The emotional stress of the role of mom and nurse all in one is another source of emotional stress [7]. Kirk et al. showed that parents felt that they had to take on the role of a nurse or medical provider when medical technology was being used in their home [8]. This stressful experience of being the parent of a technology-dependent child cannot be overlooked.

The initiatives to include parents in education and research have been limited [9]. Parent feedback was essential for us to advance care for our HMV children [10]. In addition to strengthening skills in communication, confidence in the team, and compassion, parents in a survey study identified a need for hospital staff to anticipate financial and social stressors and provide supportive resources more readily [9]. Kingston RL articulated well some of the major stressors when caring for HMV children: a change in the family's finances, the effects on the siblings and sleep deprivation, loss of usual routine, changes in social life, and marital discord [11]. Many HMV programs have considered these stresses associated with HMV children and incorporated sound recommendations in the management of their programs.

One of the priorities in the development of the home care program is the consideration of safety. Knowing that first and foremost, they are the **sole practitioners in the home**, parents do not have the luxury of different shifts of nurses and respiratory care practitioners (RCPs) and that they have to make critical decisions to triage emergencies alone.

A well-designed educational program includes the consideration of how parents could duplicate these procedures easily and fit them into their lifestyles. If parents are unable to follow the schedules, home care would be compromised. Hence, to promote adherence and continuity of care, the home schedule should be manageable. In the case of emergency training, we need to consider that parents have limited manpower in their home. They would not be able to call a code with a team of trained RCP to triage the home emergencies. Bear in mind that we turn parents into semi-paramedics in 4–6 weeks. Therefore, the training program has to include the fact that they are **non-licensed caregivers making critical decisions in the home**.

"**There is no room for error in airway management**" and "**Listen to the parents**." These beliefs offered a sound philosophy and strategy to treat the HMV children as they transitioned from ICU to home setting. Nurses played a key role in

infusing the "home care" visions in managing this population. The HMV program had to be **safe, easy, and manageable.**

The preparation to transition from hospital to home demands **seamless coordination** and collaboration among the inpatient and outpatient staff to prevent emergency room visits and readmissions. The case management model applies accurately for HMV patients: comprehensive complex condition management to proactively identity and coordinate medical and social services to optimize patient health and prevent complications and exacerbations [12].

Just being able to breathe with a ventilator was not the ultimate goal; children supported by HMV should have **a quality of life to maximize their best potential**. They require ongoing medical care from an interdisciplinary team who can address medical, developmental, psychosocial, and equipment needs. **Nurses coordinate both inpatient and outpatient services** and collaborate with social workers, RCP, durable medical equipment (DME) vendors, community resources, and outpatient colleagues to ensure continuous family support.

Many nursing quality improvement and research projects addressed clinical barriers to HMV care. Kun et al. identified learning gaps, defined the best practice by working with parents and home care colleagues, and provided clinical care based on **critical observations and nursing research** [13–15].

From a recent publication in 2020 titled "Discharge Practices for Children with Home Mechanical Ventilation Across the United States," the authors reported that many programs have similar approaches on caregiver training and independent care, discharge criteria checklists, and guidelines. A minority of institutions had a standard definition of medical stability for discharge and struggle with attaining needed DME for home care [16].

This chapter shares the vast experience and successful approaches in caring for our children supported by HMV from a nursing perspective in the United States; we will highlight how nurses conceptualized the program and executed and implemented home procedures and policies, with safety as the main goal. **Family-centered care** (FCC) has been the philosophy of care adopted by pediatric nursing: the clinician incorporates into caregiving the knowledge and conviction that family is the constant in children's lives [17]. We will share how to customize home care routines based on the individual needs of the home caregivers, placing the needs of the **families and patients** at the **center of our mission**. Nurses offered practical insight into the problem, and research guided us to quality improvement projects.

As this book is meant to be used globally, our infrastructure, regional services, and resources might be different. However, our fundamental beliefs in working with parents, making lives easier, putting their children in the center of care, and painting a brighter future for our children have universal application.

2 Parents Are Our Global Positioning System (GPS)

2.1 It Is a New World

HMV had a dual impact on parents, providing them with a sense of security and moderated stress levels. Despite the tremendous hardships, parents also reported a deep sense of personal enrichment arising from their caregiving role [18]. Parents taking a child dependent on a ventilator home are faced with the reality of a "new world"; this is an expression describing the new experiences when a home becomes a place fitted with medical machinery and a home nursing regime [19]. We observed that parents initially are **novices** in HMV care while in the hospital; learning the technology was a frightening but necessary process [19]. Later on, most parents become good **apprentices** during their in-depth home care training. Most parents become **knowledgeable and confident caregivers** [18] very quickly after having the daily practice for 6–12 months at home. Their decision-making is increasingly on target. Eventually, parents are valuable resource when they become **intuitive experts** regarding their child's care [9]. **Parental survey researches from Australia, Canada, and the United States** reported valuable input and feedback in better understanding of HMV home care adjustment and educational needs [19, 20].

2.2 Parents as Novices Before Discharge

During this post-diagnosis phase, we need to recognize that parents of NICU patients go through **a period of grieving** for the loss of the normal and healthy baby that they had hoped for [1–3]. And for those children with chronic illness, the progression to needing ventilator support would be another blow to the parents. This is a tough time for the parents; learning complex home care is difficult until they are able to move on to the acceptance phase [5]. For all parents, it is a **life-changing experience** that impacts them for the rest of their lives [18]. When grief is unresolved, it would be difficult to move to the phase of preparation for home. However, in spite of being the **novices** in HMV care, new parents were a **useful resource to identify what the needs** are in their own home setting.

An important aspect of normalizing life for parents was for the HMV children to return to school, preventing social isolation [19]. Parents were happy to see their children in the school system. Nurses took on the task of initiating **school integration program,** assisting with development of school procedures. With the implementation of care coordination programs, many unmet needs such as school integration issues had been addressed [21].

2.3 *Parents as Apprentices in Preparation for Home Care [10]*

Parents as home caregivers are required to go through a vigorous training program before discharge [16]. What are some of the practical tips we have learned during this training process? Successful caregivers were the ones who were able to spend a lot of time at the bedside, forming sustained bonds with their infants despite obstacles [22]. **Knowing the baseline** of the child is key to enhance their assessment skills. Parents whose visits are infrequent should be a red flag to the team as this is a definite barrier to learning the care. Most institutions require demonstration of independent care prior to discharge [16]. The key elements to consider when assessing the parents during their independent practice go beyond performing the home procedures correctly. We look for the skill of **integration.** Are they able to do all the home care procedures within a reasonable schedule for the day? Parents need to consider their lifestyle, work, role, and responsibilities at home to come up with a workable schedule [4]. Hence, parents attain **organizational skills** to make life easy and manageable.

2.4 *Parents as Confident Caregivers*

"Confident parents" had been described by many once they had the care routine under their belt. Most parents become **confident caregivers** who exercise good judgment and make independent decisions appropriate for their children [18]. They considered themselves as the "lifeline" to their child [18]. Therefore, when experienced parents call in as a "sick call," most of them know how their children have responded to such intermittent illnesses before and what has worked for them in the past. The team needs to **listen to the parents' stories** and provide guidance based on their history.

2.5 *Parents as Intuitive Experts*

We need to respect the knowledge of the parents and establish a relationship that welcomes parents' input: they become **intuitive experts** [9, 19]. **Listening to the parents has been our guiding principle.** Our program received tremendous support from parents over the years. They helped to develop the Tracheostomy Home Care for Children, and they were the stars of our educational home care video. When parents see themselves as partners in solving clinical problems, they too become astute observers on clinical changes. They volunteered to take HMV home setup pictures in their homes, shared past experience with near-miss situations, and offered practical advice to guide our care; parents are intuitive experts and **monitors of deviation from clinical baseline.**

3 Critical Success Factors in the Management of HMV Programs

Tamasitis J et al. described the key components of a successful hospital to home program for HMV children; the success stems from three elements: **standardization of its most basic components, orchestrated communication and interdisciplinary collaboration, and commitment from personnel.** With these factors in mind, nurses were able to provide the same comprehensive program and the same quality care to every patient, every time [23].

3.1 Family-Centered Pediatric Nursing Care

Family-centered care (FCC) has appropriately been adopted as a philosophy of care for pediatric nursing [24]. This approach is especially applicable to the management of HMV children. With the recognition that the family is the constant factor in the child's life, the model adopted to facilitate family/professional collaboration at all levels of hospital, home, and community care. FCC is the exchange of complete and unbiased information between families and professionals in a supportive manner with respect to cultural diversity [25].

As illustrated above, the preparation for a successful transition from hospital to home requires a designated team of personnel, with a comprehensive approach to standard of care, communication, and commitment, and putting the needs of the patient and family at the center. Many HMV programs operationalized the FCC approach. A designated respiratory care unit (RCU) for HMV patients had been helpful in preparing the parents for home care.

3.2 The Role of Nursing in Respiratory Care Unit Designated for the HMV Program

In our institution, the RCU nurses designed the unit to create an environment for safe and efficient care based on their nursing expertise. The staff had input on staffing selection. Nurses having **ownership of the RCU dedicated unit** impacted their commitment and success in carrying out their goals for timely and safe discharge.

The RCU nurses **possess critical thinking, knowledge, and abilities** making the program of superior quality and outcome. Daily exposure to a rapid response system trains them to have a high level of awareness to situations preventing the child needing HMV from deteriorating. They can translate the RCU care, both routine and urgent, into educational opportunities. Even when a rapid response is called, this becomes a teachable moment to caregivers so that when the situation is observed at home, caregivers will know how to react appropriately.

Another quality that RCU nurses possess is **superior communication with the multidisciplinary team.** They are active participants in multidisciplinary rounds which have broken barriers to effective communication, improved patient safety, as well as staff and patient satisfaction. They have created a group HMV email to communicate on a timely basis to the whole team, both inpatient and outpatient team members. RCU nurses lead the family-centered rounds daily. RCU nurses are active in **shared decision-making** with the whole team and the families. During the **family-centered rounds**, nurses present the patient's situation and any actions taken. They also have the family present allowing them to ask questions and seek recommendations from the team on how they could support their child's needs. They always respect and **understand the uniqueness of every caregiver** and every situation, nurturing a climate of trust. RCU nurses contribute to the success of the HMV program with a sense of accountability and autonomy.

RCU nurses receive **initial HMV training in their orientation** and a **review of the HMV skills every 6 months**. They lead **the team in the assessment of the HMV program on a quarterly basis** and modify interventions as needed. They facilitate the transition of patients and families from the PICU, CTICU, and NICCU to the RCU by providing support, clarifying expectations, defining the role of the parents upon transfer, and identifying goals from each discipline.

3.3 Collaboration and Care Coordination

Collaboration and coordination are the actions these nurses live by. These nurses demonstrate inter-professional care defined as "care provided by a team of health professionals with overlapping expertise and appreciation of the contributions of others in achieving a common goal" [26]. For these nurses, the achievement of one is an honor for the whole team; they always celebrate the completion of every caregiver's training; nurses along with the social worker provide the caregivers a **certificate of completion** once the HMV program is completed.

Nurses are one of the **greatest coordinators of care** with a holistic focus to not only the patient and parents, but also **helping siblings** with the life-changing event. They **follow up with the pharmacy**, coordinate the **caregivers' training schedules** with other disciplines, and assist caregivers to ensure that they are meeting their goals by **documenting the training checklist**. Discharge guidelines, including the use of a checklist, assurance of home care, and caregiver training, were prevalent in the United States from a 2020 survey on discharge practices across the United States [16]. The Nurses will alert the HMV team of any barriers or delays, and they also seek solutions to the pressing issues.

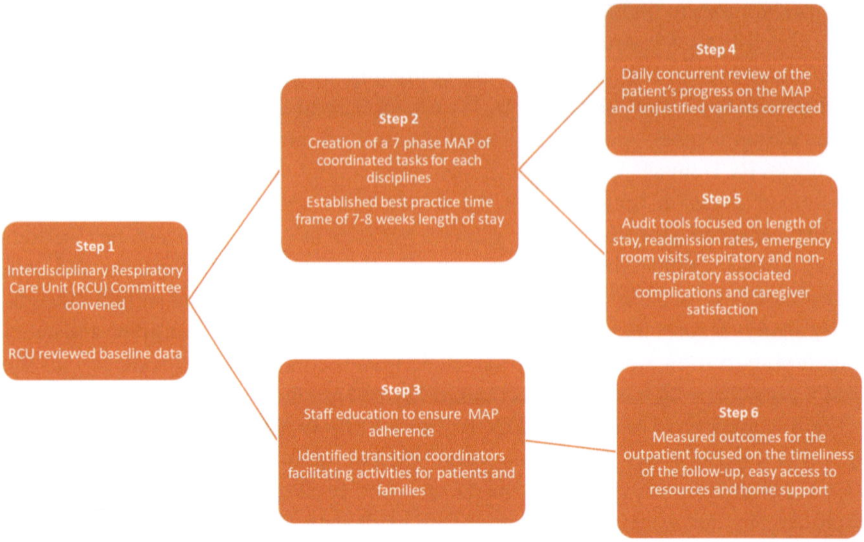

Fig. 1 The dynamic role of nursing in the HMV program

3.4 Patient/Caregiver Advocacy

Advocacy is another nurse's role that is well observed in this program. These nurses work hand-in-hand with parents, spending considerable time at bedside with parents/caregivers, and are well positioned to identify their needs in the hospital and at home. They connect the families to resources for assistance. Caregivers are encouraged to voice their concerns to the team. The RCU nurses are their best advocates!

The efficacy of a multidisciplinary action plan (MAP) in discharge planning for pediatric HMV was presented at the American Thoracic Society International Conference, May 2015 [27]. The key points described above are captured in Fig. 1.

4 How Do We Ensure Safety Measures in Inpatient and Outpatient Settings?

Nurses wear the many hats of being the educator, coordinator, researcher, advocator, and financial counselor as we walk with the parents to provide growth and the best opportunities that life can offer. **Nurses identified gaps in clinical needs and developed safety measures both for inpatient and outpatient settings through nursing research**. A few examples illustrating such effort on HMV patients are described below.

4.1 Avoiding Risk Factors for Emergency Room Visit or Readmission

Significant efforts have been made to mitigate emergency risks and readmissions. Boroughs et al. suggested decreasing accidental mortality of ventilator-dependent children at home by more vigorous training and motoring. They attributed the primary causes of preventable death in ventilator-dependent children at home to inadequate training, improper response, and a lack of vigilance by the clinicians who care for them [28].

Nursing had tuned into utilizing research to assess risk factors and work on improvement strategies. One such effort was the research in identifying rapid response team (RRT) incidence after the HMV patients were transferred from ICU to the RCU. This research noted that children on HMV preparing for their initial hospital discharge had the greatest number of RRT/code events. The **most prevalent interventions** among children with **RRT events were ventilator setting adjustments**, and among children with **code events, the most frequent actions were tracheostomy-related interventions** [13]. Knowing the risk factors for RRT/code events helped us develop **protocols on stabilizing ventilator settings for 1 week before transfer to the RCU**, and nurses paid meticulous attention to tracheostomy-related risk such as accidental decannulation and mucus plugging.

How did we **define medical stability for discharge**? Based on the nursing research on hospital readmissions for newly discharged pediatric home mechanical ventilation patients in 2012, of the ten patients that had changes made within 7 days prior to discharge, eight (80%) were readmitted shortly after discharge [14]. Therefore, the recommendation of "**no changes in home care regimen 7 days before discharge**" makes sense. The survey on discharge practices for HMV children in the United States also noted that over one-third of the respondents reported that their institutions had this standard definition of medical stability [16].

The same HMV readmission study also identified a 12-month incidence of non-elective readmission of 40%. Close to half of these readmissions occurred within the first 3 months post first HMV index discharge. Many of these readmissions were airway related, and some may have been potentially preventable [14]. Subsequent quality improvement strategies **stressed rehearsals on tracheostomy and respiratory emergency responses,** especially during parents' independent care days, and offered **simulation on emergencies** during their **three out-of-room pre-discharge excursions/walks** in the RCU unit and in the outdoor garden of the hospital. Sobotka's study [16] echoed a similar finding—almost 94% of discharge hospitals had standardized training guidelines with demonstration of independent care by primary caregivers. Improved parental performance in tracheostomy emergency simulation training was reported by Prickett el al. [29].

Another approach to mitigate barriers in the home post-discharge is to compulsively schedule newly discharged HMV patients' **outpatient follow-up** in the pulmonary clinic within **1–2 weeks post-discharge**. The goal is to catch home care problems early.

4.2 Extra Support During Transport

There was no specific guideline to capture the type of transportation used for HMV discharge. This author noted that it varied from institution to institution. Personal communication with major program clinicians noted that the use of ambulance to transport HMV patients was common. As part of the training in using the portable home ventilator, at CHLA, parents are asked to assemble the portable ventilator and circuit on the day of discharge. **Parents drive their HMV child home,** with home health nursing support and the home RCP driving behind so they are there for the homecoming. **We do not use an ambulance or other medical transportation for discharge** unless family does not have a personal vehicle. On the day of discharge, the home RCP spends hours in the home to observe and support the home ventilator setup. Within 2 days, the home RCP would verify stability of the patient and is available for any questions related to the ventilator.

4.3 Virtual Telehealth Home Visit and Assessment Within 3 Days Post-discharge

Trial of telemedicine for patients on home ventilator support noted its feasibility, confidence in clinical management, and use in medical decision-making [30].

Taking advantage of the virtual visits that became practical during the COVID pandemic, this author initiated another safety measure in 2021. A telehealth visit is conducted with the primary pulmonologist and a nurse within 3 days post-discharge. We look for home setup that promotes prompt response to emergencies. Some of the questions in our checklist are the following:

1. Pretend that an **accidental tracheal decannulation** occurred, what are you going to do? In this scenario, we look for whether suctioning and airway rescue medical durable equipment are easily available within arm's reach.
2. We ask whether the **portable ventilator unit is ready to go when emergency happens**: an assigned location for the emergency DME, with the portable unit and circuits connected. We confirm that the portable oxygen tank is on hand.
3. Based on parents' feedback, we encouraged **all respiratory DME to be on a mobile cart**. This facilitates easy access of respiratory equipment support when the child is moved to different parts of the house.
4. We visually **inspect the safety of the home**, for example, ensuring that the head of the bed is always higher than the humidifier of the ventilator.
5. When parents are **organized**, they cut down on the time when responding to emergencies. Hence, we focus on emergency DME setup, schedules for medication, and procedures.
6. Other preventive measures include a **monthly calendar** for return appointment, refill of medication, and DME supplies.

7. We always take a moment to celebrate the family's reunification in their home, and reinforce the family's capabilities and successes.

The telehealth home visit depicted above was presented at the American Thoracic Society International Conference, May 2022 [31]. Figure 2 captures some safety tips in setting up the home.

4.4 Special Quality Improvement Initiative Specific for Outpatient Clinic

How ready are we when respiratory emergencies arise in the clinic settings? In 2014, a **research study, surveying all the clinicians (physicians, fellows, nurses, and respiratory care practitioners)** was performed to identify **whether the respiratory DME setup was correct for outpatient use** [15]. This survey allowed us to identify learning needs of DME for outpatient use and standardize our approach to outpatient emergencies. A good example was the use of humidifier moisture exchange (HME) in the circuit. This is not the usual arrangement setup for the inpatient unit. In an emergency, we had seen nebulizer treatments given with the HME in the circuit. It was not surprising that the treatment was not effective because the medication was collected in the HME.

Another communication tool to identify high-risk patients in the **clinic** is the **pre-clinic huddle every morning.** Nurses, along with RCPs and administrative staff, lead the discussion of the plan of care for high-risk patients for that day. The

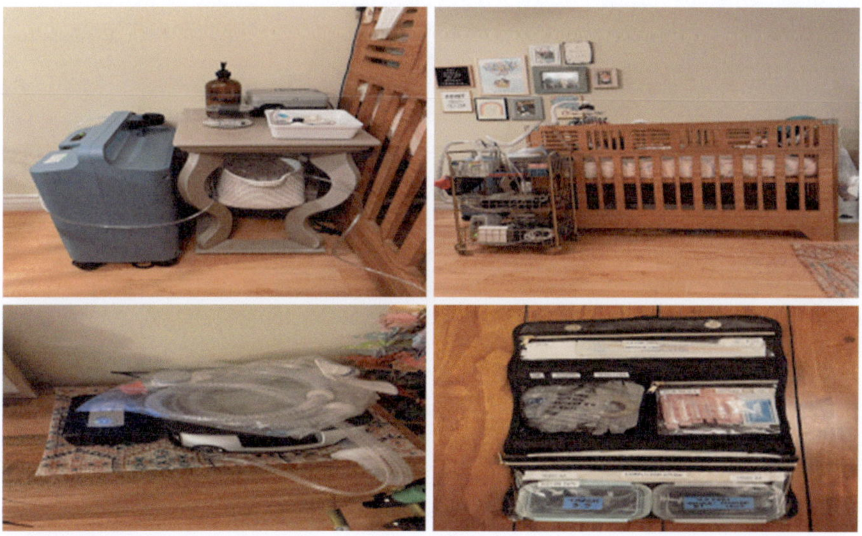

Fig. 2 HMV bedside and emergency setup. Photo courtesy of the Willis Family

team anticipates their clinical condition and proposes strategies to serve these patients, including those needing isolation or special monitoring of fragile patients. It is routine for nurses to document parents' emergency supplies on hand when they arrive for the clinic visit.

Clinic nurses ensure that **emergency DME** such as those for the nebulized treatment, oxygen therapy, and crash cart are **readily available from a designated location**. Another DME safety feature is the arrangement from vendors to **loaner oxygen tanks** and circuits for immediate use in case of a shortage during an outpatient visit.

5 Growing the HMV Program by Nursing Innovations

Medical advances with standardized comprehensive care plans enable children to thrive at home while using HMV [32]. Nurses trained in HMV care have been the innovators and credible partners for our HMV program. Nurses developed home care standards by sharing their bedside day-to-day care and extrapolated that to the home settings. Our nurses have evolved from the hospital clinical role into innovators of home care management. In addition to parent training, we found it beneficial to include **incoming new pulmonary fellows to receive education on tracheostomy and ventilator care pertinent to the home/clinic setting during their first month of training**. One of the most enjoyable training days is for the fellows to **learn the use of all respiratory equipment used in the home from a vendor RCP.**

Nurses constantly explore best practices for the children who rely on HMV—we are the **antennae** for noticing failures and the **lighthouse** to guide the smooth sailing of our precious children whose lives depend on technology and skilled caretakers.

5.1 Problem-Solving Clinical Issues Through Research

Nurses did not separate clinical care from their research and education efforts. Nurses participated in the research of clinical issues such as that ventilator low-pressure alarms do not sound with tracheostomy decannulation [33]. A retrospective review of HMV program in our institution noted 20% 5-year mortality [34] and that many of these deaths were due to tracheostomy accidents.

5.2 How Do We Improve the Knowledge of Parents and Home Health Nurses on HMV Care?

Becoming aware of the impact of tracheostomy accidents and ventilator failures, the study on how much parents and in-home nurses knew about how to respond to these emergencies was extremely helpful [20]. As there was limited data on what specific home emergencies were encountered in the home setting and how caregivers should respond, a research survey of 28 in-home nurses, RCPs, and parents of children receiving home mechanical ventilation yielded necessary information for home training [35]. The survey resulted in the creation of a curriculum on HMV emergency response providing a customized and individualized emergency lesson for each patient. Emergency review specific for an individual family has become part of the standardized discharge preparation.

5.3 Recruiting Governmental Support and Engaging Community Resources to Optimize Care

Parents cannot care for children supported by technology alone without governmental, community, and insurance services [16]. Dependent on the available resources, HMV families needed **electric discounts** and **generators during electric shortage. Other community services should be considered: financial support programs** for eligible families, **handicapped parking** applications, and **nonmedical transport services**. They can do this but not safely or sustainably.

Nurses are **at the table** with policy makers when it comes to them making decisions on health policies that impact our patients. **Being proactive** is the key to success. Legislators usually are glad to hear from scientists about regulations that impact health.

Home health nurses and school nurses are integral parts of the HMV program. Accessing home health nursing is one of the issues related to planning for home care before discharge from the hospital [36]. Assistance in the **development of school protocols and home health procedures proved to be advantageous in advancing care**. We are **partners in care across the continuum of care.**

Manufacturers seek advice from nursing when they design a new product. Thus, **membership at a state or national level in major professional organizations facilitates important changes in clinical practice.**

5.4 *Ongoing HMV Management*

Physicians, fellow nurses, and allied health and community partners can trust **nurses as the potential go-to person** when it comes to HMV management. However, there are models that utilize respiratory care practitioners or other allied healthcare providers as the key managers for HMV discharge as well. Sterni et al. suggested the medical home model as a likely successful approach to HMV care. Standardized discharge criteria are suggested. Training of primary caregivers including emergency preparation is essential to the program [32].

Nursing is one of the most valuable players in the HMV team and an irreplaceable contributor to every aspect of the HMV programs. If we were to summarize the nursing perspective on HMV in children, this phrase comes to mind: **nursing is the glue that holds the program together**.

References

1. Carter MC, Miles MS. Parental stressor scale: pediatric intensive care unit. Kansas City, KS: School of Nursing, College of Health Science, University of Kansas; 1984.
2. Miles MS, Funk SG, et al. The stress response of mothers and fathers of preterm infants. Res Nurs Health. 1992;152:61–269.
3. Board R. Father stress during a child's critical care hospitalization. J Pediatric Health Care. 2004;18:244–9.
4. Carnevale FA, Alexander R, et al. Daily living with distress and enrichment: the moral experience of families with ventilator-assisted children at home. Pediatrics. 2006;117(1):e48–60. https://doi.org/10.1542/peds.2005-0789.
5. McCubbin MA, McCubbin HI. Families coping with illness: the resiliency model of family stress, adjustment, and adaptation. In: Danielson CB, Hamel-Bissell B, Winstead-Fry P, editors. Families, health, & illness: perspectives on coping and intervention. St. Louis Mosby. p. 21–63.
6. Dunn K, Board R. Parents and technology in the inpatient pediatric setting: a beginning model for study. Pediatr Nurs. 2011;37(2):75.
7. Ratliffe C, Harrigan R, et al. Stress in families with medically fragile children. Comprehensive Pediatric Nursing. 2002;25:167–88.
8. Kirk S, Glendinning C, et al. Parent or nurse? The experience of being the parent of a technology dependent child. J Adv Nurs. 2005;51:456–64.
9. Arora G, Caliboso M, Baird J, et al. Educational priorities for providing end-of-life care: parent perspectives. Pediatrics. 2021;148(4):e2021051379. https://doi.org/10.1542/peds.2021-051379.
10. Graham RJ, Amar-Dolan L, et al. Bridging the stressful gap between ICU and home: medical stimulation for pediatric patients and their families. Pediatr Crit Care Med. 2019;20(4):e 221–4. https://doi.org/10.1097/PCC.0000000000001869.
11. Kingston RL. Home care of the ventilator dependent child. Home Health Care Manag Pract. 2007;19(6):436–41. https://doi.org/10.1177/1084822307304264.
12. Maeng DD, Snyder SR, et al. Impact of a complex care management model on cost and utilization among adolescents and young adults with special care and health needs. Popul Health Manag. 2017;20(6):435–41.

13. Kun SS, Deavenport-Saman A, Keens TG, et al. Rapid response team and code events in hospitalized children on home mechanical ventilation. Respir Care. 2019;64(12):1461–8. https://doi.org/10.4187/respcare.06402. PMID: 31641073
14. Kun SS, Edwards JD, Davidson Ward SL, et al. Hospital Readmissions for newly discharged pediatric home mechanical ventilation patients. Pediatr Pulmonol. 2012;47:409–14.
15. Kun SS, Beas VN, Davidson Ward SL, et al. Pediatric respiratory emergencies in an ambulatory setting—are we ready? Am J Respir Crit Care Med. 2014;189:A2790.
16. Sobotka SA, Dholakia A, Agrawal RK, et al. Discharge practices for children with home mechanical ventilation across the United States. Key-informant perspectives. Ann Am Thorac Soc. 2020;17(11):1424–30.
17. American Nurses Association and Society of Pediatric Nurses. Scope and standards of pediatric nursing practice. Washington, D.C: Author; 2003.
18. Mah JK, Thannhauser JE, et al. Being the lifeline: the parent experience of caring for a child with neuromuscular disease on home mechanical ventilation. Neuromuscul Disord. 2008;18(12):983–8. https://doi.org/10.1016/j.nmd.2008.09.001. Epub 2008 Oct 29.
19. Wang KK, Barnard A. Caregivers' experiences at home with a ventilator-dependent child. Qual Health Res. 2008;18(4):501–8.
20. Kun SS, Davidson Ward SL, Hulse LM, et al. How much do primary caregivers know about tracheostomy and home ventilator emergency care? Pediatr Pulmonol. 2010;45(3):270–4.
21. Boudreau AA, Perrin JM, et al. Care coordination and unmet specialty care among children with special health care needs. Pediatrics. 2014;133(6):1046–53. https://doi.org/10.1542/peds.2013-2174.
22. Black BP, Holditch-Davis D, et al. Life course theory as a framework to examine becoming a mother of a medically fragile preterm infant. Res Nurs Health. 2009;32(1):38–49. https://doi.org/10.1002/nur.20298.
23. Tamasitis J, Shesser L. A hospital to home program for ventilator dependent children sets the standard of care. AARC Times. 2012;2(10):44–51.
24. Harrison T. Family centered pediatric nursing care: state of the science. J Pediatric Nurs. 2010;25(5):335–43. https://doi.org/10.1016/j.pedn.2009.01.006.
25. Shelton TL, Stepanek JS. Family center care for children needing specialized health and developmental services. 3rd ed. Publication of Association for the Care of Children's Health; 1994. p. 106–14.
26. Donovan AL, Aldrich JM, Gross AK, et al. Inter-professional care and teamwork in the ICU. Crit Care Med. 2018;46(6):980–90.
27. Ellashek J, Barrios L, Fredlund J, et al. Determining the efficacy of a multidisciplinary action plan in discharge planning for pediatric home mechanical ventilation. Am J Respir Crit Care Med. 2015;191:A2224.
28. Boroughs D, Dougherty JA. Decreasing accidental mortality of ventilator-dependent children at home: a call for action. Home Healthc Nurse. 2012;30(2):103–11. https://doi.org/10.1097/NHH.Ob013e3182429243; quiz 112-3
29. Prickett K, Deshpande A, Paschal H, et al. Simulation-based education to improve emergency management skills in caregivers of tracheostomy patients. Int J Pediatr Otorhinolaryngol. 2019;120:157–61.
30. Casavant DW, McManus ML, Graham RJ, et al. Trial of telemedicine for patients on home ventilator support: feasibility, confidence in clinical management and use I medical decision-making. J Telemed Telecare. 2014;20(8):441–9. https://doi.org/10.1177/1357633X14555620.
31. Connelly A, Kun SS, Ellashek J, et al. Incorporating telemedicine into an established pediatric home mechanical ventilation (HMV) program. Am J Respir Crit Care Med. 2022;205:4354.
32. Sterni LM, Collaco JM, Baker CD, et al. Pediatric chronic home invasive ventilation. American Journal Respiratory Critical Medicine. 2016;193(8):e16–35.
33. Kun SS, Nakamura CT, Ripka JF, et al. Home ventilator low pressure alarms fail to detect accidental decannulation with pediatric tracheostomy tubes. Chest. 2001;119:562–4.

34. Edwards JD, Kun SS, Keens TG. Outcomes and causes of death in children on home mechanical ventilation via tracheostomy. J Pediatr. 2010;157:955–9. PMID: 2071329.
35. Kun SS, Miller C, Davidson Ward SL, et al. Pediatric home mechanical ventilation emergency responses for home caregivers and nurses. Clinical Research in Pulmonology. 2020;7:1048.
36. Elias ER, Murphy NA, the Council on Children with Disabilities. Home care of children and youth with complex health care needs and technology dependencies. Pediatrics. 2012;129:996. https://doi.org/10.1542/peds.2012-0606. Originally published online April 30, 2012.

Future Consideration

Atsushi Kawaguchi

1 Introduction

Scientific advances, population growth, reduced mortality, and increased disease complexity have led to an increase in the number of children requiring prolonged and long-term mechanical ventilation (PLMV) [1, 2]. Evidence suggests that there is a small group of children who require these high levels of healthcare resources for prolonged periods of time. Rigorous investigations are essential to optimize their care, including defining the indications for tracheotomy, evaluation of weaning processes and maintenance supports, and refinements of the healthcare environment that will promote their respiratory recovery and neurodevelopment and shorten the time needed to transfer them to home. Nevertheless, the practice for children requiring PLMV is not straightforward.

These children tend to have chronic comorbidities such as chronic lung disease related to their premature birth, cardiac complications, neuromuscular disease, and other cumulative morbidities. We also need to consider nonclinical or nonventilatory issues such as family issues, healthcare systems, and other medical conditions, to fully discuss the management of PLMV. It is also important to identify these variations and their potential causes and to develop solutions accordingly. The comprehensive interprofessional approach needed to optimize and reduce unnecessary prolongation of mechanical ventilation or improve care for PLMV may not be consistent across programs. In addition, there are significant financial and resource implications for healthcare systems and organizations for these patients, and we have seen that improving efficiency can no longer be seen as an option, but as a clinical and political imperative [2, 3].

A. Kawaguchi (✉)
Division of Pediatric Critical Care, Department of Pediatrics, St. Marianna University School of Medicine, Kawasaki, Japan
e-mail: atsushi.kawaguchi@marianna-u.ac.jp

A. Kawaguchi et al. (eds.), *Prolonged and Long-Term Mechanical Ventilation in Children*, https://doi.org/10.1007/978-981-97-8903-0_24

In this chapter, the various topics discussed in this special issue will be summarized from the perspective of what is needed to improve the care of pediatric patients with PLMV. We would like to summarize what can be done to improve the quality of management, including anticipating technological advances in acute ventilation and monitoring, and what we can do to improve the quality of care for chronically ventilated children.

2 Issues in Pediatric Acute Ventilatory Management

The management of acute respiratory distress syndrome (ARDS) in children has evolved dramatically over the last half-century, contributing to a significant reduction in mortality. However, even with the recently published pediatric acute respiratory distress syndrome (ARDS) guideline, PALICC-2, there is still a lack of high-quality pediatric studies on ventilation management itself, monitoring, and adjunctive therapies (nutrition and rehabilitation) in many cases, and high-quality clinical evidence is largely borrowed from neonates and adults [4].

In modern pediatric intensive care unit (PICU), the failure rate of tracheal tube extubation is reported to be in the single-digit percentage range [5–9]. Preparation for extubation according to the extubation readiness test (ERT) or other relevant criteria is expected to increase the success rate of the extubation [8, 10–12]. However, most of the currently proposed criteria, such as the spontaneous breathing test (SBT) criteria, are empirically based or proposed based on the knowledge of adult patients and have not necessarily been clinically validated for use in pediatric patients [8, 12–14]. There are other reasons for ventilatory support in children that cannot be measured by SBT, such as nutritional and circulatory status and the degree of need for sedation and analgesia. Therefore, careful observation, weaning according to a comprehensive protocol, and communication of this approach within the team should be warranted.

Although high-quality evidence on ventilatory support after extubation is beginning to emerge, such as the recently published FIRST-ABC trial, there is still a lack of evidence that directly relates to management policy for each detailed practice [15]. For example, evidence is still needed for each pediatric-specific event, such as assessing respiratory muscle strength and whether the patient's circulatory status can withstand extubation. In addition to strategies and settings for weaning patients from the ventilator, evidence is needed from a variety of perspectives to identify the best weaning strategy or to anticipate it early and develop strategies to improve prognosis.

3 Advancements in Technology and Management Strategy

There are ongoing advances in mechanical ventilation technology and management strategy, including the development of new devices and modes of ventilation that can improve patient outcomes and quality of life. These include lung-protective strategies and modes of ventilation such as high-frequency oscillation (HFO), neurally adjusted ventilatory assist (NAVA), and extracorporeal membrane oxygenation (ECMO). The strategies for invasive ventilation have also been accepted for pediatric patients, such as the practice of keeping the tidal volume low and not increasing the driving pressure beyond a certain level, which should improve the prognosis [4]. It is desirable to develop new parameters that can be used to interpret these parameters to replace invasive parameters such as transesophageal pressure, which is relatively difficult to measure in pediatric patients. It is also time to rethink the validation of these new modalities in pediatric patients.

In the next sections, some new indicators and methodologies will be presented that may help to address some of these issues.

4 Individualized Treatment Plans Applying New Technologies

4.1 Respiratory Monitoring

One of the approaches recently highlighted would be to seamlessly and individually assess the patient's respiratory function and take preventive or mitigating measures. The following section provides a summary of various methods and parameters used to assess respiratory functions including respiratory muscle function (RMF), which may help to develop strategies to avoid long-term mechanical ventilation or early weaning. Various data from built-in software of ICU and home ventilators would also be important information to provide an individual management plan for children with PLMV. In particular, children with PLMV usually require a transition period on home ventilators before being discharged from the hospital. The built-in software should be encouraged to be applied more to optimize the setting of parameters and to analyze the events that occurred during the transition from the ICU to the home setting. The use of these individualized data will be particularly important as there is an increasing focus on individualized treatment plans that take into account the patient's acute disease etiology, underlying medical conditions, prognosis, and goals of care.

4.2 Respiratory Muscle Function in PLMV

PLMV, itself, may contribute to the weakening and deconditioning of RMF, which may be a risk factor for difficult weaning from MV [16, 17]. In addition, mechanisms of respiratory muscle injury known as myotrauma can lead to ventilator-induced diaphragm dysfunction, including ventilator over-assistance, under-assistance, eccentric contractions, and end-expiratory shortening [18].

Physiological techniques may be useful to assess RMF and to individualize and optimize the management of PLMV, particularly in children weaned from intensive care. For example, during the weaning process of PLMV, RMF monitoring may help to adjust the level of support, optimize ventilator weaning, and predict the success of extubation or weaning from positive-pressure support. Techniques currently used clinically in the ICU may include measurement of esophageal pressure using a balloon catheter, electrical activity of the diaphragm (EAdi), and inspiratory occlusion maneuvers, all of which are relatively invasive to measure. However, none of these have been thoroughly evaluated or well documented in children, particularly in PLMV. Recent studies have proven the utility of ultrasound for diaphragmatic muscle imaging to assess diaphragmatic thickness in the zone of apposition, an echogenic layer bordered by the pleural and peritoneal membranes. However, the technique, reproducibility, and normal values have only been evaluated in a large population of healthy adults and children, not in PLMVed children. You will find more details in the next section.

4.3 Activity of Diaphragm

EAdi is a parameter used to monitor respiratory muscle unloading and patient-ventilator synchrony [19–24]. EAdi has been validated in clinical practice using technology developed for the NAVA ventilation mode. It reflects respiratory drive and correlates with other indicators such as $P_{0.1}$ [25]. EAdi has a wide range of applications in pediatric ventilator management. Visual inspection of flow and pressure waveforms with EAdi can be used to detect patient-ventilator asynchronies. An increased value of EAdi during the expiratory phase may indicate increased efforts to create a larger end-expiratory lung volume. Although currently not well supported by clinical evidence, better synchronization may reduce the need for sedation, reduce events such as aspiration, or reduce secondary lung injury in the care of children with PLMV [26, 27].

4.4 Measurement of Breathing Effort

$P_{0.1}$ is a measure of neural respiratory drive, which is often used to assess extubation readiness. The airway pressure (P_{aw}) generated in the first 100 milliseconds of inspiration has been used as an index of neural respiratory drive [28, 29]. This delay prevents any patient response to occlusion. It can be measured in most conventional mechanical ventilators and has been used successfully in ventilated children. However, the value of $P_{0.1}$ in the assessment of PLMVed children has not been investigated.

EAdi can also help us monitor respiratory muscle workload, patient-ventilator synchrony, and breathing efficiency in critically ill patients. The ratio of actual EAdi to peak EAdi, observed during 20 s of inspiratory occlusion, is a measure of the patient's ventilatory effort. A small value of the ratio indicates excessive ventilatory support, whereas a large value of the ratio indicates inadequate respiratory muscle unloading.

The ratio of tidal volume (VT) to EAdi also represents the neuroventilatory efficiency (NVE) of the diaphragm [30–32]. Improvement in NVE may indicate that a patient is generating adequate VT with a lower level of EAdi. NVE is influenced by changes in diaphragm function and the patient's respiratory load. Although not always easy to measure in children on NIV, it would be useful to measure and evaluate such indicators in children requiring positive-pressure ventilation, with or without tracheostomy, for example to discuss and optimize ventilator settings and the timing of extubation. It may be a particularly good indicator in cohorts where respiratory drive and effort are not matched, e.g., children on long-term opioids, patients with cerebral palsy, or patients with neuromuscular disease [31, 32].

The tension-time index (TTI) of the diaphragm (TT_{di}) is derived by relating the mean transdiaphragmatic pressure per breath (P_{di}) to the maximum inspiratory transdiaphragmatic pressure (P_{dimax}) and the inspiratory time (T_I) to the total respiratory cycle time (T_{tot}). It may be a fraction of the maximum effort exerted by the diaphragm during the contraction time. The difference between esophageal (P_{es}) and gastric (P_{ga}) pressures is used to calculate P_{di}. Measurement of TT_{di} requires the use of balloon catheters. A noninvasive TTI measurement (TT_{mus}) based on airway pressure has been developed and studied in children. One of the advantages of TT_{mus} is that it reflects the contribution of all inspiratory muscles rather than being specific to the diaphragm muscle. Measurement of TT_{mus} would be useful in several settings, such as optimizing the ventilatory setting and deciding on a liberation strategy from PLMV [33–35].

4.5 Ultrasound of Diaphragm

Assessment of the diaphragm has recently become a common practice in critical care, as many clinical situations require specific assessment of diaphragm function. Diaphragm thickness can be measured using M-mode ultrasound, and changes in diaphragm thickness at the end of expiration and at the end of inspiration can be measured using B-mode ultrasound. In adult patients, diaphragm thickness within 1.4 mm is considered atrophic, and changes in diaphragm thickness are associated with PLMV. In children, the diaphragm is easy to observe due to its small size and thin subcutaneous fat, and it is possible to view both sides simultaneously from the pericardial fossa. The degree of diaphragmatic atrophy is related to the use of ventilators and muscle relaxants, especially in pediatric patients. Diaphragmatic excursion, which measures the distance between respiratory cycle movements at a fixed point posterior to the diaphragm, has also been associated with ventilator weaning [36–42]. Measurement and observation over time could help to assess diaphragmatic atrophy and other factors that may be useful in the ventilatory management of PLMV, in conjunction with a global assessment of respiratory mechanics, including accessory muscles.

4.6 Phrenic Nerve Stimulation

Phrenic nerve stimulation can provide valuable information about the mechanical function of the diaphragm and how the force of its contraction is converted into pressure. It allows us to non-voluntarily assess diaphragmatic strength, measured as the magnitude of twitch transdiaphragmatic pressure or twitch airway pressure. Four techniques have been implemented; needle stimulation and implanted wire stimulation are both invasive and are no longer recommended, and transcutaneous electrical stimulation and magnetic stimulation have been more extensively studied and have minimal reported side effects. The integrity of the phrenic nerve in response to stimulation can be used to calculate the phrenic nerve conduction time, which helps us to detect phrenic nerve injury. It is currently used extensively in research [43–45]. In particular, the establishment of a noninvasive and accurate measurement method to assess the respiratory status of PLMV alongside EAdi would be useful.

4.7 Summary of Assessment of Respiratory Function in PLMV

Assessment of respiratory function, with a focus on diaphragm function, and new mechanical ventilation modes that assess respiratory drive, may reduce secondary lung injury by increasing synchrony with the ventilator or reduce various management problems caused by non-synchrony, such as increased sedation requirements, aspiration, and gastrointestinal disturbances, which may result in reduced duration of ventilation and oxygen requirements. In addition, the use of NVE and other indicators may allow earlier detection of respiratory muscle deterioration, and interventions to adjust ventilator settings and restore respiratory muscle recovery may contribute to improved respiratory outcomes in patients with PLMV. Further accumulation of data and the development of quality improvement in ventilator management based on these data are desirable in the future.

5 Other Management Indicators

5.1 Biological Markers on PLMV

Studies in critically ill patients with MV have shown that respiratory muscle weakness is associated with muscle fiber damage and loss of contractile proteins. Although a few potential candidates have been suggested, including classical plasma biomarkers such as creatine kinase, myoglobin, B-type natriuretic peptide, and troponin I, none of these have been studied in children with PLMV, which is likely to have specific structural damage in the respiratory muscles. Respiratory muscle weakness and generalized muscle weakness are two distinct processes in critically ill patients. Therefore, the evaluation of plasma biomarkers that capture all skeletal muscle damage should be carefully considered in the context of other clinical findings, such as diaphragm function on ultrasound and EAdi. Inflammatory biomarkers have also been studied in patients with PARDS, including surfactant protein D and epithelium- and endothelium-related proteins (e.g., sCIAM-1, KL-6, sRAGE). These markers may also be candidates for use in managing the care of children with PLMV [46–51].

5.2 Respiratory Variables Derived from Imaging

Selected lung injury and ventilatory oxygenation parameters that may serve as prognostic indicators or management tools for respiratory outcome in PLMV are presented, depending on future research.

5.3 Electric Impedance Tomography

Electrical impedance tomography (EIT) is a noninvasive bedside monitoring technique that allows us to assess dynamic lung volumes and changes in different lung regions in real time. EIT can only quantify relative changes in the local impedance of the lung, so normal or pathologically stable structures such as pleural effusions are functionally attenuated and cannot be visualized. In other words, the lung is a good candidate for EIT because its impedance is closely related to the stage of parenchymal inflation [35]. In children, chest EIT can typically be performed by placing an electrode belt around the chest between the third and sixth intercostal spaces. The resulting image shows the impedance changes that occur in a cross section of the thorax [52–54].

EIT has been well validated against other lung volume imaging techniques in an adult population. However, several factors can affect its performance and resolution, such as electrode position and conformational changes of the chest wall and diaphragm. Research is underway to improve image reconstruction algorithms, develop dedicated algorithms for specific clinical applications, improve communication with modern ventilators including noninvasive ventilators, and find ways to remove artifacts due to changes in chest shape. It may be useful in children with PLMV when ventilation is not easily determined by respiratory effort or auscultation, e.g., in severe scoliosis, and for changes in ventilation when ventilator conditions are changed in PLMV [55].

5.4 *Respiratory Variables Derived from Additional Monitoring*

Lung compliance is useful in assessing ventilator settings in children with PLMV, as well as in the intensive care setting, and in assessing the progression of ongoing disease. Dynamic compliance measurement (Vt (ml/kg ideal body weight)/(Pplat-PEEP (cmH_2O)), normal range 1.5–2 ml/kg/cmH_2O) is preferred to quasi-static compliance, which is more difficult to obtain. Note that plateau pressure (Pplat) is measured with end-inspiratory occlusion in volume control mode and the patient should not be actively breathing [35]. We also need to be cautious that ideal tidal volumes for the acute phase of respiratory disease such as PARDS may not be applicable in PLMV, especially in conditions that are not related to primary lung disease, e.g., neuromuscular disorders, thoracic insufficiency, or CNS conditions.

5.5 *Oxygenation and Ventilation Parameters and Severity Scores*

Oxygen index (OI) and P/F ratios are also important indicators to assess lung status in children with PLMV. However, there are problems such as the need for blood gas sampling and the inability of NIV to accurately collect the parameters required for the calculations. In the event of poor oxygenation due to respiratory infection or aspiration pneumonia during management, for example in the home environment, a simple and accurate parameter to assess respiratory status and changes in oxygenation in addition to SpO2 would be desirable [56, 57]. Other various physiological measures and scoring systems have been proposed and evaluated to assess the severity of lung injury and predict mortality. The Lung Injury Score (LIS), proposed by Murray et al., has been widely used to assess the severity of illness in studies of adult ARDS and has been validated in some PARDS studies. A higher value of LIS could indicate the possibility of needing rescue therapy. Changes in LIS over time have also been used as a primary outcome to study the efficacy of interventions in PLMV. Noninvasive LIS using S/F for the P/F ratio has also been validated in acute care settings, but not in PLMV [58–60]. Although CO2 clearance and management will not be addressed in detail here (see specific chapters), it should be added that a thorough understanding of CO2 and pH management in relation to pulmonary vascular resistance, such as pulmonary hypertension, as well as permissive hypercapnia, is important in the management of PLMV.

The next section organizes matters indirectly related to the management of PLMV.

6 ICU-Acquired Weakness

Intensive care unit (ICU)-acquired weakness, also known as critical illness myopathy or neuropathy, is a condition characterized by muscle weakness and loss of muscle mass that develops in patients who have been in the ICU for an extended period of time. This weakness can make it difficult for patients to leave the ICU, move, breathe, and perform daily activities and can significantly delay their recovery and increase their risk of death.

In pediatric patients, the problem with ICU-acquired weakness is that it is often underrecognized and undertreated. This is partly because the condition is relatively rare in children and the symptoms of weakness may be attributed to other factors, such as sedation or immobilization. There is also a lack of standardized diagnostic criteria for ICU-acquired weakness in pediatric patients, which can make it difficult to identify and quantify the severity of the condition.

Another problem is that the management of ICU-acquired weakness in pediatric patients is not well established. There are few studies on the effectiveness of interventions such as physical therapy and early mobilization in this population. In addition, many of the medications and interventions used to treat adult ICU-acquired weakness have not been studied in children and their safety and efficacy in this population are unknown. The recognition and management of ICU-acquired weakness in pediatric patients remain an important area of research and clinical practice, with a need for better diagnostic criteria and evidence-based interventions [61, 62].

7 Rehabilitation and Post-intensive Care Syndrome

Many patients require PLMV in addition to ventilatory management due to the sequelae of nutrition, analgesia, and sedation or muscle weakness caused by ventilation itself. Early respiratory and physical rehabilitation and post-intensive care syndrome (PICS) should be considered from the acute phase of treatment. While there is good-quality evidence that early rehabilitation reduces the duration of mechanical ventilation, particularly in adults, there are few good-quality prospective studies in pediatric patients. Taking these and other factors into account, each medical institution or region should seek the best interventional approach [63–65].

8 Multidisciplinary and Patient-Centered Approaches to Care

As with all medical care, there is an increasing emphasis on patient-centered care in the management of PLMV. This includes involving patients and their families in decision-making, improving communication between healthcare providers, and responding to the needs of patients and families. The management of PLMV also requires a multidisciplinary team approach involving physicians, nurses, respiratory therapists, physical therapists, social workers, psychologists, and other healthcare professionals. There is a growing emphasis on collaborative care models that improve communication and coordination among team members to optimize patient outcomes. Transitional care models such as pediatric respiratory intermediate care units (RICUs) and their role in reducing the length of stay in NICUs and PICUs and the length of transfer to home should also be monitored in the pediatric setting [66]. The effectiveness and role of these approaches need to be re-understood through future research.

9 Needs of Sharing Experience and Data

Certain pediatric patients require a transition from acute to chronic ventilation. The process of transitioning to home ventilation requires several steps, including timing of tracheostomy, selection of the ventilator mode required for home use, identification of social support resources for home use, and education and training of respiratory management staff in the receiving institution, including the home setting. Most institutions experience only a few cases of such patients per year, and it takes time to gain sufficient experience if information is shared only within the institution. Therefore, successful cases should be shared between institutions to clarify problems in each institution or region and to consider how to respond to each case.

Most databases in pediatric critical care exist for acute conditions or rare diseases and specialized therapies. As mentioned earlier, the background conditions of patients requiring PLMV are diverse, so it is necessary to collect and understand many patients with similar conditions to clarify the relationship between the conditions and the treatment plan. However, the number of patients transitioning from acute to long-term ventilation is small, and even when patients are transitioned to home ventilation, the treatment plan itself may be strongly influenced by the resources of the institution or the surrounding government and health insurance system. Considering that all pediatric patients requiring PLMV require regular visits to medical institutions for one reason or another, it is desirable to establish an inter-institutional, inter-regional, and international database based on medical institutions. The database should be linked to various real-world data, such as acute disease databases or data from different governments. This will enable the generation of evidence to support seamless medical policy.

The LongVentKids study, an international multicenter trial led by the author as a principal investigator since 2018, is currently underway. The study involved more than 200 pediatric intensive care units (PICUs) from approximately 200 children's hospitals and university medical centers in more than 30 countries and regions and collected the epidemiologic background of PICU patients requiring PLMVs. The breakthrough was the recruitment of patients from both resource-rich and resource-poor countries, and the creation of a data template that allows data from different centers to be compared. This data template could be used in the future to determine the total number of pediatric patients in each region, or to randomly select patients requiring long-term ventilation at a given time and examine the quality of care at that time. A comparison of data between regions could also be used to discuss the impact on hospital economics of pediatric patients requiring long-term ventilation, using each healthcare system as an intervention [67, 68]. It must be recognized that the sharing of experiences, problems, and case information across institutions and regions, as in this study, is particularly important when dealing with research topics such as PLMV.

10 Importance of New Modes to Monitor Breathing

To improve the quality of care for children requiring home ventilation, it is necessary to invest and maintain a high level of human resources and advanced medical equipment. Under the circumstances faced by many countries, such as an aging society with a declining birth rate and a shortage of medical personnel, new medical devices such as artificial intelligence and monitoring devices are expected to emerge to provide more advanced medical equipment in the hospital or home care setting in the future. For example, it is not easy to monitor respiratory rate or detect life-threatening events such as apnea in home-ventilated patients who are not on so-called invasive ventilators. In the hospital setting, end-tidal carbon dioxide measurements and contact impedance respiratory monitoring are commonly used.

However, these monitoring systems are far from adequate in terms of simplicity and reliability. Pediatric patients are difficult to keep still in bed, and contact-type monitoring systems may not work due to their body movements. Therefore, it is desirable to develop a monitoring system that is noninvasive and noncontact, such as a wearable type [69–71].

You have understood the wide range of issues surrounding children with PLMV. New modes of ventilation, methods of monitoring respiratory effort and drive, and technologies for monitoring breathing, including at home, are also likely to emerge. The complexity of the situation and the need to understand diverse information also make it desirable to develop a multidisciplinary approach, including family members, that is not limited to respiratory management alone. As I close this chapter, I wish the children with PLMV a bright future.

References

1. Paediatric Intensive Care Audit Network, Annual report. http://www.picanet.org.uk/Audit/Annual-Reporting/PICANet_Annual_Report_2016_Summary.pdf; 2016.
2. Zilberberg MD, Shorr AF. Prolonged acute mechanical ventilation and hospital bed utilization in 2020 in the United States: implications for budgets, plant and personnel planning. BMC Health Serv Res. 2008;8:242.
3. Lone NI, Walsh TS. Prolonged mechanical ventilation in critically ill patients: epidemiology, outcomes and modelling the potential cost consequences of establishing a regional weaning unit. Crit Care. 2011;15(2):R102.
4. Emeriaud G, Lopez-Fernandez YM, Iyer NP, Bembea MM, Agulnik A, Barbaro RP, et al. Executive Summary of the Second International Guidelines for the Diagnosis and Management of Pediatric Acute Respiratory Distress Syndrome (PALICC-2). Pediatr Crit Care Med. 2023;24(2):143–68.
5. Loberger JM, Manchikalapati A, Borasino S, Prabhakaran P. Prevalence, risk factors, and outcomes of airway versus non-airway pediatric extubation failure. Respir Care. 2023;68(3):374–83.
6. Liu Y, Wang Q, Hu J, Zhou F, Liu C, Li J, et al. Characteristics and risk factors of children requiring prolonged mechanical ventilation vs. non-prolonged mechanical ventilation in the PICU: a prospective single-center study. Front Pediatr. 2022;10:830075.
7. Badruddin SS, Clayton JA, McKee BP, Slain KN, Rotta AT, Malay S, et al. Prevalence of reintubation within 24 hours of extubation in bronchiolitis: retrospective cohort study using the virtual pediatric systems database. Pediatr Crit Care Med. 2021;22(5):474–82.
8. Loberger JM, Campbell CM, Colleti J Jr, Borasino S, Abu-Sultaneh S, Khemani RG. Pediatric ventilation liberation: a survey of international practice among 555 pediatric intensivists. Crit Care Explor. 2022;4(9):e0756.
9. Hames DL, Sleeper LA, Bullock KJ, Feins EN, Mills KI, Laussen PC, et al. Associations with extubation failure and predictive value of risk analytics algorithms with extubation readiness tests following congenital cardiac surgery. Pediatr Crit Care Med. 2022;23(4):e208–e18.
10. Tan HL, Ma YJ, Aguilan AB, Goh CY, Wong JCK, Ang LSL, et al. Respiratory therapist-driven extubation readiness testing in a single pediatric ICU. Respir Care. 2022;67(7):833–41.
11. Ista E, Redivo J, Kananur P, Choong K, Colleti J Jr, Needham DM, et al. ABCDEF bundle practices for critically ill children: an international survey of 161 PICUs in 18 countries. Crit Care Med. 2022;50(1):114–25.

12. Krasinkiewicz JM, Friedman ML, Slaven JE, Lutfi R, Abu-Sultaneh S, Tori AJ. Extubation readiness practices and barriers to extubation in pediatric subjects. Respir Care. 2021;66(4):582–90.
13. Cardinal-Fernandez P, Bougnaud J, Cour M, Argaud L, Poole D, Guerin C. Automatic tube compensation during spontaneous breathing trial. Respir Care. 2022;67(10):1335–42.
14. Shalish W, Kanbar L, Kovacs L, Chawla S, Keszler M, Rao S, et al. Assessment of extubation readiness using spontaneous breathing trials in extremely preterm neonates. JAMA Pediatr. 2020;174(2):178–85.
15. Ramnarayan P, Richards-Belle A, Drikite L, Saull M, Orzechowska I, Darnell R, et al. Effect of high-flow nasal cannula therapy vs continuous positive airway pressure following extubation on liberation from respiratory support in critically ill children: a randomized clinical trial. JAMA. 2022;327(16):1555–65.
16. Goligher EC, Brochard LJ, Reid WD, Fan E, Saarela O, Slutsky AS, et al. Diaphragmatic myotrauma: a mediator of prolonged ventilation and poor patient outcomes in acute respiratory failure. Lancet Respir Med. 2019;7(1):90–8.
17. Goligher EC, Dres M, Fan E, Rubenfeld GD, Scales DC, Herridge MS, et al. Mechanical ventilation-induced diaphragm atrophy strongly impacts clinical outcomes. Am J Respir Crit Care Med. 2018;197(2):204–13.
18. Mortamet G, Crulli B, Fauroux B, Emeriaud G. Monitoring of respiratory muscle function in critically ill children. Pediatr Crit Care Med. 2020;21(5):e282–90.
19. Crulli B, Kawaguchi A, Praud JP, Petrof BJ, Harrington K, Emeriaud G. Evolution of inspiratory muscle function in children during mechanical ventilation. Crit Care. 2021;25(1):229.
20. Mortamet G, Nardi N, Groleau V, Essouri S, Fauroux B, Jouvet P, et al. Impact of spontaneous breathing trial on work of breathing indices derived from esophageal pressure, electrical activity of the diaphragm, and oxygen consumption in children. Respir Care. 2019;64(5):509–18.
21. Fine-Goulden MR, Puppala NK, Durward A. Mechanisms of ventilator dependence in children with neuromuscular and respiratory control disorders identified by monitoring diaphragm electrical activity. Intensive Care Med. 2012;38(12):2072–9.
22. Wolf GK, Walsh BK, Green ML, Arnold JH. Electrical activity of the diaphragm during extubation readiness testing in critically ill children. Pediatr Crit Care Med. 2011;12(6):e220–4.
23. Foti G, Cereda M, Banfi G, Pelosi P, Fumagalli R, Pesenti A. End-inspiratory airway occlusion: a method to assess the pressure developed by inspiratory muscles in patients with acute lung injury undergoing pressure support. Am J Respir Crit Care Med. 1997;156(4 Pt 1):1210–6.
24. Mortamet G, Crulli B, Fauroux B, Emeriaud G. Monitoring of respiratory muscle function in critically ill children. Pediatr Crit Care Med. 2020;21(5):e282–e90.
25. Harris J, Tibby SM, Endacott R, Latour JM. Neurally adjusted ventilator assist in infants with acute respiratory failure: a literature scoping review. Pediatr Crit Care Med. 2021;22(10):915–24.
26. Beck J, Emeriaud G, Liu Y, Sinderby C. Neurally-adjusted ventilatory assist (NAVA) in children: a systematic review. Minerva Anestesiol. 2016;82(8):874–83.
27. Ducharme-Crevier L, Beck J, Essouri S, Jouvet P, Emeriaud G. Neurally adjusted ventilatory assist (NAVA) allows patient-ventilator synchrony during pediatric noninvasive ventilation: a crossover physiological study. Crit Care. 2015;19(1):44.
28. Doorduin J, van Hees HW, van der Hoeven JG, Heunks LM. Monitoring of the respiratory muscles in the critically ill. Am J Respir Crit Care Med. 2013;187(1):20–7.
29. Manczur TI, Greenough A, Pryor D, Rafferty GF. Assessment of respiratory drive and muscle function in the pediatric intensive care unit and prediction of extubation failure. Pediatr Crit Care Med. 2000;1(2):124–6.
30. Jansen D, Jonkman AH, Roesthuis L, Gadgil S, van der Hoeven JG, Scheffer GJ, et al. Estimation of the diaphragm neuromuscular efficiency index in mechanically ventilated critically ill patients. Crit Care. 2018;22(1):238.
31. Di Mussi R, Spadaro S, Mirabella L, Volta CA, Serio G, Staffieri F, et al. Impact of prolonged assisted ventilation on diaphragmatic efficiency: NAVA versus PSV. Crit Care. 2016;20:1.

32. Roze H, Repusseau B, Perrier V, Germain A, Seramondi R, Dewitte A, et al. Neuro-ventilatory efficiency during weaning from mechanical ventilation using neurally adjusted ventilatory assist. Br J Anaesth. 2013;111(6):955–60.
33. Mulreany LT, Weiner DJ, McDonough JM, Panitch HB, Allen JL. Noninvasive measurement of the tension-time index in children with neuromuscular disease. J Appl Physiol (1985). 2003;95(3):931–7.
34. Ramonatxo M, Boulard P, Prefaut C. Validation of a noninvasive tension-time index of inspiratory muscles. J Appl Physiol (1985). 1995;78(2):646–53.
35. Kawaguchi A, Jouvet P. Imaging and monitoring in pediatric acute respiratory distress syndrome. In: Pediatric acute respiratory distress syndrome. Springer Nature; 2020. p. 47–61.
36. Yeung T, Mohsen N, Ghanem M, Ibrahim J, Shah J, Kajal D, et al. Diaphragmatic thickness and excursion in preterm infants with bronchopulmonary dysplasia compared with term or near term infants: a prospective observational study. Chest. 2023;163(2):324–31.
37. Sik N, Citlenbik H, Ozturk A, Yilmaz D, Duman M. Point of care diaphragm ultrasound: an objective tool to predict the severity of pneumonia and outcomes in children. Pediatr Pulmonol. 2021;56(6):1666–72.
38. IJland MM, Lemson J, van der Hoeven JG, Heunks LMA. The impact of critical illness on the expiratory muscles and the diaphragm assessed by ultrasound in mechanical ventilated children. Ann Intensive Care. 2020;10(1):115.
39. Xue Y, Zhang Z, Sheng CQ, Li YM, Jia FY. The predictive value of diaphragm ultrasound for weaning outcomes in critically ill children. BMC Pulm Med. 2019;19(1):270.
40. Ng KWP, Dietz AR, Johnson R, Shoykhet M, Zaidman CM. Reliability of bedside ultrasound of limb and diaphragm muscle thickness in critically ill children. Muscle Nerve. 2019;59(1):88–94.
41. Glau CL, Conlon TW, Himebauch AS, Yehya N, Weiss SL, Berg RA, et al. Progressive diaphragm atrophy in pediatric acute respiratory failure. Pediatr Crit Care Med. 2018;19(5):406–11.
42. Lee EP, Hsia SH, Hsiao HF, Chen MC, Lin JJ, Chan OW, et al. Evaluation of diaphragmatic function in mechanically ventilated children: an ultrasound study. PLoS One. 2017;12(8):e0183560.
43. Skalsky AJ, Lesser DJ, McDonald CM. Evaluation of phrenic nerve and diaphragm function with peripheral nerve stimulation and M-mode ultrasonography in potential pediatric phrenic nerve or diaphragm pacing candidates. Phys Med Rehabil Clin N Am. 2015;26(1):133–43.
44. Rafferty GF, Greenough A, Manczur T, Polkey MI, Harris ML, Heaton ND, et al. Magnetic phrenic nerve stimulation to assess diaphragm function in children following liver transplantation. Pediatr Crit Care Med. 2001;2(2):122–6.
45. Garrido H, Mazaira J, Gutierrez P, Gonzalez E, Rivas J, Madrazo J. Continuous respiratory support in quadriplegic children by bilateral phrenic nerve stimulation. Thorax. 1987;42(8):573–7.
46. Dahmer MK, Flori H, Sapru A, Kohne J, Weeks HM, Curley MAQ, et al. Surfactant Protein D Is Associated with Severe Pediatric ARDS, Prolonged Ventilation, and Death in Children with Acute Respiratory Failure. Chest. 2020;158(3):1027–35.
47. Jain K. Biomarkers of pulmonary diseases. In: The handbook of biomarkers. Humana Press Inc.; 2017. p. 673–88.
48. Orwoll BE, Sapru A. Biomarkers in pediatric ARDS: future directions. Front Pediatr. 2016;4:55.
49. Sapru A, Flori H, Quasney MW, Dahmer MK, Pediatric Acute Lung Injury Consensus Conference G. Pathobiology of acute respiratory distress syndrome. Pediatr Crit Care Med. 2015;16(5 Suppl 1):S6–22.
50. Huusko JM, Karjalainen MK, Mahlman M, Haataja R, Kari MA, Andersson S, et al. A study of genes encoding cytokines (IL6, IL10, TNF), cytokine receptors (IL6R, IL6ST), and glucocorticoid receptor (NR3C1) and susceptibility to bronchopulmonary dysplasia. BMC Med Genet. 2014;15:120.
51. Moldoveanu B, Otmishi P, Jani P, Walker J, Sarmiento X, Guardiola J, et al. Inflammatory mechanisms in the lung. J Inflamm Res. 2009;2:1–11.

52. Inany HS, Rettig JS, Smallwood CD, Arnold JH, Walsh BK. Distribution of ventilation measured by electrical impedance tomography in critically ill children. Respir Care. 2020;65(5):590–5.
53. Rosemeier I, Reiter K, Obermeier V, Wolf GK. Mechanical ventilation guided by electrical impedance tomography in children with acute lung injury. Crit Care Explor. 2019;1(7):e0020.
54. Vogt B, Lohr S, Zhao Z, Falkenberg C, Ankermann T, Weiler N, et al. Regional lung function testing in children using electrical impedance tomography. Pediatr Pulmonol. 2018;53(3):293–301.
55. Zhang C, Wang Y, Liu L, Li Q, Li Y, Li N, et al. Regional ventilation distribution in patients with scoliosis assessed by electrical impedance tomography: is individual thorax shape required? Respir Physiol Neurobiol. 2022;299:103854.
56. Thomas NJ, Shaffer ML, Willson DF, Shih MC, Curley MA. Defining acute lung disease in children with the oxygenation saturation index. Pediatr Crit Care Med. 2010;11(1):12–7.
57. Flori HR, Glidden DV, Rutherford GW, Matthay MA. Pediatric acute lung injury: prospective evaluation of risk factors associated with mortality. Am J Respir Crit Care Med. 2005;171(9):995–1001.
58. Kangelaris KN, Calfee CS, May AK, Zhuo H, Matthay MA, Ware LB. Is there still a role for the lung injury score in the era of the Berlin definition ARDS? Ann Intensive Care. 2014;4(1):4.
59. Khemani RG, Patel NR, Bart RD 3rd, Newth CJL. Comparison of the pulse oximetric saturation/fraction of inspired oxygen ratio and the PaO2/fraction of inspired oxygen ratio in children. Chest. 2009;135(3):662–8.
60. Khemani RG, Thomas NJ, Venkatachalam V, Scimeme JP, Berutti T, Schneider JB, et al. Comparison of SpO2 to PaO2 based markers of lung disease severity for children with acute lung injury. Crit Care Med. 2012;40(4):1309–16.
61. Vanhorebeek I, Latronico N, Van den Berghe G. ICU-acquired weakness. Intensive Care Med. 2020;46(4):637–53.
62. Field-Ridley A, Dharmar M, Steinhorn D, McDonald C, Marcin JP. ICU-acquired weakness is associated with differences in clinical outcomes in critically ill children. Pediatr Crit Care Med. 2016;17(1):53–7.
63. Patel BK, Wolfe KS, Patel SB, Dugan KC, Esbrook CL, Pawlik AJ, et al. Effect of early mobilisation on long-term cognitive impairment in critical illness in the USA: a randomised controlled trial. Lancet Respir Med. 2023;11(6):563–72.
64. Cho J, Park H, Kang D, Park E, Chung CR, Cho J, et al. Rehabilitation in critically ill children: findings from the Korean National Health Insurance database. PLoS One. 2022;17(3):e0266360.
65. Smith HAB, Besunder JB, Betters KA, Johnson PN, Srinivasan V, Stormorken A, et al. 2022 Society of Critical Care Medicine Clinical Practice Guidelines on Prevention and Management of Pain, Agitation, Neuromuscular Blockade, and Delirium in Critically Ill Pediatric Patients with Consideration of the ICU Environment and Early Mobility. Pediatr Crit Care Med. 2022;23(2):e74–e110.
66. Curran JA, Breneol S, Vine J. Improving transitions in care for children with complex and medically fragile needs: a mixed methods study. BMC Pediatr. 2020;20(1):219.
67. A. Kawaguchi, Philippe J. Prevalence, management, health-care burden, and 90-day outcomes of prolonged mechanical ventilation in the paediatric intensive care unit (LongVentKids): an international, prospective, cross-sectional cohort study, accepted Lancet XXX in October 2024.
68. Kawaguchi A, Burren J, Fernandez A, Chiusolo F, Baudin F, Brierley J, et al. 506: prolonged mechanical ventilation in pediatric intensive care: interim report of LongVentKids Study. Crit Care Med. 2021;49(1):244.
69. Selvaraju V, Spicher N, Wang J, Ganapathy N, Warnecke JM, Leonhardt S, et al. Continuous monitoring of vital signs using cameras: a systematic review. Sensors (Basel). 2022;22(11):4097.
70. Qiu C, Wu F, Han W, Yuce MR. A wearable bioimpedance chest patch for real-time ambulatory respiratory monitoring. IEEE Trans Biomed Eng. 2022;69(9):2970–81.
71. He S, Han Z, Iglesias C, Mehta V, Bolic M. A real-time respiration monitoring and classification system using a depth camera and radars. Front Physiol. 2022;13:799621.

MIX
Papier aus verantwortungsvollen Quellen
Paper from responsible sources
FSC® C105338

If you have any concerns about our products,
you can contact us on
ProductSafety@springernature.com

In case Publisher is established outside the EU,
the EU authorized representative is:
Springer Nature Customer Service Center GmbH
Europaplatz 3, 69115 Heidelberg, Germany

Printed by Libri Plureos GmbH
in Hamburg, Germany